Ketamine Revisited - New Insights into NMDA Inhibitors

Edited by Nieves Saiz-Sapena and Manuel Granell-Gil

Published in London, United Kingdom

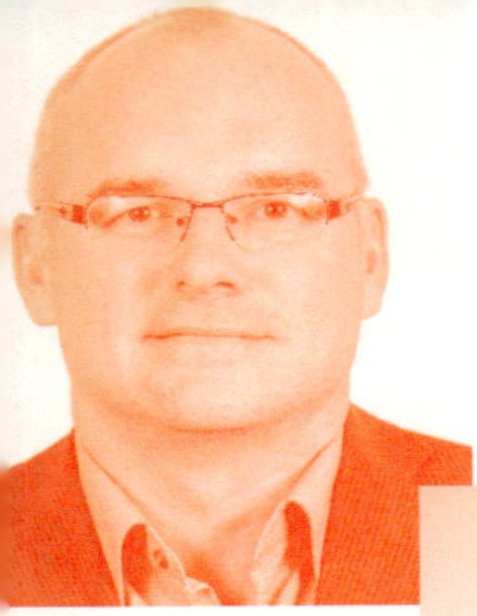
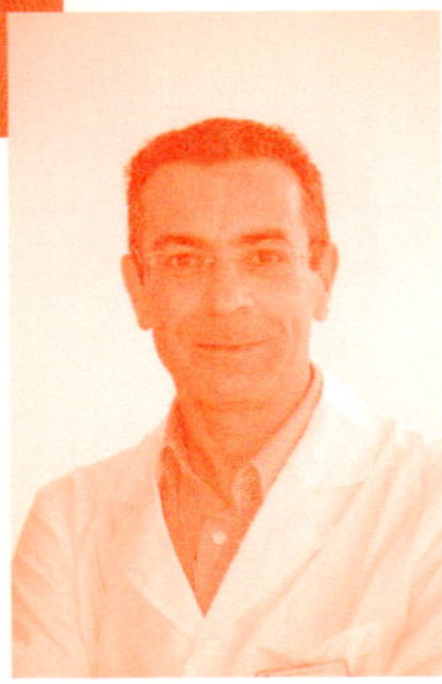
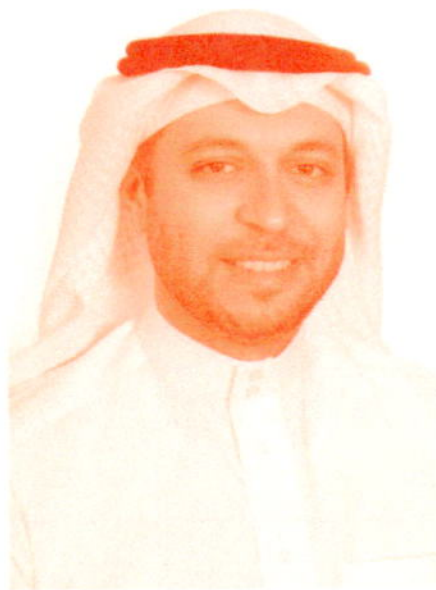
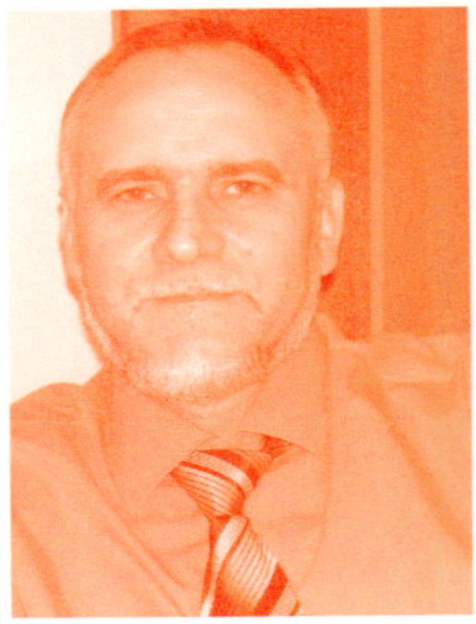
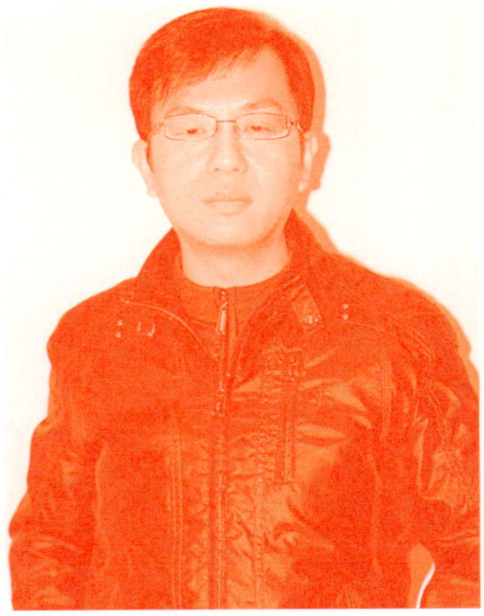
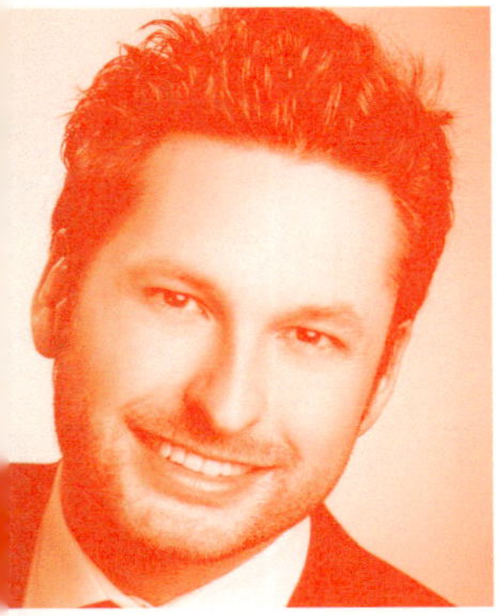
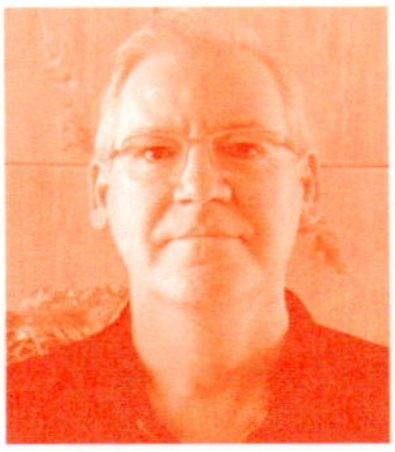

IntechOpen

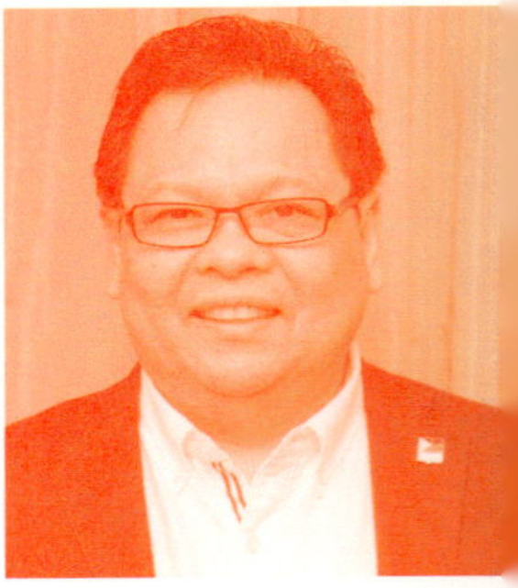
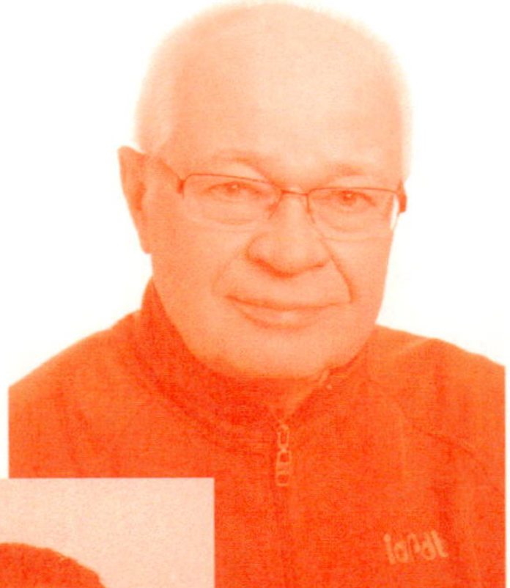
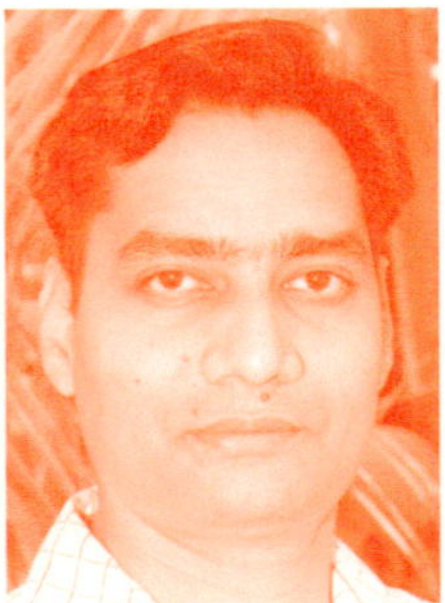
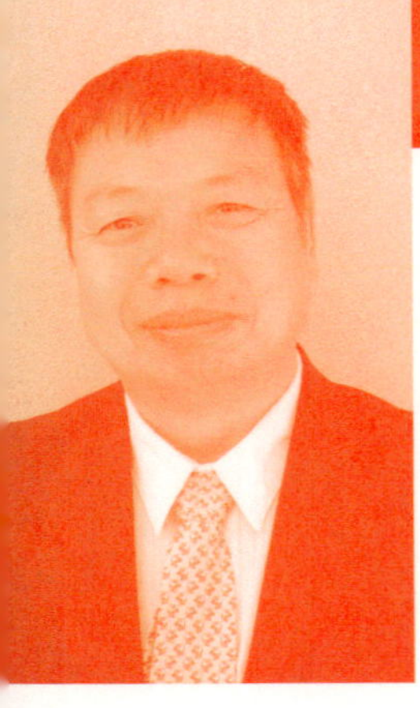
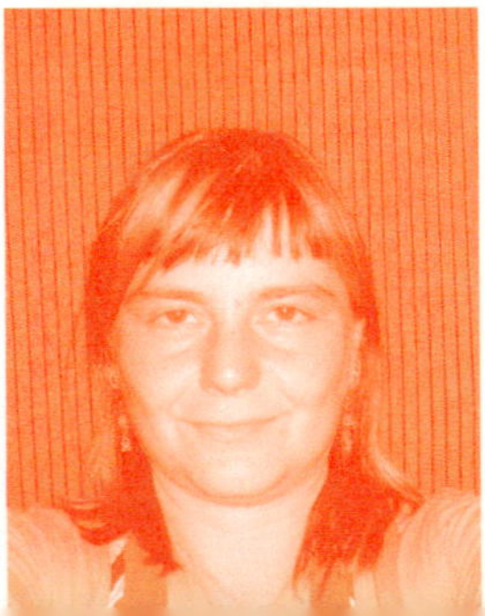
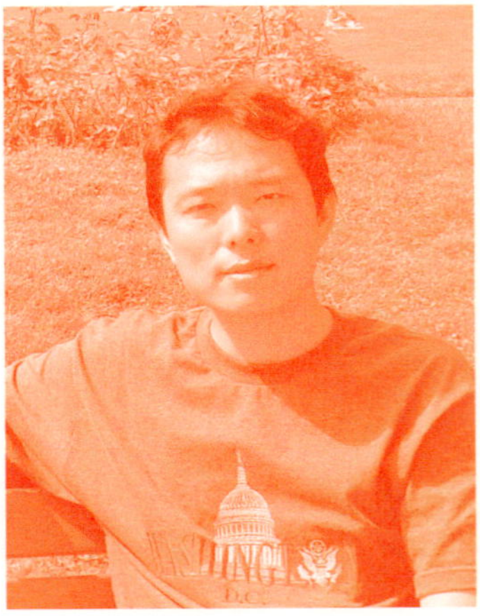

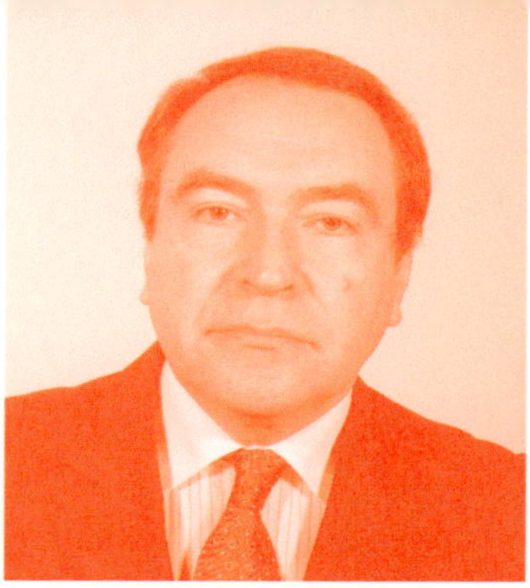

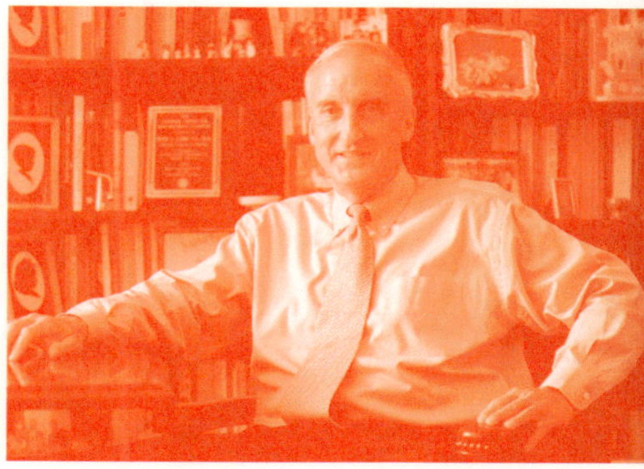

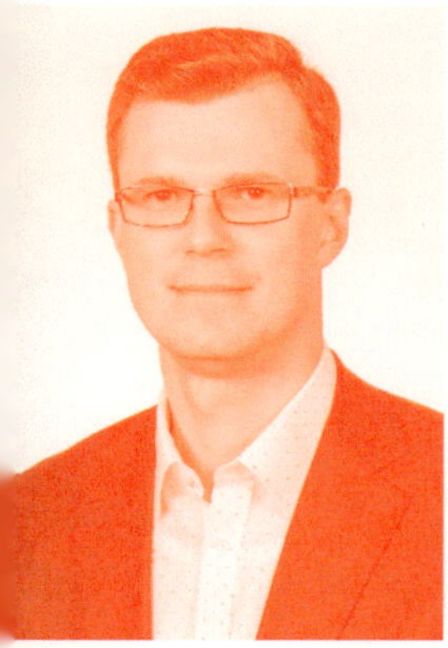

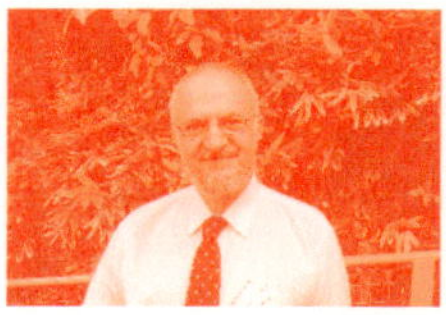

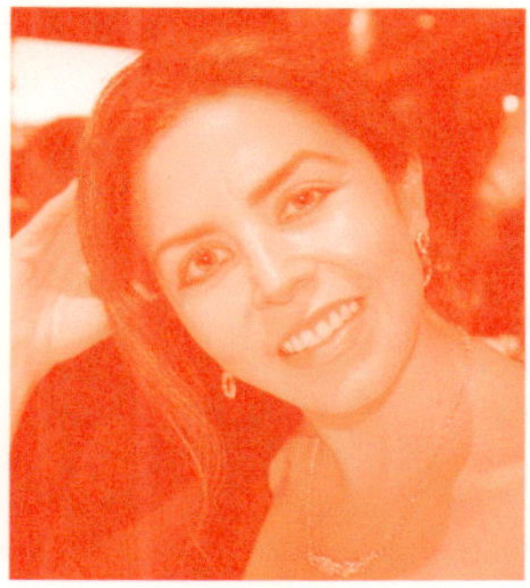

Supporting open minds since 2005

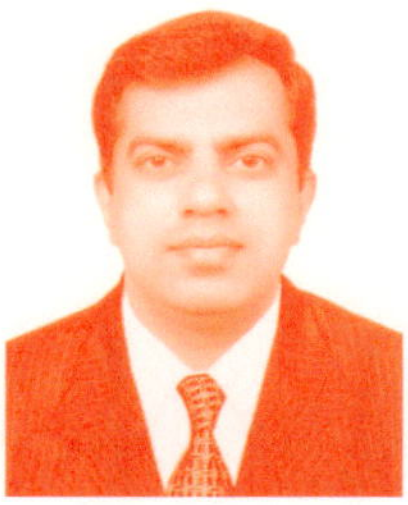

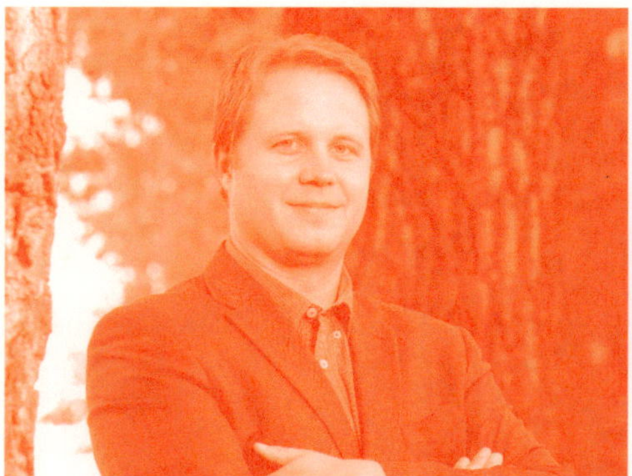

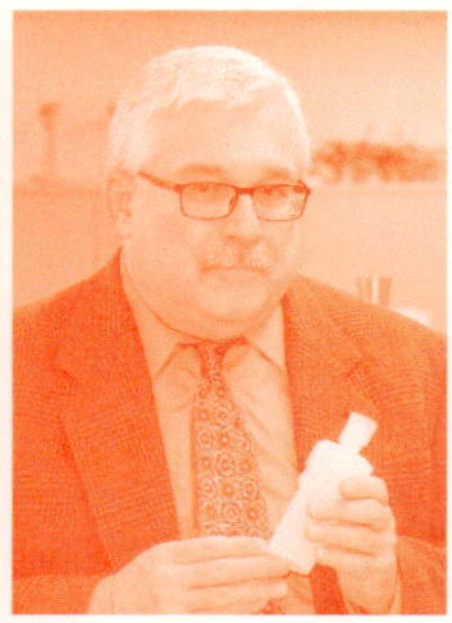

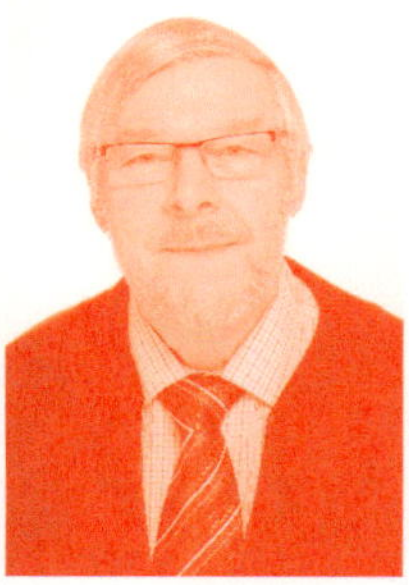

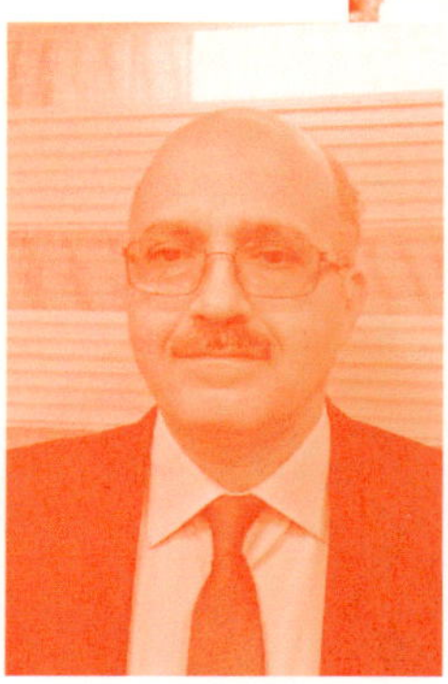

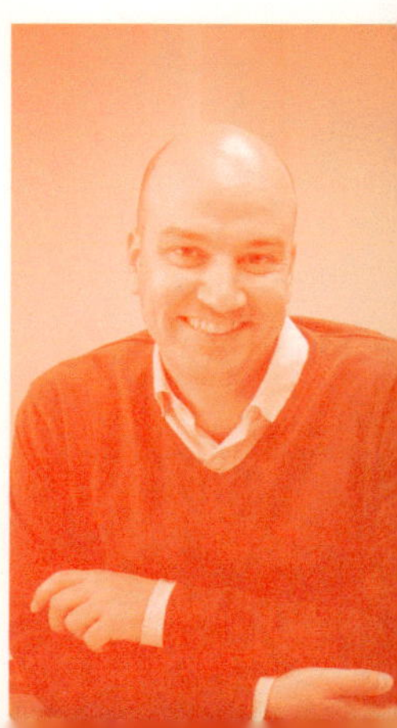

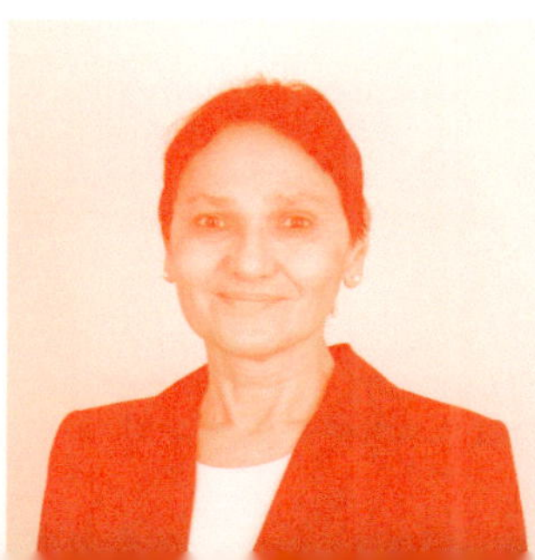

Ketamine Revisited - New Insights into NMDA Inhibitors
http://dx.doi.org/10.5772/intechopen.95733
Edited by Nieves Saiz-Sapena and Manuel Granell-Gil

Contributors
Shridevi Pandya Shah, Antony Irungu, Devanshi Patel, Tahani K. Alshammari, Sarah Alseraye, Nouf M. Alrasheed, Anfal F. Bin Dayel, Asma S. Alonazi, Jawza F. Al Sabhan, Musaad A. Alshammari, Maiko Satomoto, Cigdem Yildirim Guclu, Preet Mohinder Singh Bedi, Atamjit Singh, Guochuan Emil Tsai, Chih-Hung Lin, Po-Chang Shih, Shahla Haleem, Mateja Lopuh, Bhagyalakshmi Ramesh, Carlos Rafael Ramirez-Paesano, Claudia Rodiera Clarens, María Martínez Alberici, José Carlos Torres Mandujano, Milen Bonev Bonev, Florencia Borghetti, Karen Salazar Loaiza, Josep Rodiera Olive, Jesus Santaliestra Fierro, Bhargab Deka, Biswajit Dash, Alakesh Bharali, Ashique Ahmed, Chimaobi Tim Nnaji, Arunas Gelmanas, Migle Vitartaite, Ramunas Tamosiunas, Andrius Macas, Patrycja Kleczkowska, Malgorzata Zaremba, Mihai Octavian Botea, Erika Bimbo-Szuhai, Subbulakshmi Sundaram, Ashok Swaminathan Govindarajan, Molotchnikoff Stephane, Ouelhazi Afef, Rudy Lussiez, Nieves Saiz-Sapena, Manuel Granell-Gil

First published in London, United Kingdom, 2022 by IntechOpen
IntechOpen is the global imprint of INTECHOPEN LIMITED, registered in England and Wales, registration number: 11086078, 5 Princes Gate Court, London, SW7 2QJ, United Kingdom
Printed in Croatia

British Library Cataloguing-in-Publication Data
A catalogue record for this book is available from the British Library

Additional hard and PDF copies can be obtained from orders@intechopen.com

Ketamine Revisited - New Insights into NMDA Inhibitors
Edited by Nieves Saiz-Sapena and Manuel Granell-Gil
p. cm.
Print ISBN 978-1-83962-792-7
Online ISBN 978-1-83962-793-4
eBook (PDF) ISBN 978-1-83962-831-3

For EU product safety concerns:
IN TECH d.o.o., Prolaz Marije Krucifikse Kozulić 3, 51000 Rijeka, Croatia, info@intechopen.com or visit our website at intechopen.com.

Meet the editors

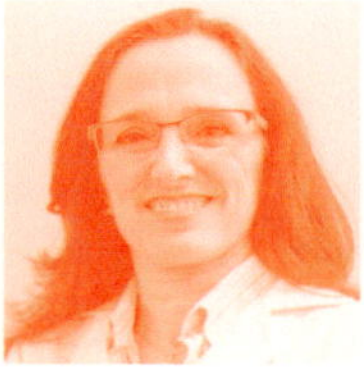

Dr. Nieves Saiz-Sapena, MD, Ph.D., is an anesthesiologist at Hospital General Universitario de Valencia, Spain. She has more than twenty-five years of experience in anesthesia in specialized fields such as neurosurgery, airway management, hostile environments, and bariatric surgery. She has numerous publications to her credit and is a member of several national and international scientific societies. Dr. Saiz-Sapena has taught at various institutions in Spain, including Universidad de Navarra, Universidad de Barcelona, Universidad Cardenal Herrera-CEU, and Universidad Catolica de Valencia, both on site and online.

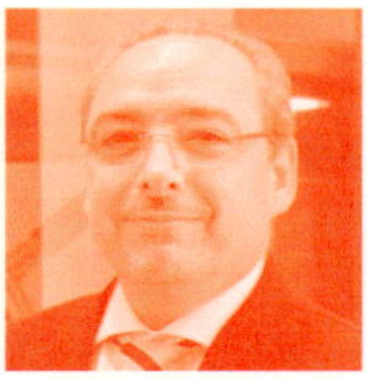

Dr. Manuel Granell-Gil, MD, Ph.D., is a Professor of Anesthesiology, at the University of Valencia, Spain. He is also the head of the Thoracic Anesthesia Section, Hospital General Universitario of Valencia, where he directs the Thoracic Anesthesia Exchange Program of the European Association of Cardiothoracic Anesthesia and Intensive Care. His most personal project is the organization of the Update Conference on Anesthesiology and Resuscitation in Thoracic Surgery, in his home city, of which he has already run nine editions, covering all aspects of the treatment of patients undergoing thoracic surgery, including acute and chronic pain.

Contents

Preface

The re-discovering of ketamine in anesthesia and other medical disciplines cannot be understood without a timeline. In the 1980s, ketamine was reserved for veterinary and experimental animal studies. During my early research years, I used ketamine for anaesthetizing rats, cats, and monkeys. Unfortunately, some people began using ketamine irresponsibly as a recreational drug. As such, ketamine was considered a dangerous substance more than a medication to be used in anesthesia.

Phencyclidine (PCP) was synthesized in 1956 and soon was used in human trials. However, sometimes its psychotic excitatory effects made patients unmanageable in the postoperative period, so it was removed from the anesthetic armamentarium for humans. Other phencyclidine derivatives were synthesized, but ketamine (a ketone plus an amine) outperformed the others, as it retained analgesic and anesthetic action with no hypnotic effects. In the 1970s, some PCP derivatives were considered illegal drugs, while ketamine, although approved, was only used by certain groups (including the military during the Vietnam War) because its psychedelic effects (e.g., hallucinations) were considered unacceptable by most of the scientific community. The introduction of diazepam, droperidol, or chlorpromazine minimized those adverse effects. However, concomitant use of those drugs did extend the use of ketamine as a drug of abuse, but not its use in regular Anesthesia. Hence its bad reputation.

In the 1990s, the arrival of new intravenous hypnotics such as propofol almost relegated ketamine to the drawer of oblivion in the clinical setting. But there were many research groups dedicated to studying NMDA calcium channels, NMDA receptor blockade drugs, and NMDA-receptor glutamatergic phenomena. Investigation of analgesia pathways and mechanisms originated new knowledge on mu and other opioid receptors, including evidence that opioids could open NMDA receptors and induce opioid-induced hyperalgesia.

In the new century, management of both acute and chronic pain has attracted great interest. Our modern society does not accept any suffering, including pain, depression, schizophrenia, or other disabling conditions, and the medical community agrees. Thus, it is the perfect time to re-examine ketamine.

The last twenty years have witnessed a renaissance of ketamine. Deep knowledge of pharmacokinetics and pharmacodynamics has led to a better understanding of different administration routes and how to manage the drug. The synthesis of isomers and derivatives has unveiled new uses, for example, in psychiatry. The usefulness of ketamine in war, in developing countries, and as premedication in children, has regained interest in other populations and situations.

This book provides a comprehensive overview of ketamine. It includes a discussion of NMDA receptors, the use of ketamine in anesthesia and pain disorders, the clinical non-anesthetic uses of ketamine (especially in depression), and special situations that will benefit from ketamine, such as palliative care and the trauma suite.

The book ends with a review on the use of ketamine in low-resource countries and examines the current illicit use of the drug.

We hope this book reaches young healthcare professionals and helps to eradicate the fear and misgivings associated with the use of ketamine.

Dr. Nieves Saiz-Sapena, MD, Ph.D. and Dr. Manuel Granell-Gil, MD, Ph.D.
Department of Anesthesiology,
Critical Care and Pain Clinic,
Consortium General University Hospital of Valencia,
Valencia, Spain

Section 1

Introduction

Chapter 1

Introductory Chapter: Is Ketamine the New Panacea of the 21st Century?

Nieves Saiz-Sapena and Manuel Granell-Gil

1. Introduction

Ketamine is an old drug with bewildering uses. Although it was initially introduced in anesthesia, its use has spread to many areas, primarily due to its properties in the pain control and antidepressant domains.

It was first described as a drug with cataleptic, analgesic, and anesthetic action without hypnosis [1]. But its adverse effects, especially in terms of hallucinations and the availability of other anesthetics, made ketamine a controversial drug whose use was almost limited to disasters, the military, and third world countries. Nevertheless, it is still on the WHO Model List of Essential Medicines-22nd List.

But the last word is not said yet. On the contrary, new potential uses are being published that broaden the horizon. Of particular interest is to realize that the two different optical isomers of this drug can have differential actions and be used for various other therapeutic purposes in different nosological conditions. Right now, ketamine research is experiencing a resurgence. The better chemical and pharmacological knowledge, and the better control over its administration, are expected to return ketamine to a prominent place in the pharmacopeia of anesthesia.

The synthesis of ketamine resulted from an investigation on phencyclidine (PCP) in the 1950s, which was considered unsuitable for human anesthesia due to severe excitatory effects. Clavin Stevens synthesized in 1962 a related compound, a ketone plus an amine, which was called ketamine [2]. It has been in clinical use since 1970. In the next 10 years, studies revealed that it is a racemic mixture comprising equal parts of two optical isomers of the 2-(2-chlorophenyl)-2-(methylamino)-cyclohexanone ketamine: S(+) ketamine or esketamine and R(−) ketamine or arketamine, with differential effects. At the same time, some drugs were proposed to limit emergence excitement, such as chlorpromazine, diazepam, or droperidol [3–5]. Although physicians initially introduced it in the anesthetic armamentarium and later almost abandoned it in favor of other anesthetics with better profiles, many more applications are returning ketamine to the present day.

2. Pharmacokinetics

Its pharmacological action is achieved through the N-methyl-d-aspartate (NMDA), opioid, muscarinic, and several voltage-gated receptors. Its anesthetic and analgesic properties are due to direct ketamine-induced inhibition of *N*-methyl-D-aspartate receptors.

Esketamine (S-Ketamine) is almost four times more potent than arketamine (R-Ketamine) to induce anesthesia and analgesia due to the higher affinity of the former for the NMDA receptors [6, 7], but also more prone to cause side effects [6].

Because it is both water and lipid-soluble, it can be administered to most routes (oral, sublingual, transmucosal, intravenous, intramuscular, subcutaneous, intranasal, and rectal) [8], providing an excellent distribution in the whole body [9].

It induces bronchodilatation and sympathetic nervous and cardiovascular system stimulation [9], two characteristics that give ketamine an interesting role in shock and anesthesia-related cardiovascular depression.

Ketamine is a well-tolerated drug in the short term, but it induces an increase in salivation, arterial and intracranial pressure [10, 11], cardiorespiratory [10, 12], neuropsychiatric, dissociative, and psycho-mimetic effects with delirium [7, 10, 11, 13], and psychodysleptic, cognitive, and peripheral side effects [14, 15]. The most common are the psycho-mimetic side effects [9, 11]. Nevertheless, in the long-term, it can induce neurocognitive and urologic toxicity [7, 16] and has the potential of abuse [13], same as its predecessor, phencyclidine (PCP). Therefore, experts recommend not to administer this drug to patients suffering from arterial hypertension or coronary artery disease [17].

It is metabolized in the liver primarily to norketamine, which is an active metabolite [18]. This characteristic makes it a good option when considering the oral route (although this is not approved). Other metabolites are dehydronorketamine, hydroxyketamine, and hydroxynorketamine [19], all of which, but particularly the last one, has antidepressant effects [20].

3. Clinical uses

Today it is relatively simple to control its side effects. Hence, its clinical uses have escalated from only anesthesia, to its use in the pain clinic, neurology, psychiatry, palliative care, and others.

It is well known that it induces dissociative anesthesia, which means that although the sensory inputs reach the cortical receiving areas, these inputs are not perceived at the association cortex. The lack of loss of consciousness together with the preservation of ventilation and cardiovascular stability made it a drug of choice in wars and disasters, and in third world countries.

Thus, it is useful for premedication, sedation, and induction and maintenance of general anesthesia, particularly esketamine.

Additionally, the analgesic action is present with plasma levels 10 times lower than those required for hypnotic purposes [18], which confers ketamine a high interest in acute and chronic pain treatment. Also, anti-inflammatory and even antidepressant properties have been described. Finally, at subanesthetic doses, this form of ketamine is helpful in postoperative analgesia and sedation [21].

It has excellent potential in trauma patients [22–24], even in children [2], hypovolemic or septic shock, and pulmonary diseases.

Its use in ICU patients is also increasing, usually combined with midazolam or propofol, and particularly in patients with sepsis or cardiovascular instability [25]. It also has excellent potential in short anesthetic procedures, particularly in pediatric patients [26] and endoscopic diagnostic procedures [27].

Because of its anti-hyperalgesic and anti-inflammatory properties, ketamine is currently used to treat acute and chronic pain [28]. It is gaining a role in acute pain treatment. In the postoperative period, it not only controls the pain [29, 30] but also improves patients' mood and depression [31].

Moreover, patients suffering from chronic pain, particularly of oncologic origin [14, 32], may benefit from a treatment that includes ketamine, either used as a single drug or combined with others, or as a substitute when other medications are not well tolerated [9]. An additional bonus is that it can be administered orally, both in adults and children [8]. The effects of this drug on chronic pain patients might be due, at least in part, to the modulation of the effective aspects [33] and to the fact that it can help to fight depression in chronic pain patients [8].

Sub-anesthetic doses of ketamine have antidepressant action [12, 34, 35], particularly in major depressive and bipolar disorders [36, 37] and resistant depression [12, 38]. Its antidepressant action starts within 2 hours of administration, and this effect is sustained for about 7 days on average and reduces suicidal ideation [39, 40] and suicidal attempts [7, 8, 14]. It has also been recommended as an anesthetic agent in electroconvulsive therapy to treat chronic depressive disorders [12, 38, 41]. Although low doses of intranasal esketamine are very effective and approved by the FDA (March 5, 2019) [6, 7, 42] and Europe (December 19, 2019) [43], the intravenous route is more potent [44, 45]. The oral route, although not yet approved, has also been used [8, 38, 46]. However, other researchers have found that arketamine is more effective and has more lasting antidepressant effects [47], at least in animal models [36, 48], and fewer side effects [47].

A new whole area of research is being explored in Psychiatry. It has a potential application in treatment-resistant generalized anxiety and social anxiety disorders [49]. Lately, some have started to use ketamine successfully to treat posttraumatic stress disorder (PTSD) both from military and civilian origin [50].

Other uses are to treat alcohol abuse and drug addiction (like heroin and cocaine) [42], asthma [51], and even prevent cancer growth [14].

4. Ketamine side effects

As it happened with phencyclidine, which was finally placed on the Schedule I list of illegal drugs in the 1970s, ketamine use has also been associated with abuse, particularly among young people using this drug for recreational purposes and spiritual seekers seeking schizophrenia-like symptoms and mental dissociation (i.e., out-of-body experience) [47].

The long-term consequences of chronic high ketamine dose administration are unknown, although neuronal apoptosis has been seen in animal models, particularly in the neonatal and pediatric periods [18]. What is known is that frontal white matter changes with cognitive deterioration happen in chronic ketamine abusers [18]. However, at this moment, there is not that much experience concerning the chronic use in the clinical setting, as in clinical praxis it is restricted to chronic pain of neuropathic or oncogenic origin.

5. Benefits versus harm: the panacea effect

Although ketamine has been living a real genuine revival in the last 10 years, clear boundaries have not been established yet. The situation looks like the rediscovery of a hidden germ. We are now on an upward learning curve, same as with any *new* drug when it is used for several different clinical situation trying to explore the whole set of benefits and the most secluded of latent *cons* that could overcome those *pros*.

Even if not a panacea, perhaps will ketamine in this 21st century, more than 60 years after it was synthesized, reach its full clinical potential. It seems that the last century was not prepared for it.

6. Conclusion

Ketamine is a drug with many possible uses and abuses. Physicians need to know all its potential to use it for the patients' best benefit but also be careful to avoid unwanted side effects. More research is needed to clearly establish boundaries on indications based on its clinical benefits.

Conflict of interest

The authors declare no conflict of interest.

Author details

Nieves Saiz-Sapena* and Manuel Granell-Gil
Department of Anesthesia, Intensive Care and Pain Treatment, Consorcio Hospital General Universitario, Valencia, Spain

*Address all correspondence to: nssapena@hotmail.com

References

[1] Mccarthy DA, Chen G, Kaump DH, Ensor C. General anesthetic and other pharmacological properties of 2-(O-chloropheny)-2-methylamino cyclohexanone HCL (CI-58L). The Journal of New Drugs. 1965;**5**:21-33

[2] Domino EF. Taming the ketamine tiger. 1965. Anesthesiology. 2010;**113**:678-684

[3] Erbguth PH, Reiman B, Klein RL. The influence of chlorpromazine, diazepam, and droperidol on emergence from ketamine. Anesthesia and Analgesia. 1972;**51**:693-700

[4] Muhlmann-Weill M, Mangeney F, Gauthier-Lafaye JP. Ketamine-diapezam association in anesthesia. Anesthesia and Analgesia. 1972;**29**:355-363

[5] Sadove MS et al. Clinical study of droperidol in the prevention of the side effects of ketamine anesthesia: A preliminary report. Anesthesia and Analgesia. 1971;**50**:388-393

[6] Andrade C. Ketamine for depression, 3: Does chirality matter? The Journal of Clinical Psychiatry. 2017;**78**:e674-e677

[7] Molero P et al. Antidepressant efficacy and tolerability of ketamine and Esketamine: A critical review. CNS Drugs. 2018;**32**:411-420

[8] Andrade C. Oral ketamine for depression, 1: Pharmacologic considerations and clinical evidence. The Journal of Clinical Psychiatry. 2019;**80**:19f12820

[9] Sinner B, Graf BM. Ketamine. Handbook of Experimental Pharmacology. 2008;**182**:313-333. DOI: 10.1007/978-3-540-74806-9_15

[10] Szarmach J, Cubała WJ, Włodarczyk A, Wiglusz MS. Short-term ketamine administration in treatment-resistant depression: Focus on cardiovascular safety. Psychiatria Danubina. 2019;**31**:585-590

[11] Mihaljević S, Pavlović M, Reiner K, Ćaćić M. Therapeutic mechanisms of ketamine. Psychiatria Danubina. 2020;**32**:325-333

[12] Fond G et al. Ketamine administration in depressive disorders: A systematic review and meta-analysis. Psychopharmacology. 2014; **231**:3663-3676

[13] Iqbal SZ, Mathew SJ. Ketamine for depression clinical issues. Advances in Pharmacology. 2020;**89**:131-162

[14] Nowacka A, Borczyk M. Ketamine applications beyond anesthesia - a literature review. European Journal of Pharmacology. 2019;**860**:172547

[15] Zanos P et al. Ketamine and ketamine metabolite pharmacology: Insights into therapeutic mechanisms. Pharmacological Reviews. 2018;**70**:621-660

[16] Ng J et al. Ketamine-induced urological toxicity: Potential mechanisms and translation for adults with mood disorders receiving ketamine treatment. Psychopharmacology. 2021;**238**:917-926

[17] Zielmann S, Kazmaier S, Schnüll S, Weyland A. S-(+)-ketamine and circulation. Anaesthesist. 1997; **46**(Suppl. 1):S43-S46

[18] Mion G, Villevieille T. Ketamine pharmacology: An update (pharmacodynamics and molecular aspects, recent findings). CNS Neuroscience & Therapeutics. 2013;**19**:370-380

[19] Kamp J et al. Pharmacokinetics of ketamine and its major metabolites

norketamine, hydroxynorketamine, and dehydronorketamine: A model-based analysis. British Journal of Anaesthesia. 2020;**125**:750-761

[20] Aleksandrova LR, Phillips AG, Wang YT. Antidepressant effects of ketamine and the roles of AMPA glutamate receptors and other mechanisms beyond NMDA receptor antagonism. Journal of Psychiatry & Neuroscience. 2017;**42**:222-229

[21] Motov S, Rosenbaum S, Vilke GM, Nakajima Y. Is there a role for intravenous subdissociative-dose ketamine administered as an adjunct to opioids or as a single agent for acute pain Management in the Emergency Department? The Journal of Emergency Medicine. 2016;**51**:752-757

[22] Nichols KA, Paciullo CA. Subdissociative ketamine use in the emergency department. Advanced Emergency Nursing Journal. 2019;**41**:15-22

[23] Sheikh S, Hendry P. The expanding role of ketamine in the emergency department. Drugs. 2018;**78**:727-735

[24] Lee EN, Lee JH. The effects of low-dose ketamine on acute pain in an emergency setting: A systematic review and Meta-analysis. PLoS One. 2016;**11**:e0165461

[25] Erstad BL, Patanwala AE. Ketamine for analgosedation in critically ill patients. Journal of Critical Care. 2016;**35**:145-149

[26] Jamora C, Iravani M. Unique clinical situations in pediatric patients where ketamine may be the anesthetic agent of choice. American Journal of Therapeutics. 2010;**17**:511-515

[27] Wang J et al. Pharmacokinetics and safety of Esketamine in Chinese patients undergoing painless gastroscopy in comparison with ketamine: A randomized, open-label clinical study. Drug Design, Development and Therapy. 2019;**13**:4135-4144

[28] Noppers I et al. Ketamine for the treatment of chronic non-cancer pain. Expert Opinion on Pharmacotherapy. 2010;**11**:2417-2429

[29] Wang X, Lin C, Lan L, Liu J. Perioperative intravenous S-ketamine for acute postoperative pain in adults: A systematic review and meta-analysis. Journal of Clinical Anesthesia. 2021;**68**:110071

[30] Allen CA, Ivester JR. Low-dose ketamine for postoperative pain management. Journal of PeriAnesthesia Nursing. 2018;**33**:389-398

[31] Reinert J, Parmentier BL. Effect of perioperative ketamine on postoperative mood and depression: A review of the literature. Expert Review of Clinical Pharmacology. 2021;**14**:25-32

[32] Gao M, Rejaei D, Liu H. Ketamine use in current clinical practice. Acta Pharmacologica Sinica. 2016;**37**:865-872

[33] Yang Y, Maher DP, Cohen SP. Emerging concepts on the use of ketamine for chronic pain. Expert Review of Clinical Pharmacology. 2020;**13**:135-146

[34] Zanos P, Gould TD. Mechanisms of ketamine action as an antidepressant. Molecular Psychiatry. 2018;**23**:801-811

[35] McIntyre RS et al. The effect of intravenous, intranasal, and oral ketamine in mood disorders: A meta-analysis. Journal of Affective Disorders. 2020;**276**:576-584

[36] Hashimoto K. Rapid-acting antidepressant ketamine, its metabolites and other candidates: A historical overview and future perspective. Psychiatry and Clinical Neurosciences. 2019;**73**:613-627

[37] Kraus C et al. Administration of ketamine for unipolar and bipolar depression. International Journal of Psychiatry in Clinical Practice. 2017;**21**:2-12

[38] Ritter P, Findeis H, Bauer M. Ketamine in the treatment of depressive episodes. Pharmacopsychiatry. 2020;**53**:45-50

[39] Das J. Repurposing of drugs-the ketamine story. Journal of Medicinal Chemistry. 2020;**63**:13514-13525

[40] Bartoli F, Wlkinson ST. Ketamine and esketamine for suicidal ideation: Recent progress and practical issues. The Australian and New Zealand Journal of Psychiatry. 2020;**54**:206-207

[41] Cobb K, Nanda M. Ketamine and electroconvulsive therapy: So happy together? Current Opinion in Anaesthesiology. 2018;**31**:459-462

[42] Ivan Ezquerra-Romano I, Lawn W, Krupitsky E, Morgan CJA. Ketamine for the treatment of addiction: Evidence and potential mechanisms. Neuropharmacology. 2018;**142**:72-82

[43] Wei Y, Chang L, Hashimoto K. A historical review of antidepressant effects of ketamine and its enantiomers. Pharmacology, Biochemistry, and Behavior. 2020;**190**:172870

[44] Bahji A, Vazquez GH, Zarate CA. Comparative efficacy of racemic ketamine and esketamine for depression: A systematic review and meta-analysis. Journal of Affective Disorders. 2021;**278**:542-555

[45] Witt K et al. Ketamine for suicidal ideation in adults with psychiatric disorders: A systematic review and meta-analysis of treatment trials. The Australian and New Zealand Journal of Psychiatry. 2020;**54**:29-45

[46] Smith-Apeldoorn SY et al. Oral esketamine for treatment-resistant depression: Rationale and design of a randomized controlled trial. BMC Psychiatry. 2019;**19**:375

[47] Hashimoto K. Molecular mechanisms of the rapid-acting and long-lasting antidepressant actions of (R)-ketamine. Biochemical Pharmacology. 2020;**177**:113935

[48] Chang L et al. Comparison of antidepressant and side effects in mice after intranasal administration of (R,S)-ketamine, (R)-ketamine, and (S)-ketamine. Pharmacology, Biochemistry, and Behavior. 2019;**181**:53-59

[49] Glue P et al. Effects of ketamine in patients with treatment-refractory generalized anxiety and social anxiety disorders: Exploratory double-blind psychoactive-controlled replication study. Journal of Psychopharmacology. 2020;**34**:267-272

[50] Feder A, Rutter SB, Schiller D, Charney DS. The emergence of ketamine as a novel treatment for posttraumatic stress disorder. Advances in Pharmacology. 2020;**89**:261-286

[51] Jørgensen BG. Ketamine as a broncholytic agent in status asthmaticus and as an anesthetic for patients with bronchial asthma. Ugeskrift for Laeger. 1992;**154**:2132-2135

Section 2

NMDA and NMDA Antagonists

Chapter 2

Ketamine: More than Just NMDA Blocker

Bhargab Deka, Biswajit Dash, Alakesh Bharali and Ashique Ahmed

Abstract

Ketamine has been extensively used in the medical field for more than 50 years, but its exact mechanism of action remains unknown. It's used to induce dissociative anesthesia (a state of profound analgesia, amnesia with light sleep, immobility, and a sense of disassociation from one's own body and surroundings). Clinical studies on ketamine as a dissociative anesthetic, a model for psychosis, and as a rapidly acting antidepressant have sparked great interest in understanding its effects at the molecular and cellular level. It exerts uncompetitive inhibitory effects on NMDARs (N-Methyl-D-asperate) and may preferentially affect the function of NMDARs in interneurons. The hypnotic effects of this drug are attributed to its blocking action on NMDA and HCN1 receptors; however, both positive and negative modulation of choline, amine, and opioid systems appears to occur. It is likely that ketamine's effect on chronic pain and depression far outlasts its actual levels. This could be due to the hyperglutamatergic state induced by ketamine causing a secondary increase in structural synaptic connectivity. The authors of this review have attempted to highlight the action of ketamine not only on NMDA receptors but also on a variety of biochemical processes and functions found in intercellular environments, which may explain its diverse role in many diseases.

Keywords: ketamine, NMDA, antidepressant, analgesia, anesthesia

1. Introduction

Ketamine is an anesthetic drug that has been used for around more than 50 years in the medical field. In contrast to more traditional volatile-based anesthesia, it produces a broader range of anesthetic effects, resulting in a qualitatively different type of anesthesia [1]. This state is known as "dissociative anesthesia". These include: (a) hypnosis with psychotomimetic properties at low doses, accompanied by increased sedation and unconsciousness at higher doses; (b) analgesic properties (or antinociception); (c) sympathetic stimulation; and (d) maintenance of intrapulmonary pressure and respiratory regulation. Research has found that ketamine inhibits the N-methyl-D-aspartate (NMDA) receptor in a dose-dependent manner and that this blocking of excitatory synaptic activity [2]. It is responsible for the loss of responsiveness associated with clinical ketamine anesthesia. However, later scientific research has revealed that it has a wide array of molecular effects that have a clinically beneficial effect on many illnesses, including acute and chronic pain, and recently as an antidepressant with a rapid onset [3]. It is intriguing to note that many of these therapeutically beneficial effects appear long after the drugs are almost fully eliminated from the body. The link between drug binding and therapeutic outcomes is more intricate than previously understood.

Researchers and Clinicians are increasingly keen to understand the exact mechanism of action by which ketamine and other N-methyl-D-aspartate receptors (NMDAR) antagonists affect the brain [4]. Pioneering investigations by Krystal and colleagues in the early 1990s established that a 40-minute subanesthetic infusion of ketamine (0.5 mg/kg) produced temporary psychotic symptoms in otherwise healthy subjects. As a result of ketamine infusions, sensory illusions, persecutory ideas, and altered cognition, including difficulties with attention, word-finding, and acute learning difficulties were observed. A few hours after cessation of the infusion, these symptoms disappeared [5]. Researchers discovered that in patients with major depression, the same ketamine infusion produces a slower but still rapid antidepressant effect. In some patients, this effect began within a few hours of ketamine infusion and lasted for a week or more [6]. Additionally, it has shown antidepressant effects, including rapid improvements in suicidal thoughts in patients with treatment-resistant depression [7]. Ketamine does not bind closed NMDAR channels; instead, it requires them to open before it can cause antagonistic effects. In a similar manner to phencyclidine and MK-801, ketamine also causes an open channel block that involves binding to an electrically deep part within the channel, which stops ion flow, persisting within the channel until the channel closes. The latter attribute is responsible for an extended block relieved by channel opening [8]. In the membrane depolarization theory, the dissociation of drugs is accelerated, but an electrostatic model of voltage dependence does not fully explain the mechanism by which it decreases block. Ketamine is less effective than phencyclidine and MK-801 due to its quicker dissociation from the open channel [9]. Despite the fact that it is not selective for NMDARs, and recent research has called into question the significance of NMDAR antagonism as an antidepressant, the effects of ketamine on NMDARs appear to contribute significantly to its analgesic, anesthetic, and psychotomimetic, if not antidepressant, properties [10]. The research is yielding a plethora of innovative hypotheses about mood and psychotic illnesses, including the possible function of NMDARs in these diseases and the application of novel therapeutic approaches. In this review, we will provide a wide overview of the available data on ketamine's effects and possible repercussions [11].

2. Ketamine and its molecular effects

2.1 Immediate effects

It is now known that ketamine directly influences a wide range of cellular processes in clinical doses. In this case, as shown in **Figure 1**, the effects include blocking NMDA channels, hyperpolarization-induced cationic currents (also known as hyperpolarization-activated cyclic nucleotide channels (HCN1)), nicotinic acetylcholine channels, delta, opioid receptor agonists and potentiators [12], the nitric oxide (NO)–cyclic guanosine-mono-phosphate (cGMP) system, non-NMDA glutamate receptors (α-amino-3-hydroxy-5-methylisoxazole-4-propionic acid (AMPA)), and metabotropic glutamate receptors (mGluR), decreased activity of cholinergic neurons, stimulation of aminergic neurons (dopamine and noradrenaline), L-type Ca^{2+} channels, and neurosteroids. Each of these systems is a component of the integrated nervous system, and they interact at all levels [13, 14].

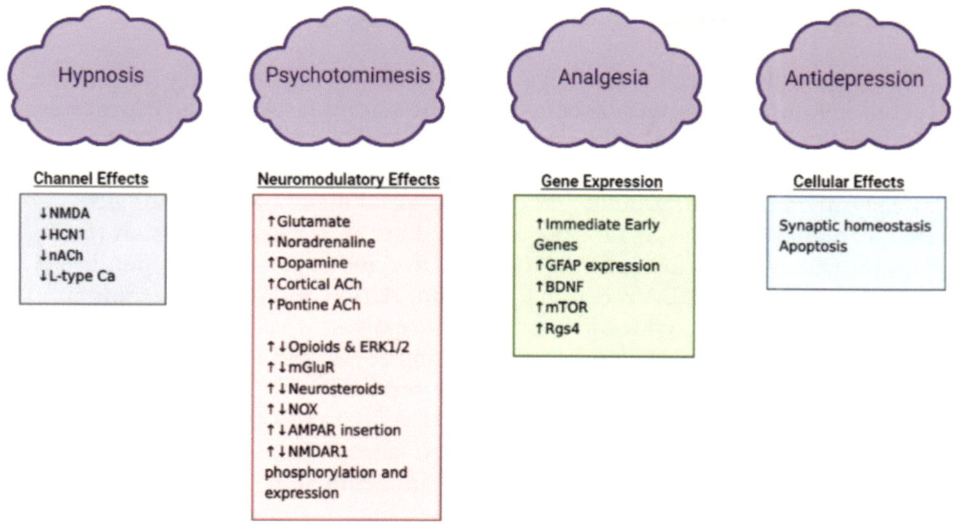

Figure 1.
*There are immediate effects and actions on the left, and delayed and prolonged ones on the right. [**NMDA:** N-methyl-d aspartate, **HCN1:** Hyperpolarization-activated cyclic nucleotide channels, **ACh:** Acetylcholine, **nACh:** Nicotinic acetylcholine receptors, AMPA: α-amino-3-hydroxy-5-methylisoxazole-4-propionic acid, **mGluR:** Metabotropic glutamate receptors, **ERK1/2:** Extracellular signal-regulated kinases, **NOX:** NADPH oxidase, **BDNF:** Brain-derived neurotrophic factor, mTOR: Mammalian target of rapamycin, **Rgs4:** Regulator of G protein signaling 4, **L-type Ca^{2+}:** L-type calcium channels, **GFAP:** Glial fibrillary acidic protein].*

2.2 Disruption of NMDA channel functions by ketamine

There is a great deal of complexity in the way in which several groups of compounds affect NMDA receptor function at the level of chemical binding, and this is explored in great detail in this review. Many compounds have been shown to influence the action of NMDA. Generally, they fall into the following categories: (a) open channel blockers (ketamine is one of the least potents), (b) competitive antagonists, and (c) allosteric modulators, (d) non-competitive antagonists [12, 15]. In all of these compounds, the relative potency of their action on the various NMDA receptor subtypes is different (commonly termed GluN1, GluN2A, GluN2B, GluN2C, and GluN2D – but also called NR1, NR2A-D) [16]. The distributions of these subtypes in the brain are markedly heterogeneous, which may explain why different NMDA blocking compounds produce different clinical effects. GluN2A is reported to be present throughout the brain, while GluN2B is present mainly in limbic systems, thalamus, and spinal cord. The thalamus and cerebellum contain GluN2C, whereas the brain stem, diencephalon, and spinal cord contain GluN2D. The off-rate of the compound is another important reason for the variation in effect. The phenomenon is known as "trapping block" [17]. High-trapping antagonists with a slow off-rate include compounds such as ketamine (86% trapping) and MK-801 (almost 100% trapping) [18]. After glutamate has dissociated from its binding site on the NMDA receptor, ketamine remains trapped in the closed ion channel, disrupting both physiological and pathological functions. Conversely, low-trapping (fast off-rate) antagonists escape the channel before it closes, preserving NMDA function at some level, and having fewer side effects. As an example, the compound memantine (50–70%) has minimal psychotomimetic or sedative effects. This is a slow-off-rate, low-affinity open-channel blocker. Thus, it blocks NMDA channels only when they are pathologically open, but not when they are temporarily open as in most physiological states [19]. In many ways, this mechanism is similar to persistent sodium channel blockers used in antiepileptic drugs. The end result is an NMDA blocker without any apparent anesthetic effects.

2.3 Ketamine possesses delayed effects

The functions of a cell go far beyond ion channels. Almost every immediate effect of ketamine disrupts subsequent and more long-lasting cellular processes, including gene expression and protein metabolism. It is not surprising since NMDA is largely responsible for calcium entry into cells, and calcium ions play a significant role in protein and mitochondrial metabolism. In subjects with mechanical injuries, it suppresses immediate early gene expression (fosB, c-jun, junD, zif/268, c-fos, junB,) [20]. A rat and mouse model of hyperalgesia have shown altered NMDA receptor1 phosphorylation and NMDA receptor1 mRNA expression [21], which has reduced the expression of the glial fibrillary acidic protein (GFAP) and also reduction in astrocytic and microglial activation [22, 23], an effect that is associated with reduced neuropathic pain. These chronic pain models represent complex patterns of nociception, but they may also encompass acute pain. A study found that ketamine can affect the number and function of synaptic connections in rat hippocampal regions by increasing brain-derived neurotrophic factor (BDNF) and mammalian target of rapamycin (mTOR) [24, 25] protein levels.

3. Psychotomimetic effects of ketamine

Aside from encouraging illegal usage, the psychotomimetic effects of ketamine can lead to distressing psychic disturbances, particularly in children, with the risk of experiencing nightmares, hallucinations, and delirium. Recent studies reveal that ketamine disrupts synaptic homeostasis - either by altering the release or uptake of neurotransmitters or by modifying neuromodulator activity. In addition, one intriguing possibility is that ketamine might inhibit NADPH oxidase (NOX2) from controlling glutamate release. There has been an association between psychosis and an excess of glutamate activity [26]. Alternatively, or perhaps simultaneously, ketamine may disrupt RGS4 (Regulator of G protein signaling 4). This particular protein regulates the G protein-coupled receptors such as opiate and muscarinic receptors [27]. Historically, ketamine's effects in increasing dopamine production [28] along with a possible decrease in acetylcholine activity [14] will be responsible for aggravating delirium.

The oral formulation of ketamine offers an effective analgesic for patients with chronic pain. In a study of 21 patients with chronic neuropathic pain in the central and peripheral nerves, the starting dose of oral ketamine was 100 mg/day, which was gradually increased by 40 mg/day every 2 days until the desired effect was achieved. Nine of the 21 patients stopped using ketamine because of unpleasant side effects, including psychotomimetic effects such as dissociative experiences, somatic sensations, sleep, and taste abnormalities [26]. During a double-blind, randomized placebo-controlled study, 73 traumatized participants with severe acute pain (expressed on a visual analog pain scale) were administered either ketamine 0.2 mg/kg or placebo (isotonic saltwater) along with morphine 0.1 mg/kg followed by 3 mg every 3 minutes [29]. There was a significant reduction in consumption of morphine with ketamine (0.20 mg/kg versus 0.15 mg/kg), even though no differences were noted in the pain scores. It showed a greater degree of adverse effects, including increased incidences of neuropsychiatric symptoms. Patients in both groups found their treatments satisfactory and no adverse reactions were requiring additional treatment [30]. Due to the short study period (30 minutes), it is possible that adverse reactions were not identified as a result of this, although a power study was not designed to explore this.

Again, in a randomized, double-blind, placebo-controlled study involving 120 people who underwent elective laparotomy, the effects of administering ketamine 0.1 mg/kg/hour along with tramadol 0.2 mg/kg/hour were evaluated. The ketamine group consumed 54% less morphine compared with the placebo group, resulting in superior analgesia. No differences were found in nausea and use of antiemetic drugs, mental performance, sleep difficulties, or non-disturbing hallucinations. However, there were three patients, receiving ketamine who opted out of the study because they experienced disconcerting hallucinations [31].

A linear relationship between plasma ketamine concentrations of 50–200 ng/ml and psychotomimetic effects was observed in a placebo-controlled experiment on 10 healthy young men. The psychedelic effects were similar to those reported in an earlier study of dimethyltryptamine, an illegal LSD-25 type of drug. Additionally, the effects were proportional to plasma concentrations rather than simply one of emergence. In clinical studies, plasma levels of 100–200 ng/ml resulted in useful analgesia. Observations of lateral nystagmus were consistent across subjects at 200 ng/ml plasma concentrations. Large doses of ketamine rapidly cause patients to become unconscious, and therefore the effects that were observed in this study are usually only evident afterward [32, 33].

Ketamine is a racemic mixture consisting of two enantiomers, R- and S-ketamine. Both of the enantiomers displays similar pharmacological effect but there is a question regarding the psychotomimetic effects of these enantiomers. Earlier research findings reported S-ketamine to be less prone to psychotomimetic side effects as compared to R-ketamine. While recent studies reported R-Ketamine to cause fewer psychotomimetic side effects. In a recent study with 11 participants, the pharmacological and psychotomimetic effect of R- and S-enantiomeric ketamine has been tested. The participants received 0.5 mg R-ketamine and then 0.15 mg S-ketamine separately for 1 week [34]. Using a nerve stimulator placed on the right central incisor tooth, these subjects were exposed to painful stimulation before and after the administration of each drug. Both drugs were equally effective in suppressing pain. The subjects reported that S-ketamine produced less pleasant psychotomimetic effects than R-ketamine. Of the 11 subjects, seven preferred R-ketamine to S-ketamine [35]. Based on these results, it is considered that ketamine may have a significant neuropsychiatric effect predominantly due to its S-enantiomer, making R-ketamine an ideal alternative. In contrast to earlier research suggesting that the most serious neuropsychiatric side effects are caused by R-ketamine, this study finds no evidence of this.

4. Hypnosis

Ketamine loses its vulnerability when the concentration is about 20 times higher (about 2000 ng/ml) than the concentration required inducing psychotropic effects. Because it has an elimination half-life of approximately 3 hours, there is a prolonged period during which drug levels are near the concentrations required to produce psychomimetic effects [36]. It should also be noted that the duration of hypnosis strictly corresponds to changes in drug concentration in the blood (and the site of action), indicating that the slow side effects in hypnosis/anesthesia do not have a significant causal effect. Ketamine is anomalous among commonly used anesthetics in that it has a strange combination of tranquilizers (such as NMDA antagonism) and stimulants (increasing amines, excess glutamate, and increasing AMPA receptor administration), as well as molecular effects. As a result, achieving complete anesthesia is difficult. Ketamine is typically used in conjunction with 2-adrenergic agonists to achieve surgical anesthesia in many animal species and veterinary anesthesia. It causes central nervous system depression because the NMDA receptors on the dendrites of inhibitory neurons are less sensitive to the effects of ketamine than the receptors on excitatory neurons [37].

In hypnosis, other molecular effects may play significant roles in addition to NMDA blockade. Numerous sources provide evidence on this point. As a first point, the hypnotic effect is unrelated to NMDA blockade effectiveness. Numerous NMDA blocker compounds, including dizocilpine maleate (MK801) and dextrorphan, have weak hypnotic effects. This difference may be explained by ketamine having a considerably stronger effect on GluN2C receptors which would theoretically cause more thalamic hyperpolarization than drugs that are more effective on GluN2A or B receptors (such as MK801) [38]. The counterexample is memantine, which has an affinity for GluN2C receptors similar to ketamine but does not cause clinical sedation. Memantine and ketamine have a markedly different trapping blocks, which may explain this difference in results.

NMDAR knockout animals should be completely resistant to ketamine. Petrenko and colleagues discovered that knockout mice lacking the NMDA receptor GluE epsilon1 subchain are resistant to ketamine hypnosis. Furthermore, these animals cannot be sedated by anesthetics or pentobarbital, which do not directly block NMDA, implying that their excitatory effects are nonspecific. Based on their findings, the authors concluded that the decreased ketamine sensitivity of animals was due to a compensatory increase in monoaminergic tone, which would help reduce hypnotic tendencies rather than a genetic knockout of NMDA receptors [39].

Furthermore, ketamine has been shown to hypnotize by interacting with other receptor types. Its hypnotic activity was reduced by 30% in a mouse model with conditional forebrain knockout of the HCN1 channel [40, 41]. Rather, it promotes wakefulness by increasing aminergic [42] and cholinergic activity in the neocortex [43].

5. Pain

In concentrations similar to that which produces psychotomimetic effects (200 ng/ml), ketamine reduces pain scores. In addition to producing hypnotic, analeptic, and anti-nociceptive effects, it also exhibits an unusual mix of anti- and pro-nociceptive properties. It is still largely debated whether ketamine is a useful analgesic in clinical practice or not. A careful examination of its analgesic effects is required, with the analgesic effects being compared to the specific pain syndrome [42] in question [44, 45]. Notably, norketamine has been reported to have anti-analgesic effects [46], while ketamine can facilitate endogenous pain pathways under certain conditions. Because the drug's analgesic effects are often accompanied by excessive sedation or psychotomimetic effects, its widespread use is somewhat limited. In many cases, the mechanism of direct receptor-mediated analgesia is dependent on drug levels for their analgesic effect. Long post-drug analgesia has been shown to outlast the effective drug levels in chronic neuropathic pain syndromes, which indicates that downstream mechanisms are involved [46–48].

Ketamine also directly stimulates opioid mu-receptors, acting as an opioid mu-receptor agonist, and is considered to have the strongest anti-nociceptive effect [49]. It undoubtedly alters opioid receptor responsiveness [50]. A series of studies using G protein-coupled inwardly rectifying potassium channels (GIRK2s) knockout mice have provided evidence for the hypothesis that opioids and clonidine exert a significant portion of their analgesic effects via the influence of these channels. In contrast to opioids, ketamine's analgesic effects have been associated with increased dopamine activity in mice [46]. Among the patients suffering from chronic pain, ketamine probably reduces opioid tolerance more than other opioid antagonists.

A recent study by Gupta and colleagues showed that ketamine has anti-desensitization effects in vitro, acting by reducing ERK1/2 phosphorylation and reverses opioid receptor desensitization [51].

A potential mechanism through which ketamine augments endogenous antinociceptive systems might be its stimulation of aminergic pathways (serotonin and noradrenergic) and inhibition of its reuptake [52]. The analgesic effects of Ketamine may also be related to its inhibition of nitric oxide synthase [53], although the relative importance of these mechanisms has not been determined to date.

5.1 Control of chronic pain

Ketamine can have long- and short-term effects on chronic neuropathic pain. Low-dose analgesics (250 mg/kg) can reduce ongoing pain, allodynia, and hyperalgesia symptoms quickly (within 5 minutes) and transiently (within 2 to 3 hours) [54]. The latter could be explained by an NMDA-mediated "wind-up" reduction [55]. Nonetheless, these effects do not follow a consistent pattern from one person to the next. Even within the same subject group, there is the possibility of temporary (<2 hours), long-lasting (6–24 hours), and no analgesic effects [48]. Ketamine has even been shown to reduce chronic postsurgical pain for up to 180 days after a single infusion around the time of surgery [56].

In clinical studies, ketamine was found to be capable of producing long-lasting analgesic effects. According to the literature, some of these indicators may contradict clinical observations. In this case, ketamine's antidepressant effect may explain why the drug has a preemptive effect on neuropathic pain that lasts long after the drug is no longer present [57, 58]. Although the cause of the causal link between depression and chronic pain is more often unknown, pain and depression are closely tied. Furthermore, its ability to inhibit gradual pathophysiological changes may help to prevent the development of chronic pain by inducing signaling cascades [59]. According to the previous section, ketamine affects several gene expression pathways that may affect the etiology of chronic pain, including the expression of NMDA receptors and astrocytic activity. This drug's effects would last much longer than its detectable presence.

6. Antidepressant effects of ketamine

Recent studies have shown that ketamine can be a powerful antidepressant that works quickly. This time-of-onset, however, lasts for about a week, and the antidepressant effect lasts about 2 hours. This is indicative of ketamine-induced signaling cascades that happen long after the substance has been eliminated [60]. By reviewing all the putative mechanisms, Duman and colleagues suggest [4] that ketamine at low doses increases glutamate neurotransmission by both increasing glutamate release and increasing insertion of the AMPA receptors into synaptic vesicles. This leads to increased BDNF release and thus activation of ERK signaling, which then stimulates mammalian targets of rapamycin (mTOR). A protein translation kinase stimulates synaptic protein synthesis (GluR1) and increases synaptic density and insertion through a complex signal pathway. Furthermore, it increases structural connectivity between neurons, slowing down the aging process.

7. Conclusion

Ketamine affects a range of neuronal processes within cells, including the well-known NMDA receptor blockade. According to the results, blockage of NMDA and HCN1 channels likely causes hypnotic effects to occur. On the other hand, the antidepressant-induced long-term effects are likely a result of its post-therapeutic effect. Ketamine's analgesic effects appear to be mediated by both short- and long-term changes in cellular function. Analgesic effects are probably mediated primarily through opioid system activation and the antinociceptive effects of the amine, whereas neuropathic pain is suppressed through receptor-mediated mechanisms and sustained cell signaling pathways.

Funding

There was no funding for this project from any government, commercial, or non-profit organization.

Declaration of interest

The authors state that they have no conflicts of interest that could impede the impartiality of this review.

Author details

Bhargab Deka[1*], Biswajit Dash[2], Alakesh Bharali[3] and Ashique Ahmed[4]

1 Department of Pharmacology, Pratiksha Institute of Pharmaceutical Science, Guwahati, Assam, India

2 Department of Pharmaceutical Chemistry, NEPEDS College of Pharmaceutical Sciences, Guwahati, Assam, India

3 Department of Pharmaceutics, Girijananda Chowdhury Institute of Pharmaceutical Sciences, Guwahati, Assam, India

4 Department of Pharmacology, NEPEDS College of Pharmaceutical Sciences, Guwahati, Assam, India

*Address all correspondence to: bhargavdeka98@gmail.com

References

[1] Domino EF, Chodoff P, Corssen G. Pharmacologic effects of CI-581, a new dissociative anesthetic, in man. Clinical Pharmacology & Therapeutics. 1965; **6**(3):279-291

[2] MacDonald J, Miljkovic Z, Pennefather P. Use-dependent block of excitatory amino acid currents in cultured neurons by ketamine. Journal of Neurophysiology. 1987;**58**(2):251-266

[3] Hirota K. Special cases: ketamine, nitrous oxide and xenon. Best Practice & Research. Clinical Anaesthesiology. 2006;**20**(1):69-79

[4] Duman RS, Li N, Liu R-J, Duric V, Aghajanian G. Signaling pathways underlying the rapid antidepressant actions of ketamine. Neuro pharmacology. 2012;**62**(1):35-41

[5] Krystal JH, Karper LP, Seibyl JP, Freeman GK, Delaney R, Bremner JD, et al. Subanesthetic effects of the noncompetitive NMDA antagonist, ketamine, in humans: psychotomimetic, perceptual, cognitive, and neuro endocrine responses. Archives of General Psychiatry. 1994;**51**(3):199-214

[6] Berman RM, Cappiello A, Anand A, Oren DA, Heninger GR, Charney DS, et al. Antidepressant effects of ketamine in depressed patients. Biological Psychiatry. 2000;**47**(4):351-354

[7] Zarate CA, Singh JB, Carlson PJ, Brutsche NE, Ameli R, Luckenbaugh DA, et al. A randomized trial of an N-methyl-D-aspartate antagonist in treatment-resistant major depression. Archives of General Psychiatry. 2006;**63**(8):856-864

[8] Huettner JE, Bean BP. Block of N-methyl-D-aspartate-activated current by the anticonvulsant MK-801: selective binding to open channels. Proceedings of the National Academy of Sciences. 1988;**85**(4):1307-1311

[9] Johnson JW, Kotermanski SE. Mechanism of action of memantine. Current Opinion in Pharmacology. 2006;**6**(1):61-67

[10] Lavender E, Hirasawa-Fujita M, Domino EF. Ketamine's dose related multiple mechanisms of actions: Dissociative anesthetic to rapid antidepressant. Behavioural Brain Research. 2020;**390**:112631

[11] Heifets BD. Piercing the ketamine cloud. Anesthesiology. 2020;**133**(5): 970-972

[12] Zhang K, Hashimoto K. Lack of opioid system in the antidepressant actions of ketamine. Biological Psychiatry. 2019;**85**(6):e25-ee7

[13] Jonkman K. Ketamine pharmacology revisited [Doctoral thesis]. Leiden University Scholarly Publications. Available at https://hdl.handle.net/1887/83274-29LeidenUniversity; 2020

[14] Lydic R, Baghdoyan HA. Ketamine and MK-801 decrease acetylcholine release in the pontine reticular formation, slow breathing, and disrupt sleep. Sleep. 2002;**25**(6):615-620

[15] Weigt HU, Adolph O, Georgieff M, Georgieff EM, Föhr KJ. Evidence that xenon does not produce open channel blockade of the NMDA receptor. Journal of Neurophysiology. 2008;**99**(4): 1983-1987

[16] Vance KM, Simorowski N, Traynelis SF, Furukawa H. Ligand-specific deactivation time course of GluN1/GluN2D NMDA receptors. Nature Communications. 2011;**2**(1): 1-11

[17] Bolshakov K, Gmiro V, Tikhonov D, Magazanik L. Determinants of trapping block of N-methyl-d-aspartate receptor

channels. Journal of Neurochemistry. 2003;**87**(1):56-65

[18] Lanthorn T, Mealing G, Morley P. Differences in degree of trapping between AR-R15896 and other uncompetitive NMDA receptor antagonists. Amino Acids. 2000; **19**(1):173-175

[19] Lipton SA. Pathologically-activated therapeutics for neuroprotection: mechanism of NMDA receptor block by memantine and S-nitrosylation. Current Drug Targets. 2007;**8**(5):621-632

[20] Belluardo N, Mudo G, Dell'Albani P, Hang X, Condorelli D. NMDA receptor-dependent and-independent immediate early gene expression induced by focal mechanical brain injury. Neurochemistry International. 1995;**26**(5):443-453

[21] Ohnesorge H, Feng Z, Zitta K, Steinfath M, Albrecht M, Bein B. Influence of clonidine and ketamine on m-RNA expression in a model of opioid-induced hyperalgesia in mice. PLoS One. 2013;**8**(11):e79567

[22] Hayashi Y, Kawaji K, Sun L, Zhang X, Koyano K, Yokoyama T, et al. Microglial Ca2+–activated K+ channels are possible molecular targets for the analgesic effects of S-ketamine on neuropathic pain. Journal of Neuroscience. 2011;**31**(48):17370-17382

[23] Mei X, Wang W, Wang W, Li Y, Zhang H, Wu S, et al. Inhibiting astrocytic activation: A novel analgesic mechanism of ketamine at the spinal level? Journal of Neurochemistry. 2009;**109**(6):1691-1700

[24] Garcia LS, Comim CM, Valvassori SS, Réus GZ, Barbosa LM, Andreazza AC, et al. Acute administration of ketamine induces antidepressant-like effects in the forced swimming test and increases BDNF levels in the rat hippocampus. Progress in Neuro-Psychopharmacology and Biological Psychiatry. 2008;**32**(1): 140-144

[25] Yang C, Hu Y-M, Zhou Z-Q, Zhang G-F, Yang J-J. Acute administration of ketamine in rats increases hippocampal BDNF and mTOR levels during forced swimming test. Upsala Journal of Medical Sciences. 2013;**118**(1):3-8

[26] Sorce S, Schiavone S, Tucci P, Colaianna M, Jaquet V, Cuomo V, et al. The NADPH oxidase NOX2 controls glutamate release: A novel mechanism involved in psychosis-like ketamine responses. Journal of Neuroscience. 2010;**30**(34):11317-11325

[27] Stratinaki M, Varidaki A, Mitsi V, Ghose S, Magida J, Dias C, et al. Regulator of G protein signaling 4 is a crucial modulator of antidepressant drug action in depression and neuropathic pain models. Proceedings of the National Academy of Sciences. 2013;**110**(20):8254-8259

[28] Wang M, Wong AH, Liu F. Interactions between NMDA and dopamine receptors: A potential therapeutic target. Brain Research. 2012;**1476**:154-163

[29] Radvansky BM, Shah K, Parikh A, Sifonios AN, Le V, Eloy JD. Role of ketamine in acute postoperative pain management: A narrative review. BioMed Research International. 2015;**2015**:1-10

[30] Jabbour H, Jabbour K, Abi Lutfallah A, Abou Zeid H, Nasser-Ayoub E, Abou Haidar M, et al. Magnesium and ketamine reduce early morphine consumption after open bariatric surgery: A prospective randomized double-blind study. Obesity Surgery. 2020;**30**(4):1452-1458

[31] Wilkinson ST, Ostroff RB, Katz RB, Krystal JH. Ketamine: A promising rapid-acting antidepressant. In: Kim Y-K,

editor. Understanding Depression, Vol 2. Clinical Manifestations, Diagnosis and Treatment. Singapore: Springer Singapore; 2018. pp. 223-239

[32] Peltoniemi MA, Hagelberg NM, Olkkola KT, Saari TI. Ketamine: a review of clinical pharmacokinetics and pharmacodynamics in anesthesia and pain therapy. Clinical Pharmacokinetics. 2016;**55**(9):1059-1077

[33] Sellers EM, Romach MK, Leiderman DB. Studies with psychedelic drugs in human volunteers. Neuropharmacology. 2018;**142**:116-134

[34] Balmer CN. Anaesthesia Recovery Quality and Immediate Postoperative Analgesia After Racemic Ketamine or S-Ketamine Administration to Male Cats Undergoing Routine Neutering Surgery. University of Zurich Main Library Strickhofstrasse 39 CH-8057 Zurich; 2008. www.zora.uzh.ch

[35] Fawkner-Corbett J, Hall A. General anesthetics and therapeutic gases. In: Ray S, editor. Side Effects of Drugs Annual. Vol. 39. Amsterdam, New York, Oxford: Elsevier; 2017. pp. 111-121

[36] Mion G, Villevieille T. Ketamine pharmacology: An update (pharmacodynamics and molecular aspects, recent findings). CNS Neuroscience & Therapeutics. 2013; **19**(6):370-380

[37] Homayoun H, Moghaddam B. NMDA receptor hypofunction produces opposite effects on prefrontal cortex interneurons and pyramidal neurons. Journal of Neuroscience. 2007;**27**(43): 11496-11500

[38] Kelland MD, Soltis RP, Boldry RC, Walters JR. Behavioral and electrophysiological comparison of ketamine with dizocilpine in the rat. Physiology & Behavior. 1993;**54**(3): 547-554

[39] Petrenko AB, Yamakura T, Fujiwara N, Askalany AR, Baba H, Sakimura K. Reduced sensitivity to ketamine and pentobarbital in mice lacking the N-methyl-D-aspartate receptor GluRε1 subunit. Anesthesia & Analgesia. 2004;**99**(4):1136-1140

[40] Chen X, Shu S, Bayliss DA. HCN1 channel subunits are a molecular substrate for hypnotic actions of ketamine. Journal of Neuroscience. 2009;**29**(3):600-609

[41] Zhou C, Douglas JE, Kumar NN, Shu S, Bayliss DA, Chen X. Forebrain HCN1 channels contribute to hypnotic actions of ketamine. Anesthesiology. 2013;**118**(4):785-795

[42] Rabben T, Øye I. Interindividual differences in the analgesic response to ketamine in chronic orofacial pain. European Journal of Pain. 2001;**5**(3): 233-240

[43] Kubota T, Anzawa N, Hirota K, Yoshida H, Kushikata T, Matsuki A. Effects of ketamine and pentobarbital on noradrenaline release from the medial prefrontal cortex in rats. Canadian Journal of Anaesthesia. 1999;**46**(4):388-392

[44] Dahan A, Olofsen E, Sigtermans M, Noppers I, Niesters M, Aarts L, et al. Population pharmacokinetic–pharmacodynamic modeling of ketamine-induced pain relief of chronic pain. European Journal of Pain. 2011;**15**(3):258-267

[45] Niesters M, Martini C, Dahan A. Ketamine for chronic pain: Risks and benefits. British Journal of Clinical Pharmacology. 2014;**77**(2):357-367

[46] Olofsen E, Noppers I, Niesters M, Kharasch E, Aarts L, Sarton E, et al. Estimation of the contribution of norketamine to ketamine-induced acute pain relief and neurocognitive impairment in healthy volunteers. The

Journal of the American Society of Anesthesiologists. 2012;**117**(2):353-364

[47] Noppers I, Niesters M, Aarts L, Smith T, Sarton E, Dahan A. Ketamine for the treatment of chronic non-cancer pain. Expert Opinion on Pharmacotherapy. 2010;**11**(14): 2417-2429

[48] Rabben T, Skjelbred P, Øye I. Prolonged analgesic effect of ketamine, anN-Methyl-d-aspartate receptor inhibitor, in patients with chronic pain. Journal of Pharmacology and Experimental Therapeutics. 1999; **289**(2):1060-1066

[49] Petrenko AB, Yamakura T, Baba H, Shimoji K. The role of N-methyl-D-aspartate (NMDA) receptors in pain: A review. Anesthesia & Analgesia. 2003;**97**(4):1108-1116

[50] Sarton E, Teppema LJ, Olievier C, Nieuwenhuijs D, Matthes HW, Kieffer BL, et al. The involvement of the μ-opioid receptor in ketamine-induced respiratory depression and antinociception. Anesthesia & Analgesia. 2001;**93**(6):1495-1500

[51] Gupta A, Devi LA, Gomes I. Potentiation of μ-opioid receptor-mediated signaling by ketamine. Journal of Neurochemistry. 2011;**119**(2):294-302

[52] Koizuka S, Obata H, Sasaki M, Saito S, Goto F. Systemic ketamine inhibits hypersensitivity after surgery via descending inhibitory pathways in rats. Canadian Journal of Anesthesia. 2005;**52**(5):498-505

[53] Gordh T, Karlsten R, Kristensen J. Intervention with spinal NMDA, adenosine, and NO systems for pain modulation. Annals of Medicine. 1995;**27**(2):229-234

[54] Backonja M, Arndt G, Gombar KA, Check B, Zimmermann M. Response of chronic neuropathic pain syndromes to ketamine: A preliminary study. Pain. 1994;**56**(1):51-57

[55] Warncke T, Stubhaug A, Jørum E. Ketamine, an NMDA receptor antagonist, suppresses spatial and temporal properties of burn-induced secondary hyperalgesia in man: A double-blind, cross-over comparison with morphine and placebo. Pain. 1997;**72**(1-2):99-106

[56] Remérand F, Le Tendre C, Baud A, Couvret C, Pourrat X, Favard L, et al. The early and delayed analgesic effects of ketamine after total hip arthroplasty: A prospective, randomized, controlled, double-blind study. Anesthesia & Analgesia. 2009;**109**(6):1963-1971

[57] Romero-Sandoval EA. Depression and pain: does ketamine improve the quality of life of patients in chronic pain by targeting their mood? The Journal of the American Society of Anesthesiologists. 2011;**115**(4):687-688

[58] Wang J, Goffer Y, Xu D, Tukey DS, Shamir D, Eberle SE, et al. A single subanesthetic dose of ketamine relieves depression-like behaviors induced by neuropathic pain in rats. Anesthesiology. 2011;**115**(4):812-821

[59] Zimmermann M. Pathobiology of neuropathic pain. European Journal of Pharmacology. 2001;**429**(1-3):23-37

[60] Liu R-J, Lee FS, Li X-Y, Bambico F, Duman RS, Aghajanian GK. Brain-derived neurotrophic factor Val66Met allele impairs basal and ketamine-stimulated synaptogenesis in prefrontal cortex. Biological Psychiatry. 2012; **71**(11):996-1005

Chapter 3

Cortical Plasticity under Ketamine: From Synapse to Map

Ouelhazi Afef, Rudy Lussiez and Molotchnikoff Stephane

Abstract

Sensory systems need to process signals in a highly dynamic way to efficiently respond to variations in the animal's environment. For instance, several studies showed that the visual system is subject to neuroplasticity since the neurons' firing changes according to stimulus properties. This dynamic information processing might be supported by a network reorganization. Since antidepressants influence neurotransmission, they can be used to explore synaptic plasticity sustaining cortical map reorganization. To this goal, we investigated in the primary visual cortex (V1 of mouse and cat), the impact of ketamine on neuroplasticity through changes in neuronal orientation selectivity and the functional connectivity between V1 cells, using cross correlation analyses. We found that ketamine affects cortical orientation selectivity and alters the functional connectivity within an assembly. These data clearly highlight the role of the antidepressant drugs in inducing or modeling short-term plasticity in V1 which suggests that cortical processing is optimized and adapted to the properties of the stimulus.

Keywords: cortical plasticity, functional connectivity, ketamine, orientation selectivity, synchrony

1. Introduction

Natural animal surroundings provide a variety of external sensory stimuli. Consequently, the brain must dynamically integrate each presented feature with changes in internal patterns of responses which manifests as a change in an animal's behavioral state [1, 2]. For instance, many studies suggest that visual processing should be optimized and adapted to the properties of the stimulus. Thus, visual object representation arises from the activation of functional domains in the cerebral cortex that encodes feature-specific information such as orientation, color, and motion direction [3–8]. Such feature-specific units have specific parallel networks [9] and therefore visual processing is based on the activation of multiple circuits. Many manipulations such as visual adaptation or antidepressant applications such as ketamine can alter the neuron's inherent proprieties, and this might result in a change in correlated and uncorrelated neural activity through changes in firing rates. The effect of ketamine results in NMDAR (*N*-methyl-D-aspartate receptor) blocking, thus it can be used as a read-out informing visual NMDAR dependent processing or activity mediated processing.

2. Cortical plasticity

Plasticity phenomena in the adult cerebral cortex are known to be heavily correlated to the brain's capacity for recovery after injuries [10–13], memory storage [14, 15], and learning [16–19]. In addition, throughout an animal's life, cortical representations are continuously modified by experience. In experimental animals, alterations in cortical representations appear following manipulations of inputs and depending on the information locally and globally available to the cortical cells [20–22]. Many investigations show that the properties of visual cortical neurons are not fixed and can be altered in adulthood [20, 23, 24]. This neuroplasticity has been well documented, as a modification that occurs at many levels from system to molecular, going through the network, cellular and synaptic levels. In this chapter, the experimental electrophysiological work was done in the primary visual cortex of adult cat and mouse so that the responses of visual cortical cells as well as the modification of the cell's output under different manipulations, particularly antidepressant application, was measured. This has made the visual system a preferred field for experimentation and analysis. Investigations suggest that the enormous architecture of the visual cortex is genetically preprogrammed, however, a minor proportion is shaped by experience and subject to the brain's plasticity.

2.1 Organization of the visual cortex and visual processing

We do not yet know exactly the ultrastructural connectome of the primary visual cortex and how it processes information. However, there are some general principles of V1 architecture and processing. Visual inputs reach V1 from the lateral geniculate nucleus (LGN). The thalamocortical connections terminate mainly in layer 4 (L4) and less in supra-(L5/6) and infragranular layers (L2/3). This flow of sensory information is common to all the sensory areas. In contrast to this classic scheme, a recent investigation in mouse using an intersectional viral tracing method for ultrastructural connectivity described labeled thalamocortical synapses in all cortical layers with prevalence in L2/3 [25]. The principal vertical flow of information through the cortical layers may be from the granular layer to infragranular (L2/3) to supragranular (L5/6) [26, 27]. Considering that each layer is a level of cortical processing, one might have expected that a proportion of complex cells with larger receptive fields and more complex responses are outside of L4. Hence, at a given stage, each unit is a sampling from a broader input extent, receiving convergent information from the preceding stage, diverging out to the following stage, and in this process, establishing larger and more complex integrated receptive fields, with emerging sharper response properties [28, 29]. In parallel to this vertical flow of information, there is a horizontal connectivity. At each layer, most excitatory projections seem to originate from intra- and interlaminar pyramidal cells. The horizontal connectivity arises from L2/3 and L5 and project to infra- and supragranular levels [30, 31].

The brain processes complex visual information along with different feature aspects, such as orientation, visual motion, color or curvature [32]. Hence, visual inputs are parceled out to different extrastriatal cortical areas for further analysis. The extrastriate visual cortex receives strong direct projections from primary visual cortex which leads to a first-pass computation in the visual processing. The main outputs of V1 are to V2, V3, V4, and V5 (MT). The assumption is that the extrastriate areas which connect with V1 are in lower positions in the processing hierarchy than the extrastriate areas which connect with other extrastriate areas. This idea is superimposed on a recent concept of parallel pathways of visual areas that are implicated in some common dimensions of visual processing, i.e., "what" processing (ventral pathway), or "where" processing (dorsal pathway). From these extrastriate areas, visual inputs are then transferred back by feedback connections to areas V1 and V2 [33]. Visual object recognition depends on developing during processing across a hierarchy of visual areas both selectivity and invariance at each stage. Both simple and complex cells are selective but only complex cells are invariant to a range of object transformations. This invariance allows an object to be recognized even when some of its features (size, orientation, position, etc.) change [34].

In addition to this classical visual cortical hierarchy, it was shown that the stimulus context modulates a cell's response which suggests the implication of other [33] areas in addition to the higher order of the visual cortical hierarchy [35, 36]. Since a big number of stimuli are present in the visual field at the same time, bottom-up and top-down mechanisms, as visual spatial attention, bias the processing toward a particularly salient stimuli [37].

2.1.1 Primary visual cortex

A key element in the role V1 plays in visual perception is the ability of V1 neurons to integrate information over larger parts of the visual field, since most of them are activated by stimulation of each eye. It was shown that a single oriented bar can induce a V1 neuron to fire. This property of orientation tuning selectivity, first described by Hubel and Wiesel (1968), is an emergent property of V1, seen in an optimal response of a given neuron to a single preferred orientation of the line segment or gratings. Although, orientation selectivity (OS) was shown in retinal ganglion cells, this tuning preference has received much less attention then in the cortex because most retinal ganglion cells are selective only to cardinal orientations: horizontal (pigeon retina) [38], and vertical (rabbit retina) [39]. It was reported that zebrafish retina contains cells with oblique preference in addition to the cardinal types [40].

In addition to the orientation tuning, neurons in primary visual cortex are highly sensitive to other visual stimulus properties such as contrast, the direction of movement, and temporal and spatial frequency. These stimulus properties can interact and influence neuronal responses. For example, it was revealed in ferret visual cortex, that a cell's orientation-tuning is not affected by contrast level and the temporal-frequency of the visual stimulus. However, direction selectivity decreases, and sometimes reverses, at nonpreferred temporal frequencies [41, 42]. These investigations might support the idea that invariance of OS is a prime aspect of visual processing. However, in the next section, we will see that manipulation and the use of ketamine can alter this intrinsic propriety of V1.

2.1.1.1 Orientation selectivity in cat

OS is a salient propriety of V1. In anesthetized cats, electrophysiological studies using extracellular recordings of V1 cells reveal that neurons are orientation selective (**Figure 1**). To study OS of neurons, stimulation can be accomplished using blocks of 25 trials of each of eight black–white oriented sine gratings placed in the cat receptive field and covering a span of 157.5° equally spaced at 22.5° (**Figure 1a**). Spike sorting method allows the separation of a cell's spikes from multi-unit activity. First, spike-waveforms have to be verified qualitatively by visual control, then the spike sorting is continued by cluster-isolation using first principal components analyses, autocorrelograms (AG) showing absence of events at 0 s on the time-scale (refractory period), peri-stimulus time histograms, (PSTH) and raster plots (RP), denoting for each trial the cell's spontaneous activity (before the 0 s:

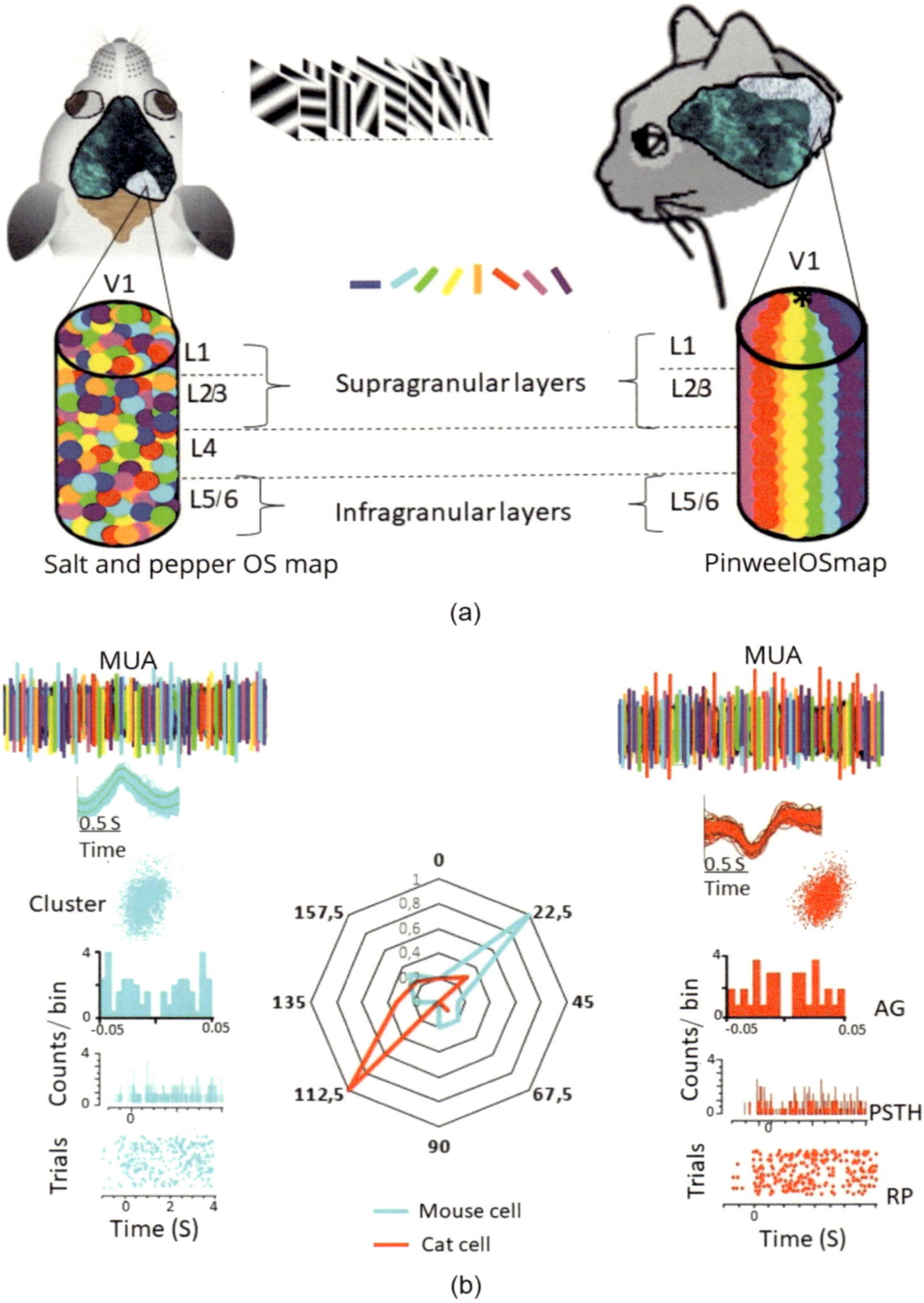

Figure 1.
Experimental procedures and spike sorting method. (a) V1 stimulation (shown as black and white gratings) and V1 architecture in mouse and cat (shown as cylinders, the black star shows the convergence of different orientations in cat). (b) Spike sorting process on the left for mouse and on the right for cat (from top to bottom): Multiunit activity (MUA), spike wave forms (cyan in mouse and red in cat), principal component analysis of the dissociated waveforms, auto-correlograms, peri-stimulus time histograms, and raster plots for the separated single units.

stimulus trigger time) and its response to the stimulus presentation (**Figure 1b**). Based on the raw data, neurons' responses are determined using Gaussian function that allows precise determination of the preferred orientation of each isolated neuron [43]. Whereas the strength of the OS can be measured by the orientation selectivity index (OSI), whose value is between 0 (orientation-nonselective) and 1(strongest OS) [44, 45], the sharpness of the tuning curve around its peak is measured by the orientation bandwidth from the Gaussian fit based on the full width at half height [46]. In cats, most V1 cells show a strong OS and sharp tuning curves. It was reported that over 82% of V1 neurons were well-tuned to stimulus orientation [47], and all the orientations were represented covering the full 180° [48]. In cats, V1 neurons with similar OS preferences are assembled in orientation columns. This columnar organization, where all cells through all six cortical layers have the same orientation preference, is a well-known characteristic that is shared by cats with ferrets and primates. Such cortical architecture, suggesting a vertical integration of feature selectivity through V1 layers, could reduce cable length, economizing the volume, and maintenance cost of V1 [49, 50]. OS is embedded in a retinotopic map in which information from neighboring locations in the visual field is coded in neighboring locations in the brain onto a two-dimensional surface that retains the image's spatial organization. In addition, the cortical organization of cats and primates is known as a pinwheel OS map because different orientations columns are organized radially around a central point (showed by a star in **Figure 1a**) in the retinotopic map.

2.1.1.2 Orientation selectivity in mouse

Unlike cats and primates where the columnar organization is an apparent characteristic of the neocortex, rodents and rabbits have a salt-and-pepper OS map, that is a random distribution of orientation-selective neurons. Hence, cells with different orientation preferences are juxtaposed horizontally across the retinotopic map and vertically through the six cortical layers in a random fashion [51–55] (**Figure 1**). Despite the lack of the columnar organization, it was shown, using extracellular recordings, that neurones in V1 of mice are sharply tuned to orientation of drifting gratings but the percentage of orientation-nonselective cells, whose orientation tuning curves were not unimodal, was bigger (63,33% of sorted cells) than in cats (18%) [24, 47]. Therefore, neuronal feature selectivity might be related to the activation of a specific cortical cell's subtype more than the cortical architecture. Indeed, it was reported that optogenetic activation of parvalbumin-positive (PV^+) interneurons in the mouse primary visual cortex (V1), that is, the increase of their firing rate, markedly sharpened OS and enhanced perceptual discrimination of nearby neurons [46]. Even in V1, neurons' responses are well known for their orientation tuning, the results of a recent study in mice seemed to leave little doubt that, in vision, the prominent role of V1 is encoding simple visual stimuli as oriented bars or gratings. It seems that in addition to a simple discrimination between light and dark oriented bars, V1 is involved in learning processes such as categorizing visual stimuli based on perceptual features, functional (semantic) relations, or a combination of both. Hence, the formation of a neuronal category representation in mice occurs in the first stages of visual information processing in the neocortex together with higher cortical association areas [56]. Despite the notion that the salt-and-pepper map is considered the most likely ancestral state, neurons can maintain high values of OS, and they are involved in complex visual processing, such as categorization. It seems that this organization in rodents was favored by their small brain size, that is in this case, the reduced visual field coverage might outweigh the potential advantage of a pinwheel OS map. However, recent studies show that cortical orientation columns perhaps are miniaturized in mouse V1 since orientation preference maps with pinwheel arrangement comparable to the macaque were described in mouse lemur [49, 57]. Hence, the V1 of rodents might represent micro-scale precursors of primate-type functional orientation columns [57]. It is likely that the relative thickness of cortical layers was a predictor for the functional organization. Indeed, an anatomical study showed that layers 2/3 are thicker in carnivores and primates than in rodents, while layers 5/6 are thicker in rodents than in carnivores and primates. The study exhibited that out of the total cortical thickness on average 44% in primates and 35% on average in carnivores were occupied by layers 2/3, but only 26% on average in rodents. In contrast, 34% of the total cortical thickness in primates and 39% in carnivores were occupied by layers 5/6, but 54% in rodents [49] . These anatomical differences between these species might affect intralaminar and cross-laminar networks and the visual cortex organization which evolved to be different in rodents versus primates and carnivores. The question that arises is whether the mechanisms of cortical plasticity, which operate at the level of single cells and the network are similar in mice and cats' V1, and so independent of the presence of columnar organization. In the next section, we will try to investigate the effect of ketamine on the OS and the synaptic weight between cells in V1 in cats and mice.

2.2 Induction of plasticity by ketamine

Antidepressant drugs are often used to treat mental and affective disorders such as maladaptive responses to stress. Although the drugs have different mechanisms of action, the "monoaminergic hypothesis" is commonly accepted to underline the antidepressant effect [58]. Ketamine is a rapidly-acting antidepressant, and its effect is profound and sustainable [59, 60]. It is used for treatment-resistant symptoms of mood disorders in patients who are resistant to typical antidepressants [45, 59, 61]. Ketamine is a blocker of glutamatergic NMDAR (N-methyl-D-aspartate receptor) activity as it acts as a non-competitive antagonist. Many findings reveal that ketamine, in addition to its antidepressant effect, induces visual cortical plasticity. It was shown, in adult mouse, that single-dose ketamine promotes functional recovery of visual acuity from amblyopia [62]. Another investigation provided evidence that ketamine enhanced visual sensory-evoked Long-Term Potentiation (LTP) in depressive patients [63]. By contrast, other investigations showed that ketamine altered or blocked some visual processing and disturbed cortical plasticity. For example, it was reported that ketamine blocked the induction of LTP in layer 2/3 of the adult rat visual cortex in vitro [64]. In addition, in kitten, it prevented the ocular dominance shift toward the open eye which suggests a retrograde effect on cortical plasticity [65]. Moreover, in humans, ketamine interfering with top-down processes distorted object recognition [66], and it altered the neuronal processing of facial emotion recognition due to the reduced activity in visual brain regions involved in emotion processing [67]. The effect of ketamine on the brain remains uncertain and sometimes contradictory according to investigations. This might be due to several variables such as the region of interest in the brain, the dose administrated, the administration mode (local, intraveinal, acute, or chronic, etc.) or the animal model. The effect of ketamine on the OS of V1 cells was tested in cat and mice and is explained in the next section.

2.2.1 Under ketamine influence cortical cells exhibit neuroplasticity by acquiring new selectivity

To examine the impact of the antidepressant on the orientation preferences of V1 cells, the drug can be applied locally over the animal's cortex. Ketamine application can be executed using a strip of filter paper (1 × 1 mm) impregnated with the drug (10 mM) and placed next to the recording sites. Test orientations can be presented, and recordings can be performed in the control conditions and ten minutes after ketamine administration [68]. As a result, cortical neurons selectively responding to the exposed orientations were altered by ketamine in that the cells acquired a new preference and showed a shift in the peak of their tuning curve. Based on the simulation results, we obtained evidence that ketamine induced orientation plasticity in mice (**Figure 2a**) and cat V1. It is shown that the ketamine effect on V1 cells is local

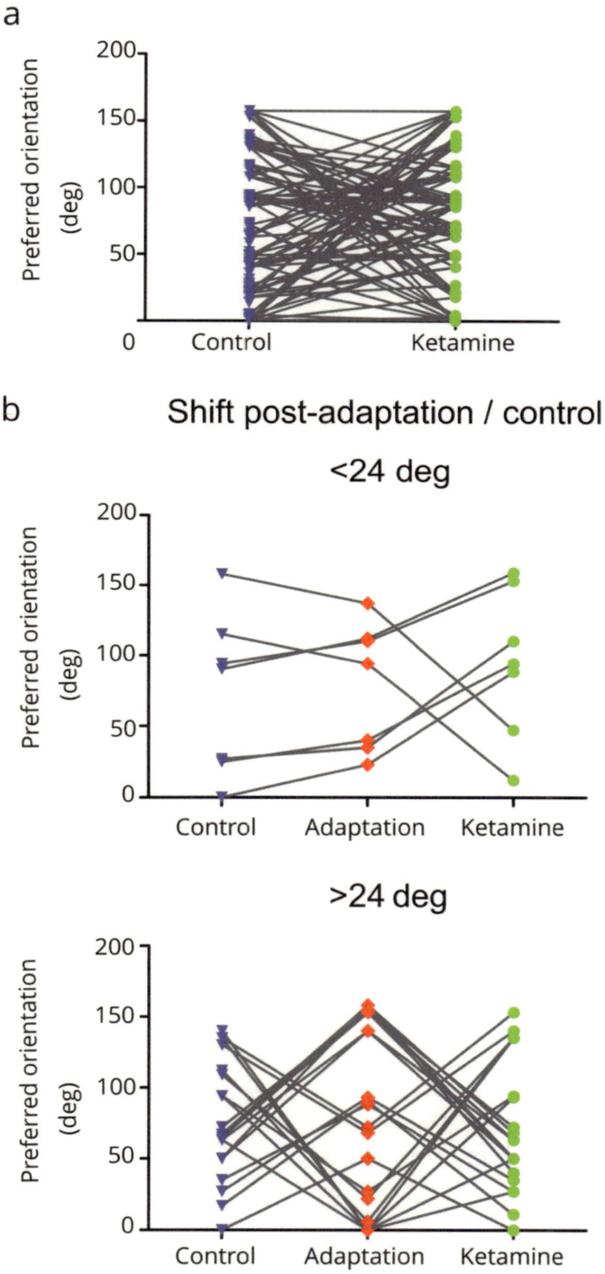

Figure 2.
Effect of ketamine on orientation selectivity in the mouse. (a) The control preferred orientation of cells changes after ketamine application. (b) The effect of ketamine on post-adaptation preferred orientation depends on the post-adaptation shifts. Shifts inferior to 24° are amplified under ketamine while shifts superior to 24° are reduced, that is, ketamine favors cells' recovery.

since it does not exceed 0.7 mm, and transient since a recovery state was observed [68]. The question is whether the observed changes of the cells' tuning properties were observed after visual adaptation, that is, could ketamine alter the adaptation effects? To implement adaptation, an imposed orientation can be exposed for several minutes. Results showed that restricted exposure of V1 cells to vertical orientation (90°) for 12 minutes shifted their original preferred orientations toward the exposed orientation (attractive shift). Contrarily, the tuning curve peaks of a few cells shifted away from the original preferred orientation (repulsive shift). Dual mechanisms have been proposed for repulsive and attractive shifts in cat. While the repulsive shift results in a decrease of excitation at the adapted flank of the tuning curve, the attractive shift is the result of the parallel facilitation of responses on the adapted flank and a depression on the opposite flank [69]. This effect of adaptation is known as a push–pull mechanism [69, 70]. In cats, Dragoi et al. [23] reported larger repulsive shifts near the pinwheels of orientation maps than in an iso-orientation domain in cats. This systematic change in V1 was attributed to a higher degree of plasticity near pinwheels because of the convergence of a broad spectrum of orientation inputs [23]. Comparing the cells' orientation preferences in control, post-adaptation, and post-ketamine, the collected data showed that ketamine abolished the adaptation effects, that it changes the new preferred orientation. Apart from this general effect, electrophysiological studies reveal a more varied scenario. Indeed, the effect of ketamine categorizes cells into two groups according to the amplitude of the adaptation-induced shift: for cells exhibiting large shifts (superior to 24°), ketamine decreases the post-adaptation shift amplitude in that it alters their new preferred orientations toward the original preference, but for cells exhibiting small shifts (inferior to 24°), ketamine increases the post-adaptation shifts. Thus, while ketamine facilitates the cell's recovery for large shifts, it potentiates the small shifts (**Figure 2b**). This might suggest that ketamine application leads to weakening or amplifying the adaptation effects according to the amplitude of the adaptation-induced shift.

Because the results are similar in mouse and cat, we assumed that the mechanisms of cortical plasticity induced by ketamine, which operate at the level of single cells, are similar, independent of the presence of columnar organization.

2.2.2 Crosscorrelation analyses

Cross-correlogram (CCG) analysis is an efficient tool to reveal the putative functional coupling between neurons that display time relationships between their respective spike trains [71–75]. The stimulus-dependent synchrony should be suppressed in the shift-corrected cross-correlation histograms [76]; this allowed the measurement of synchrony excluding latencies evoked by stimuli onset. The CCG is performed between simultaneously recorded spike trains of two neurons where one cell is set as reference and the second as target. In CCGs, the time axis (X axis) is divided into bins of 1 ms and the *Y*-axis corresponds to the probability (p) of a neuron firing in the small bin of the size b considering the spike train is a Poisson process [77]; this probability p is calculated as follows:

$$p = F \times b \tag{1}$$

$$F = N / T \tag{2}$$

where F is the neuronal firing rate, b is the bin size of the calculated firing of the neuron, T is the total time interval and N is the number of spikes in that interval. The functional connection between neuron-pairs is illustrated by a significant peak of at least one bin [78] within a window of 5 ms offset from zero. The statistical threshold for the significance peak was set at 95% and presented by the red line in **Figure 3a**. Cross-correlation function can also reveal neuronal synchrony which is generated when units receive a common input from other cells embedded in the network. In neuronal synchrony, the central peak of the

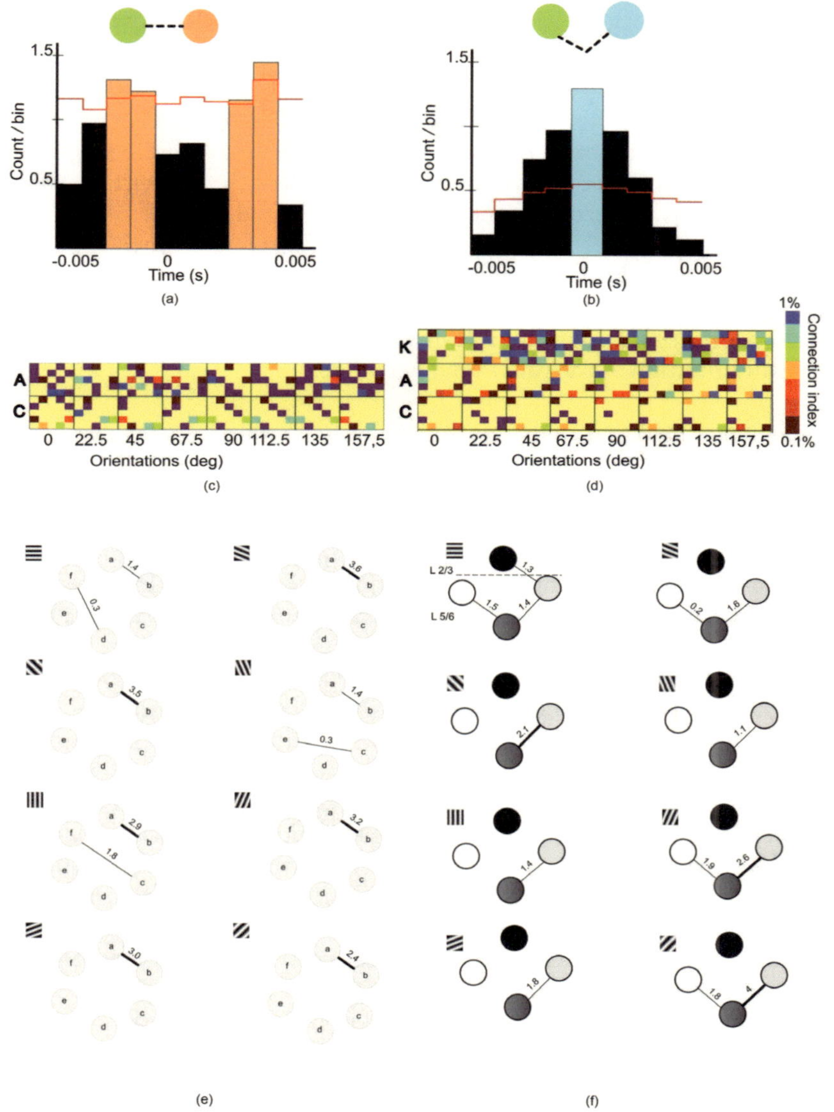

Figure 3.
Cell assembly dynamics. (a) The functional network between a reference cell (green) and a target cell (orange on the left and cyan on the right) revealed by CCG analysis. (b) Neuronal synchrony revealed by a significant bin within the time window −1 to +1 ms adjoining the central zero point. In (a) and (b) the confidence limit is shown by the red curved line. (c and d) Strength matrices of a cells (6 × 6 cells simultaneously) in mouse, at all the tested gratings and in all conditions: Control (C), and post-ketamine (K) in c, and control (C), post-adaptation (a), and post-ketamine (K) in d. the colored scale (to the right) represents normalized peaks-strengths of connections. (e and f) Functional network between neurons according to the presented orientation in mouse (e) and in cat (f). The number above the black line indicates the probability of the connection between two units. For cat, cells were simultaneously recorded from two layers (L2/3) and (L5/6) separated in the scheme by the interrupted black line.

CCG is significant within the time window −1 to +1 ms bin adjoining the central zero point (**Figure 3b**).

2.2.3 Ketamine reorganizes the cortical network

In cat and mouse, CCG analysis performed before and following ketamine application shows that this drug alters the putative synaptic links between neurons following visual adaptation. Thus, ketamine modulates the neuronal assembly by strengthening or weakening synaptic weight and/or adding new cells to connectomes (**Figure 3c**). The redistribution of synaptic weights between neurons after ketamine application suggests a reassignment of functions of each neuron pair inside the microcircuits. Ketamine not only enables altering the original network but also the post-adaptation microcircuits. This implies that when a single unit changes its selectivity after experience-dependent plasticity, its wiring changes according to its new preferred orientation (**Figure 3c** and **d**).

Ketamine might disturb cells' activity which in turn redeploys the strength of projections between cells to restructure the entire wiring-dynamic of the neuronal assembly. We conclude that, despite the organizational difference between mouse and cat, ketamine remaps the connectivity of visual cortex microcircuits, and leads to a new configuration of the functional networks.

2.2.4 Functional connectivity within an assembly changes in response to different orientations

In this section, the network-dynamics of the assembly are related to the orientation changes in each condition (control, post-adaptation, post-ketamine). Thus, we investigated whether the strength of connections between units in an assembly is related to stimulus orientation. Results, in cat and mouse, show a unique network was activated at every orientation whatever the condition. Therefore, feature-specific connectivity was generated for each input stimulus. Thus, connections are activated or deactivated depending on the feature stimulus. **Figure 3c-e** illustrates the dynamic interactions between neurons within an assembly in response to different orientations in cat and mouse. In short, in mouse, as shown in **Figure 3d**, some connections were largely maintained despite the change in orientation, whereas, and independently of the condition, other links emerged specifically for some orientations (e.g., unit (e)—unit (c) at 67.5°). The connection disclosed between (f) and (d) units at 0° disappeared at other grating orientations. Furthermore, some connections were characterized by a change in their peak-strength (p) from one orientation to another as depicted by the changing colors in the connectivity matrices (**Figure 3d**) and the weights numbers over connecting lines (**Figure 3e**). For instance, the connection between unit (a) and unit (b) (p = 3.5% at 45°) weakens (p = 1.4% at 67.5°) as shown in **Figure 3e**.

Similarly, in cat, some links were maintained at all presented orientations, implying the stability of distinctive connections between specific neurons (dark and light gray units), others were activated (black cell—light gray cell at 0°) or deactivated only at some orientations (the connectivity between dark gray cell—white cell disappeared at 45°, 67.5° and 90° (**Figure 3f**). All previous examples were drawn from the control condition. However, similar results were observed following adaptation and ketamine, depending on the orientation applied. We conclude that the functional links between pairs at a particular orientation (here 0°) show a unique network activated by a particular condition. Thus, adaptation changes the initial network and induces a new one; in addition, these cellular relationship modifications occur in both supra- and infra-granular layers (separated by the dotted horizontal black lines). This network acquired following adaptation was modified after ketamine application and a new pattern of connections emerges. It is worth mentioning that the effect of ketamine on the network dynamics is reversible since after recovery the connections between reference and targets return to the original pattern.

The change in the probabilities of connection (p) from one grating to another reflects a modification of synaptic weights between neurons in the assembly [78], wherein new neurons join and others leave in relation to the presented orientation. Accordingly, the unit output is the result of synaptic weights distributed over its dendritic tree for each grating. It was reported that within a cell-assembly, some connections are weak, therefore their feeble activation might confer flexibility to the assembly as the stimulus changes [79]. Thus, in the cortex, the functional units are neuronal ensembles rather than individual cells [80] and because of the synaptic flexibility of these neuronal groups, a dynamic salient microcircuit is involved for each visual stimulus. In line with a previous report [81], the encoding sensory stimuli might require a coordinated activity of specific groups of neurons that represent the building block of visual processing. Conclusively, all the above findings imply that the flexibility of the neuronal circuit keeps it permanently ready to receive the input efficiently and that the output is related to the assembly organization. In mouse, the proximity of neurons with different orientation preferences (salt-and-pepper organization) may favor each orientation grating, the activation of a specific group of synapses, and thus the emergence of a specific functional microcircuit. It is worth noting the activation of a specific functional network between co-active neurons as the orientation changes is a general property of stimulus processing that would be applicable to all mammals. It must be underlined that connectivity weights are independent of firing rates [79].

2.2.5 Ketamine affects the pair-wise synchrony

To investigate the effect of ketamine on the pair-wise synchrony, a computation of the number of connections and the CCG magnitudes of all summed pairs was performed at all presented orientations and compared between control, post-adaptation, and post-ketamine conditions. Results show that, contrasting with adaptation, under ketamine, the magnitude and the number of synchronous inputs was increased in cat but not in mouse. This increase might reflect a more coordinate activity of the recipient units with each other [82], which might lead to expand and upgrade the cortical processing and thus more efficient information transfer. Synchrony is energy demanding. Indeed, neuronal synchrony requires resources to time firing initiation accurately, aligned anatomical pathways to transfer the spikes, and energy expenditures for redundant action potentials [83]. Since in biological systems, the costs should not outweigh benefits, these energy costs should be counterbalanced by an information rate increase and more efficient information transfer. Moreover, it has been shown previously that in addition to the firing rate, the precise timing of firing potentially encoded visual information (the visual information is encoded in temporal patterns of firing) [84–86]. It seems that columnar, and not salt-pepper organization where cells with different orientation preferences are locally intermixed, favors the pair-wise synchrony. In the cat visual cortex, neurons with similar features are clustered together, forming columns, and are likely to be interconnected [78, 87, 88]. Thus, it is more likely to encounter close neurons with similar tuning then in mouse and this organization favors synchronization since it was shown that the latter is due in part to specific horizontal connections between cortical domains having similar tuning properties. Indeed, it was reported that cells exhibiting similar orientation preference showed a significant pair-wise synchrony [89].

2.2.6 Ketamine affects downstream signaling events and leads to plasticity

Antidepressants, in particular ketamine, influence neurotransmission since it blocks NMDAR activity. Investigators have made many important strides toward understanding the molecular mechanisms governing the induction of plasticity by ketamine in stimulus processing.

It was reported that excitation (*E*) inhibition (*I*) ratios (*E/I*) are equalized across visual cortical neurons [90] and that matched inhibition is mediated by PV interneurons [91]. Since it was demonstrated that ketamine alters the neurochemical phenotype of PV cells [92], and modulates cortical circuit *E/I* ratios [93, 94], a new equilibrium of *E/I* ratios might be a putative explanation for the neuronal microcircuits' dynamics observed following ketamine administration. E/I ratio is activity-dependent [90], and the blockage of NMDA mediated activities might rebalance it. The effects of ketamine could also be explained by the increase in the expression of several molecules involved in neuronal plasticity, in particular, the neurotrophin BDNF, and its receptor TrkB. Thus, reactivation of activity-dependent and BDNF-mediated cortical plasticity by ketamine leads to the alteration of neuronal networks to better adapt to environmental challenges [95]. Furthermore, ketamine increases neurogenesis [96–98] and synaptogenesis [60, 99–101].

3. Conclusion

In the primary cortical areas, cells are fed by the feedforward thalamic drive while their intrinsic properties are further shaped through the local recurrent network. The most striking effects of ketamine are the imposition of new intrinsic properties of individual neurons and the abolition of adaptation effects. The core of the representational question is whether the changes in synaptic strengths, under ketamine, constitute an engram of a new encoding of inputs in the visual processing. Experimental findings show that in parallel to tuning shifts of V1 orientation-selective cells, ketamine reorganizes the connectomes, that is, cells modifying their synaptic weight, and therefore a change of the synaptic links between units was observed. These results might implicitly provide that synaptic rewiring plasticity underlies cortical map reorganization and that the modification of a cell's selectivity by ketamine may be better viewed in relationship to neuronal connections. In the cat primary visual cortex, it was reported that long-range horizontal axons preferentially bind to distant columns of similar tuning preferences which favors synchrony of cells' activity under ketamine. This could suggest that ketamine through activity-dependent synaptic plasticity can redistribute connections to preferentially link neurons with similar response properties.

Acknowledgements

We acknowledge the Conseil de Recherche en Sciences Naturelles et en Genie du Canada (CRSNG) to support the completion of this study and Steve Itaya for his comments on the early version of the manuscript.

Conflict of interest

Authors declare that they have no conflict of interest

DOI: http://dx.doi.org/10.5772/intechopen.104787

Author details

Ouelhazi Afef, Rudy Lussiez and Molotchnikoff Stephane*
Université de Montréal, Quebec, Canada

*Address all correspondence to: stephane.molotchnikoff@umontreal.ca

References

[1] Calhoun AJ, Pillow JW, Murthy M. Unsupervised identification of the internal states that shape natural behavior. Nature Neuroscience. 2019;**22**(12):2040-2049

[2] Salay LD, Ishiko N, Huberman AD. A midline thalamic circuit determines reactions to visual threat. Nature. 2018;**557**(7704):183-189

[3] Chen G, Lu HD, Roe AW. A map for horizontal disparity in monkey V2. Neuron. 2008;**58**(3):442-450

[4] Hu J et al. Visual motion processing in macaque V2. Cell Reports. 2018;**25**(1):157-167. e5

[5] Li P et al. A motion direction preference map in monkey V4. Neuron. 2013;**78**(2):376-388

[6] Lu HD et al. A motion direction map in macaque V2. Neuron. 2010;**68**(5):1002-1013

[7] Lu HD, Roe AW. Functional organization of color domains in V1 and V2 of macaque monkey revealed by optical imaging. Cerebral Cortex. 2008;**18**(3):516-533

[8] Tanigawa H, Lu HD, Roe AW. Functional organization for color and orientation in macaque V4. Nature Neuroscience. 2010;**13**(12):1542-1548

[9] Roe AW et al. Toward a unified theory of visual area V4. Neuron. 2012;**74**(1):12-29

[10] Hosp JA, Luft AR. Cortical plasticity during motor learning and recovery after ischemic stroke. Neural Plasticity. 2011;**2011**:871296

[11] Kolb B, Gibb R, Gorny G. Cortical plasticity and the development of behavior after early frontal cortical injury. Developmental Neuropsychology. 2000;**18**(3):423-444

[12] Nudo RJ. Recovery after brain injury: mechanisms and principles. Frontiers in Human Neuroscience. 2013;**7**:887

[13] Spolidoro M et al. Plasticity in the adult brain: lessons from the visual system. Experimental Brain Research. 2009;**192**(3):335-341

[14] Hebscher M et al. Rapid cortical plasticity supports long-term memory formation. Trends in Cognitive Sciences. 2019;**23**(12):989-1002

[15] Merzenich MM, Sameshima K. Cortical plasticity and memory. Current Opinion in Neurobiology. 1993;**3**(2):187-196

[16] Gilbert CD, Li W. Adult visual cortical plasticity. Neuron. 2012;**75**(2):250-264

[17] Karni A, Bertini G. Learning perceptual skills: behavioral probes into adult cortical plasticity. Current Opinion in Neurobiology. 1997;**7**(4):530-535

[18] van Wassenhove V, Nagarajan SS. Auditory cortical plasticity in learning to discriminate modulation rate. Journal of Neuroscience. 2007;**27**(10):2663-2672

[19] Li Voti P et al. Correlation between cortical plasticity, motor learning and BDNF genotype in healthy subjects. Experimental Brain Research. 2011;**212**(1):91-99

[20] Bachatene L et al. Reprogramming of orientation columns in visual cortex: a domino effect. Scientific Reports. 2015;**5**(1):1-11

[21] Chang JT, Whitney D, Fitzpatrick DJN. Experience-dependent reorganization drives development of a binocularly unified cortical representation of orientation. Neuron. 2020;**107**(2):338-350. e5

[22] Siucinska E, Kossut MJN. Experience-dependent changes in cortical whisker representation in the adult mouse: a 2-deoxyglucose study. Neuroscience. 2004;**127**(4):961-971

[23] Dragoi V, Sharma J, Sur M. Adaptation-induced plasticity of orientation tuning in adult visual cortex. Neuron. 2000;**28**(1):287-298

[24] Jeyabalaratnam J et al. Adaptation shifts preferred orientation of tuning curve in the mouse visual cortex. PloS One. 2013;**8**(5):e64294

[25] Sampathkumar V et al. An ultrastructural connectomic analysis of a higher-order thalamocortical circuit in the mouse. European Journal of Neuroscience. 2021;**53**(3):750-762

[26] Bolz J, Gilbert CD, Wiesel TN. Pharmacological analysis of cortical circuitry. Trends in Neurosciences. 1989;**12**(8):292-296

[27] Douglas RJ, Martin KA, Whitteridge D. A canonical microcircuit for neocortex. Neural Computation. 1989;**1**(4):480-488

[28] Chapman B, Stryker MP. Development of orientation selectivity in ferret visual cortex and effects of deprivation. Journal of Neuroscience. 1993;**13**(12):5251-5262

[29] Gilbert CD. Laminar differences in receptive field properties of cells in cat primary visual cortex. The Journal of Physiology. 1977;**268**(2):391-421

[30] Abeles MJC. Neural Circuits of the Cerebral Cortex. Cambridge, United Kingdom: Cambridge University Press; 1991

[31] Tanifuji M, Sugiyama T, Murase K. propagation of excitation in rat visual cortical slices revealed by optical imaging. Science. 1994;**266**(5187): 1057-1059

[32] Yue X et al. Curvature-processing network in macaque visual cortex. Proceedings of the National Academy of Sciences. 2014;**111**(33):E3467-E3475

[33] Bullier J. Integrated model of visual processing. Brain Research Reviews. 2001;**36**(2-3):96-107

[34] Kravitz DJ et al. The ventral visual pathway: an expanded neural framework for the processing of object quality. Trends in Cognitive Sciences. 2013;**17**(1):26-49

[35] Li W, Piëch V, Gilbert CD. Learning to link visual contours. Neuron. 2008;**57**(3):442-451

[36] McManus JN, Li W, Gilbert CD. Adaptive shape processing in primary visual cortex. Proceedings of the National Academy of Sciences. 2011;**108**(24):9739-9746

[37] McMains S, Kastner S. Interactions of top-down and bottom-up mechanisms in human visual cortex. Journal of Neuroscience. 2011;**31**(2):587-597

[38] Maturana HR, Frenk S. Directional movement and horizontal edge detectors in the pigeon retina. Science. 1963;**142**(3594):977-979

[39] Bloomfield SA. Orientation-sensitive amacrine and ganglion cells in the rabbit retina. Journal of Neurophysiology. 1994;**71**(5): 1672-1691

[40] Antinucci P et al. Neural mechanisms generating orientation selectivity in the retina. Current Biology. 2016;**26**(14):1802-1815

[41] Alitto HJ, Usrey WM. Influence of contrast on orientation and temporal frequency tuning in ferret primary visual cortex. Journal of Neurophysiology. 2004;**91**(6): 2797-2808

[42] Moore BD IV, Alitto HJ, Usrey WM. Orientation tuning, but not direction selectivity, is invariant to temporal frequency in primary visual cortex. Journal of Neurophysiology. 2005;**94**(2):1336-1345

[43] Swindale NV. Orientation tuning curves: empirical description and estimation of parameters. Biological Cybernetics. 1998;**78**(1):45-56

[44] Liao DS et al. Recovery of cortical binocularity and orientation selectivity after the critical period for ocular dominance plasticity. Journal of Neurophysiology. 2004;**92**(4): 2113-2121

[45] Ramoa AS et al. Suppression of cortical NMDA receptor function prevents development of orientation selectivity in the primary visual cortex. Journal of Neuroscience. 2001;**21**(12):4299-4309

[46] Ringach DL, Shapley RM, Hawken MJ. Orientation selectivity in macaque V1: Diversity and laminar dependence. Journal of Neuroscience. 2002;**22**(13):5639-5651

[47] Bachatene L et al. Adaptation-induced plasticity and spike waveforms in cat visual cortex. Neuroreport. 2012;**23**(2):88-92

[48] Cattan S et al. Comparative analysis of orientation maps in areas 17 and 18 of the cat primary visual cortex following adaptation. European Journal of Neuroscience. 2014;**40**(3):2554-2563

[49] Kaschube M. Neural maps versus salt-and-pepper organization in visual cortex. Current Opinion in Neurobiology. 2014;**24**:95-102

[50] Keil W et al. Response to comment on universality in the evolution of orientation columns in the visual cortex. Science. 2012;**336**(6080):413-413

[51] Bonin V et al. Local diversity and fine-scale organization of receptive fields in mouse visual cortex. Journal of Neuroscience. 2011;**31**(50): 18506-18521

[52] Espinosa JS, Stryker MP. Development and plasticity of the primary visual cortex. Neuron. 2012;**75**(2):230-249

[53] Ohki K et al. Functional imaging with cellular resolution reveals precise micro-architecture in visual cortex. Nature. 2005;**433**(7026):597-603

[54] Reid RC. From functional architecture to functional connectomics. Neuron. 2012;**75**(2):209-217

[55] Van Hooser SD et al. Orientation selectivity without orientation maps in visual cortex of a highly visual mammal. Journal of Neuroscience. 2005;**25**(1): 19-28

[56] Goltstein PM et al. Mouse visual cortex areas represent perceptual and semantic features of learned visual categories. Nature Neuroscience. 2021;**24**(10):1441-1451

[57] Ho CLA et al. Orientation preference maps in Microcebus murinus reveal size-invariant design principles in primate visual cortex. Current Biology. 2021;**31**(4):733-741. e7

[58] Krystal JH et al. Ketamine: a paradigm shift for depression research and treatment. Neuron. 2019;**101**(5):774-778

[59] Berman RM et al. Antidepressant effects of ketamine in depressed patients. Biological Psychiatry. 2000;**47**(4):351-354

[60] Duman RS et al. Signaling pathways underlying the rapid antidepressant actions of ketamine. Neuropharmacology. 2012;**62**(1):35-41

[61] Zarate CA et al. A randomized trial of an N-methyl-D-aspartate antagonist in treatment-resistant major depression. Archives of General Psychiatry. 2006;**63**(8):856-864

[62] Grieco SF et al. Subanesthetic ketamine reactivates adult cortical plasticity to restore vision from amblyopia. Current Biology. 2020;**30**(18):3591-3603. e8

[63] Sumner RL et al. Ketamine enhances visual sensory evoked potential long-term potentiation in patients with major depressive disorder. Cognitive Neuroscience and Neuroimaging. 2020;**5**(1):45-55

[64] Salami M et al. Effects of ketamine on synaptic transmission and long-term potentiation in layer II/III of rat visual cortex in vitro. European Journal of Pharmacology. 2000;**390**(3):287-293

[65] Rauschecker JP, Hahn S. Ketamine—xylazine anaesthesia blocks consolidation of ocular dominance changes in kitten visual cortex. Nature. 1987;**326**(6109):183-185

[66] van Loon AM et al. NMDA receptor antagonist ketamine distorts object recognition by reducing feedback to early visual cortex. Cerebral Cortex. 2016;**26**(5):1986-1996

[67] Abel KM et al. Ketamine alters neural processing of facial emotion recognition in healthy men: An fMRI study. Neuroreport. 2003;**14**(3):387-391

[68] Ouelhazi A et al. Effects of ketamine on orientation selectivity and variability of neuronal responses in primary visual cortex. Brain Research. 2019;**1725**:146462

[69] Ghisovan N et al. Long adaptation reveals mostly attractive shifts of orientation tuning in cat primary visual cortex. Neuroscience. 2009;**164**(3):1274-1283

[70] Shapley R, Hawken M, Ringach DL. Dynamics of orientation selectivity in the primary visual cortex and the importance of cortical inhibition. Neuron. 2003;**38**(5):689-699

[71] Fujisawa S et al. Behavior-dependent short-term assembly dynamics in the medial prefrontal cortex. Nature Neuroscience. 2008;**11**(7):823

[72] König P et al. How precise is neuronal synchronization? Neural Computation. 1995;7(3):469-485

[73] Patterson CA et al. Similar adaptation effects in primary visual cortex and area MT of the macaque monkey under matched stimulus conditions. Journal of Neurophysiology. 2014;**111**(6):1203-1213

[74] Schwindel CD et al. Long-term recordings improve the detection of weak excitatory–excitatory connections in rat prefrontal cortex. Journal of Neuroscience. 2014;**34**(16):5454-5467

[75] Vizuete JA et al. Monosynaptic functional connectivity in cerebral cortex during wakefulness and under graded levels of anesthesia. Frontiers in Integrative Neuroscience. 2012;**6**:90

[76] Perkel DH, Gerstein GL, Moore GP. Neuronal spike trains and stochastic point processes: I. the single spike train. Biophysical Journal. 1967;7(4):391-418

[77] Abeles M. Quantification, smoothing, and confidence limits for single-units' histograms. Journal of Neuroscience Methods. 1982;5(4):317-325

[78] Alloway K, Roy S. Conditional cross-correlation analysis of thalamocortical neurotransmission.

Behavioural Brain Research. 2002;**135**(1-2):191-196

[79] Bharmauria V et al. Network-selectivity and stimulus-discrimination in the primary visual cortex: Cell-assembly dynamics. European Journal of Neuroscience. 2016;**43**(2):204-219

[80] Miller JEK et al. Visual stimuli recruit intrinsically generated cortical ensembles. Proceedings of the National Academy of Sciences. 2014;**111**(38):E4053-E4061

[81] Molotchnikoff S et al. The function of connectomes in encoding sensory stimuli. Progress in Neurobiology. 2019;**181**:101659

[82] Yu J, Ferster D. Membrane potential synchrony in primary visual cortex during sensory stimulation. Neuron. 2010;**68**(6):1187-1201

[83] Wang H-P et al. Synchrony of thalamocortical inputs maximizes cortical reliability. Science. 2010;**328**(5974):106-109

[84] Dan Y et al. Coding of visual information by precisely correlated spikes in the lateral geniculate nucleus. Nature Neuroscience. 1998;**1**(6):501-507

[85] Kumbhani RD, Nolt MJ, Palmer LA. Precision, reliability, and information-theoretic analysis of visual thalamocortical neurons. Journal of Neurophysiology. 2007;**98**(5):2647-2663

[86] Reinagel P, Reid RC. Temporal coding of visual information in the thalamus. Journal of Neuroscience. 2000;**20**(14):5392-5400

[87] Alonso J-M, Usrey WM, Reid RC. Precisely correlated firing in cells of the lateral geniculate nucleus. Nature. 1996;**383**(6603):815-819

[88] Barthó P et al. Characterization of neocortical principal cells and interneurons by network interactions and extracellular features. Journal of Neurophysiology. 2004;**92**(1):600-608

[89] Denman DJ, Contreras D. The structure of pairwise correlation in mouse primary visual cortex reveals functional organization in the absence of an orientation map. Cerebral Cortex. 2014;**24**(10):2707-2720

[90] Xue M, Atallah BV, Scanziani M. Equalizing excitation–inhibition ratios across visual cortical neurons. Nature. 2014;**511**(7511):596-600

[91] Anderson JS, Carandini M, Ferster D. Orientation tuning of input conductance, excitation, and inhibition in cat primary visual cortex. Journal of Neurophysiology. 2000;**84**(2):909-926

[92] Behrens MM et al. Ketamine-induced loss of phenotype of fast-spiking interneurons is mediated by NADPH-oxidase. Science. 2007;**318**(5856):1645-1647

[93] Li N et al. mTOR-dependent synapse formation underlies the rapid antidepressant effects of NMDA antagonists. Science. 2010;**329**(5994):959-964

[94] Zanos P et al. NMDAR inhibition-independent antidepressant actions of ketamine metabolites. Nature. 2016;**533**(7604):481-486

[95] Castrén E, Rantamäki T. The role of BDNF and its receptors in depression and antidepressant drug action: Reactivation of developmental plasticity. Developmental Neurobiology. 2010;**70**(5):289-297

[96] Choi M et al. Hippocampal VEGF is necessary for antidepressant-like behaviors but not sufficient for antidepressant-like effects of ketamine in rats. Biochimica et Biophysica Acta (BBA)-Molecular Basis of Disease. 2016;**1862**(7):1247-1254

[97] Keilhoff G et al. Increased neurogenesis in a rat ketamine model of schizophrenia. Biological Psychiatry. 2004;**56**(5):317-322

[98] Lu Y et al. Pretreatment with minocycline restores neurogenesis in the subventricular zone and subgranular zone of the hippocampus after ketamine exposure in neonatal rats. Neuroscience. 2017;**352**:144-154

[99] Liu R-J et al. Brain-derived neurotrophic factor Val66Met allele impairs basal and ketamine-stimulated synaptogenesis in prefrontal cortex. Biological Psychiatry. 2012;**71**(11):996-1005

[100] Moda-Sava R et al. Sustained rescue of prefrontal circuit dysfunction by antidepressant-induced spine formation. Science. 2019;**364**(6436):eaat8078

[101] Zunszain P et al. Ketamine: Synaptogenesis, immunomodulation and glycogen synthase kinase-3 as underlying mechanisms of its antidepressant properties. Molecular Psychiatry. 2013;**18**(12):1236-1241

Section 3

Clinical Use in Anaesthesia

Chapter 4

Application of Ketamine in Current Practice of Anesthesiology

Shridevi Pandya Shah, Devanshi Patel and Antony Irungu

Abstract

Ketamine was discovered in 1964 by merging a ketone with an amine. Patients described feeling disconnected like they were floating in outer. Thus, it was characterized as a dissociative anesthetic. It is a unique drug that expresses hypnotic, analgesic, and amnesic effects. No other drug used in clinical practice produces these three important effects at the same time. Its newly found neuroprotective, anti-inflammatory, antitumor effects and low dose applications have helped to widen the clinical profile of ketamine. Ketamine as an analgesic adjunct in chronic pain patients is currently being researched. Combined use of ketamine and an opiate analgesic has been found to provide good perioperative pain control with reduction in symptoms such as nausea and vomiting, sedation, and respiratory insufficiency.

Keywords: ketamine, pain, dissociative anesthesia, NMDA receptors, ketamine physiology, ketamine side effects, ketamine as induction agent, ketamine for maintenance of anesthesia, ketamine contraindications, perioperative analgesia, anti-inflammation, sub anesthetic dose of ketamine

1. Introduction

The story of ketamine began in the 1950s in Park-Davis and Company's Laboratories as the search for a cyclohexylamine that would serve as an "ideal" anesthetic agent. This new agent would also have analgesic properties. In March 1956, Dr. Harold Maddox synthesized a compound [N-(1-phenyl-cyclohexyl)-piperidine] known as phencyclidine (PCP) using a new chemical organic Grignard reaction [1]. Several experiments were performed at Parke-Davis labs and Wayne State University; both on animals and in human trials. These experiments made it clear that phencyclidine was capable of producing a potent analgesic and cataleptic state defined as a "characteristic akinetic state with a loss of orthostatic reflexes, but without impairment of consciousness, in which the extremities appear to be paralyzed by motor and sensory failure" [2, 3]. After administering the drug, patients had an increase in blood pressure, respiratory rate, and minute volume while corneal and laryngeal reflexes were conserved. However, increased salivation and nystagmus were noted. With these findings, PCP was deemed to be a useful agent in the setting of anesthesia. However, with further studies, it became apparent that there was a profound and prolonged state of emergence delirium. This discovery would hinder the widespread use of PCP and begin the search for a new related compound [1, 3].

Finally, in 1962, Dr. Calvin Stevens was successfully synthesized a derivative of PCP – CI-581 or ketamine – which was selected to undergo human trials. On August 3 1964, the first human intravenous subanestheic dose of ketamine was successfully administered to volunteer prisoners at Jackson prison in Michigan [1]. About one-third of the patients had reported adverse effects of psychotic reactions which they described as a feeling of floating in outer space and having no feelings in their limbs. Due to this effect, Domino's wife Toni termed it "dissociative anesthesia" originating the concept of dissociative anesthesia [1, 4]. Dissociative anesthesia would later bed deifined as a state of electrophysiological and functional dissociation between thalamocortical and limbic systems. It was then concluded that ketamine is a potent analgesic and anesthetic with lower potency and shorter duration of action than PCP. Finally, in 1969, ketamine hydrochloride became available as a prescription drug under the name of Ketalar and a year later was approved by the US Food and Drug Administration [2, 3].

Unfortunately, the popularity of ketamine declined as it caused hallucinations and psychotic reactions that were an unpleasant experience for patients. However, in the early 1990s, ketamine made a come-back due to the peak of high-dose opioid anesthesia [3]. Ketamine is becoming widely used among anesthesiologists for both induction and maintenance in anesthetic and subanesthetic doses. Commonly it is used in combination with diazepam, midazolam, or propofol to help reduce hallucinations, psychotic reactions, and emergence delirium [1]. A recent interest has also sparked in opioid free anesthesia using ketamine. Contrary to yesteryears practice, today ketamine is widely used for a variety of different procedures for its valuable anesthetic, analgesic, and even amnestic properties, as we will discuss throughout this chapter.

2. Chemistry and pharmacology

Ketamine's chiral carbon center allows for the existence of two different steric configurations - S(+) and R(−) isomers. Each isomer has varying anesthetic, analgesic, dysphoric, and sympathomimetic properties. Several studies have shown that the S(+) isomer is more potent and has a higher NMDA affinity when used intraoperatively for anesthesia compared to the R(−) isomer. In addition, the S(+) isomer causes lower cardiac stimulation, less spontaneous motor activity, better analgesia, faster recovery, fewer psychotomimetic side effects, and decreased incidence of emergence delirium [1, 2].

Ketamine primarily works by inhibition of NMDA receptors and has two different mechanisms through which it exerts its function. NMDA receptors are excitatory amino acid receptors that have been implicated in pain [5]. The first mechanism of NMDA antagonism is as a channel blocker. The second mechanism is through an allosteric mechanism that decreases the opening frequency of the NMDA channel. It can also exert its effect through a variety of other mechanisms such as inhibition of L-type calcium channels, BK channels, HCN channels, and voltage-gated sodium channels. Other mechanisms of actions include monoamine blockade and inhibition of serotonin reuptake [2].

Ketamine has a slow off-rate compared to other anesthetic agents. This means that it continues to exert its effect even after glutamate; the substrate for NMDA receptors, has dissociated. This allows for a better anesthetic effect.

Ketamine has a high lipid solubility allowing it be rapidly taken up by the brain and redistributed to highly perfused tissue with a distribution half-life between 10 and 15 minutes [2]. Its metabolism is highly dependent on the liver using the cytochrome P450 system. Ketamine can be converted into active or inactive metabolites,

Intravenous	
Induction	1–4.5 mg/kg (60s)
Maintenance (general)	1–6 mg/kg/hr
Maintenance (sedation)	0.4–1 mg/kg/hr
Subanesthetic	0.2–0.8 mg/kg
Intramuscular	
Anesthetic	6.5–13 mg/kg
Subanesthetic	2–4 mg/kg

Table 1.
Doses of ketamine.

which are then further hydroxylated to increase water solubility through various CYP450 enzymes. The metabolites are then renally eliminated [1, 6].

Research has shown that ketamine has a dose dependent effect. In this chapter, we will focus on anesthesia and analgesia. Analgesic effects are seen at levels of 100–160 ng/ml. Induction of anesthesia is usually achieved at 9000–25000 ng/ml and can be maintained with 2000–3000 ng/ml. Ketamine's half-life at anesthetic doses is approximately 79 minutes, and its actions decrease when the drug redistributes from the brain into other tissue. The threshold between consciousness and emergence from anesthesia is 1000 ng/ml. The psychic state is usually seen with doses between 50 and 200 ng/ml. The onset and duration of these psychedelic effects varies based on the route of administration [1, 6].

Because ketamine is both water and lipid soluble, it can be administered intravenously, intramuscularly, orally, and sublingually. However, due to its significant first pass metabolism oral administration yields very little bioavailability. Intravenous administration is the preferred route of administration as it allows for 100% bioavailability. Recommended doses, shown in **Table 1**, are between 1 and 4.5 mg/kg over the course of 60 seconds for induction. For general maintenance 1–6 mg/kg/hr. and 0.4–1 mg/kg/hr. for continuous sedation is recommended [6]. Ketamine can be given intramuscularly that has a 93% bioavailability and is useful in emergencies, uncooperative patients and burn patients. When administered intramuscularly higher doses, between 6.5–13 mg/kg, are needed. For subanesthetic doses the intravenous dose is between 0.2–0.8 mg/kg and 2–4 mg/kg if given intramuscularly [2].

Table 1 summarizes the various suggested doses of ketamine administration depending on route, phase and administration method of anesthesia.

For review, Induction is the transition from an awake state to an anesthetized state with a sole agent such as ketamine or propofol or a combination of drugs [2]. Maintenance involved sustaining this anesthetic [7]. The role of ketamine in induction and maintenance in the practice of anesthesia will be discussed later in this chapter.

3. Use of ketamine in anesthesia

In the first ever human trial done with ketamine, a 1–2 mg/kg dose was given to patients, which resulted in analgesia and anesthesia with an onset time of one minute and lasted for about five to ten minutes. Within one to two hours the patients were back to their initial state. An increase in blood pressure and heart rate, hyperactive reflexes, and increase in lacrimation was noticed. A transient respiratory depression was also seen but returned to baseline within seven minutes. Even so, reflexes were preserved throughout. No labs were significantly affected. However, during the recovery period, as with PCP, psychic reactions, mood and affect alterations were observed but laster for a shorter duration and were less severe than the reaction with PCP that subsided within 30 mins after awakening. Many of the effects that were seen with ketamine were not seen with the anesthetics used commonly during that time period [4]. This led to the conclusion that ketamine results in a short-acting and effective induction of anesthesia and analgesia.

Ketamine has been shown to be safe and effective for maintenance sedation in several studies. It decreases airway resistance, improves dynamic compliance, preserves functional residual capacity, tidal volume, and minute ventilation [7]. Another advantage observed was that with ketamine, pharyngeal and laryngeal reflexes were conserved. In addition, ketamine provides an additional benefit in patients with refractory bronchospasms as it decreases audible wheezes, bronchodilator requirements, and hypercarbia making it the drug of choice in patients with bronchospasms [7]. Furthermore, in patients with refractory status asthmasticus, it helps reduce the need for initiation of mechanical ventilation [8]. Ketamine is also a popular induction agent [2]. For induction, ketamine is usually used in combination with other agents such as propofol or diazepam for reduction in emergence excitement, or dissociative effects that often result when ketamine is used [8].

Since ketamine is known for its ability to cause dissociative anesthesia, it has been hypothesized to be particularly beneficial for painful or distressing procedures. For example, endotracheal intubation using ketamine has been successful in some cases with the added advantage of maintaining or even increasing cardiorespiratory tone. We will discuss four methods for endotracheal intubation that have been evaluated. In delayed sequence intubation, dissociative doses of ketamine are given to allow the patient to enter an unconscious state so that proper preparation and pre-oxygenation can be taken before a paralytic is given. With this method, there were reduced adverse events and improved oxygen saturation. In ketamine-only breathing intubation, a dissociative dose of ketamine monotherapy is used in spontaneously breathing patients. This strategy seems to be useful in patients with anatomically difficult airways, physiologic limitations and profound acidosis. With traditional rapid sequence intubation, ketamine was given with the traditional rapid sequence intubation protocol. In review, rapid sequence intubation is when an induction agent and a paralytic are administered simultaneously during endotracheal intubation without the need for bag mask ventilation. This method has an advantage when apnea caused by the paralytic agent is not a concern. Finally, in ketamine for post-intubation analgesia and sedation, ketamine given after intubation provides two benefits - stimulating heart rate and blood pressure and analgesic and sedative properties. This allows for the reduction of conventional sedative use which has been linked to prolonged ICU stay and delirium. Although advantages have been noted, using ketamine for airway management using these strategies should be done with careful planning and caution, as there still is limited evidence [9].

4. Effects of ketamine use

A major advantage of ketamine, unlike many other anesthetic agents, is hemodynamic stability. It is also generally well tolerated in both pediatric and geriatric patients. As mentioned previously, ketamine when given in a combination with propofol for induction significantly improves hemodynamic stability within the first ten minutes [10]. This advantage makes ketamine extremely beneficial in managing hemodynamically unstable patients such as those who have suffered severe trauma. For example, in which ketamine has been useful is in the management of burn patients especially during the acute phase of injury. During the acute phase, the burn victims are undergoing significant fluid shifts leading to cardiovascular and respiratory insufficiency [11].

4.1 Anti-inflammatory effect

Inflammation is a normal mechanism that the body uses to fight infection caused by viruses and bacteria. This mechanism is initiated by pro-inflammatory cytokines that are released by the immune cells. These pro-inflammatory cytokines (IL-1, IL-6, IL-8, IL-12, IFN-γ, IL-18, and Tumor Necrosis Factor (TNF) [12]. However, inflammation can also be disadvantageous in that it can lead to pain and swelling in the acute setting. Concentrations of proinflammatory cytokines during the perioperative period may significantly impact surgical outcome. Ketamine has been shown to modulate the perioperative cytokine response and plays a significant anti-inflammatory role. It inhibits the systemic response without affecting the healing process that is necessary during the postoperative state [12]. One such mechanism is the reduction of leukocyte migration through endothelial monolayers. It is well studied that neutrophils play a key role in defense against foreign pathogens. Upon activation, neutrophils need to cross endothelial cell layers. Researchers investigated the effects of ketamine on leukocytes and endothelial cells independently and together. In a dose-dependent fashion, ketamine suppressed migration when leukocytes alone were treated. Interestingly, when the endothelial cells were treated with ketamine, there was no significant reduction in migration. However, when both leukocytes and endothelial cells were treated, the suppression in migration was much higher than when only leukocytes were treated [13]. One possible mechanism that may achieve this is is the inhibition of the up-regulation of CD18 and CD26L on neutrophils. CD18 and CD26L are stimulated during inflammation and are important cell surface markers for adhesion of neutrophils to endothelial cells promoting neutrophil migration [14].

It has also been suggested that this effect might be mediated by the suppression of microglial activation in the CNS or the inhibition of large conductance calcium activated potassium channels in the microglia. Specifically, there is a reduction in postoperative pro-inflammatory cytokines such as serum IL-6, TNF-a, nuclear factor kb, CRP and nitric oxidase synthase [15]. In addition, an increase in postoperative serum IL-10 levels, an anti-inflammatory cytokine. Ketamine was also shown to impair neutrophil chemotaxis, inhibit superoxide radical production, inhibit differentiation of immature dendritic cells, and increase Treg cell concentration [16]. Ketamine may also alter the oxidative stress response in patients. When ketamine was administered, patients had lower total thiol molecules and a lower total antioxidant capacity. They also had higher lipid peroxidation, and higher superoxide dismutase and glutathione peroxidase activity [17].

4.2 Psycho modulator effects

Ketamine has several effects on brain activity that can be monitored by EEG. When subanesthetic doses are given, the complexity of EEG changes is elevated relative to the baseline. At anesthetic doses the pattern alternates between a high and low complexity. Eventually the pattern stabilizes at a high complexity that is similar to baseline. This shows that ketamine can induce a fragmented state that shows alternating patterns of conscious and anesthetic states. A bolus of ketamine induces unconsciousness causing a change from slow waves to a gamma-burst wave pattern on the EEG, which later evolved into a stable gamma pattern most likely due to decreasing plasma ketamine levels [18]. In addition, in hippocampal and cortical neurons, ketamine can increase activity of extrasynaptic GABA-a receptors which generate tonic inhibitory currents. Ketamine has been shown to increase potency of low concentration of GABA at these receptors as well [19]. Secondary effects on the dopamine system due to ketamine alters the firing rate of mesocortical and mesolimbic dopamine neurons causing an increase in extracellular dopamine in the striatum and prefrontal cortex which has been hypothesized to be a contributing factor the psychotic-like behaviors observed with ketamine [20].

Another interesting aspect of ketamine is that its effect varies depending on other anesthetic agents used with it or if it is used as a sole agent. For example, in a study done with rats it was found that when ketamine was added to ongoing sevoflurane or propofol, on EEG there was either no change or a shift to higher frequencies. However, when ketamine was given alone there was a simultaneous increase in both lower and higher frequencies. Also, when ketamine is used as a sole anesthetic agent patients can experience dissociative effects. However, at the same time ketamine is also found to be neuroprotective in preventing or mitigating postoperative delirium. This might explain why ketamine is being used both as an experimental model of psychiatric diseases as well as a proposed treatment for psychiatric diseases [21].

Ketamine's unusual cataplectic properties make it a dissociative anesthetic. At low doses, it causes alteration in visual and auditory stimuli and feelings of detachment from one's surroundings that manifest themselves as delirium, hallucinations, delusions, and confusion [20]. This leads to a potential for abuse and explains why ketamine is a class III-controlled substance and often referred to as "Special K". Long term effects of repeated ketamine use may lead to flashbacks, attentional and other cognitive dysfunctions, and decreased sociability. On the other hand, its continued use is reinforced by the other psychotropic effects. Therefore, some anesthesiologist may choose to avoid ketamine especially when it comes to patients with Post Traumatic Stress Disorder (PTSD) [15]. However, a recent study presented a trial of repeated intravenous ketamine administration for patients with PTSD. Infusion of ketamine demonstrated a clear superiority in reduction of symptoms compared to midazolam. More research on this aspect of ketamine is needed to help guide its use in anesthesia in patients with PTSD [10]. Caution should also be used when using ketamine for anesthesia in schizophrenic patients. This is because ketamine has been found to induce hallucinations, delusions and thought disorders, resembling an active schizophrenic episode of their illness. These episodes are also resistant to haloperidol, the drug traditionally used to treat active episodes [22].

Interestingly, ketamine and its metabolites modulate distinct neural circuits to produce dissociation and analgesia. The channel blocking effect of ketamine at the NMDA receptors may partially explain its dissociative properties. This is because ketamine blocks excitatory NMDA receptors on fast-spiking cortical interneurons more effectively than those on pyramidal neurons. This results in markedly dysregulated pyramidal neuronal activity. The relative inactivity of cortical interneurons leads to glutamate-mediated pyramidal–pyramidal neuronal facilitation. Consistent with this notion, lamotrigine, an antiepileptic medication that reduces cortical glutamate release and pyramidal neuron facilitation, suppresses the dissociative properties of ketamine. In the same fashion, midazolam reduces pyramidal neuron facilitation by downstream activity resulting from binding at gamma amino-butyric acid receptors on pyramidal neurons [23]. This could explain why ketamine causes a feeling of dissociation when it is used as an anesthetic agent.

4.3 Neuroprotective effects

There is also evidence that ketamine has neuroprotective effects. It is thought that this occurs due to the inhibition of calcium influx that occurs with ketamine administration. This calcium influx inhibition helps prevent ischemia and apoptosis providing a protective benefit to neurons. When ketamine was compared with other anesthetic agents such as midazolam, fentanyl, and propofol there was a reduction of spreading depolarizations with ketamine administration. Spreading depolarizations can cause neurovascular decoupling and potentiate the secondary phase of brain damage. Therefore, it is hypothesized that when ketamine is used, the suppression of these spreading depolarization allows for the maintenance of the electrochemical gradient and prevents neurovascular decoupling. This works together to have neuroprotective effects. However, the opposite effects could occur if repeated high doses are given as ketamine has the potential to cause neurotoxicity particularly in the developing brain. When ketamine is given in repeated high doses, there is an increase in a subunit of NMDA receptors, NR1. This allows the opposite effect, increasing the influx of calcium leading to apoptosis [8].

Traditionally, it was thought that ketamine increased intracranial pressure. In recent years, this theory has been rejected. Ketamine has successfully been used to reduce intracranial pressure. One study examined the effects of ketamine on intubated and sedated pediatric population at a regional trauma center with elevated ICP >18 mmHg resistant to first tier therapies. The results of 82 ketamine administrations in 30 patients were analyzed. Overall, following ketamine administration, ICP decreased by 30% (from 25.8 ± 8.4 to 18.0 ± 8.5 mm Hg) ($p < 0.001$) and Cerebral Perfusion Pressure (CPP) increased from 54.4 ± 11.7 to 58.3 ± 13.4 mm Hg ($p < 0.005$). In Group 1, ICP decreased significantly following ketamine administration and increased by >2 mm Hg during the distressing intervention in only 1 of 17 events. In Group 2, when ketamine was administered to lower persistent intracranial hypertension, ICP decreased by 33% (from 26.0 ± 9.1 to 17.5 ± 9.1 mm Hg) ($p < 0.0001$) following ketamine administration. They concluded that in ventilator-treated patients with intracranial hypertension, ketamine effectively decreased ICP and prevented untoward ICP elevations during potentially distressing interventions, without lowering blood pressure and CPP. In addition, these results refute the notion that ketamine increases ICP. Ketamine is a safe and effective drug for patients with traumatic brain injury and intracranial hypertension, and it can be used safely in trauma emergency situations [24].

4.4 Hemodynamic and respiratory effects

Ketamine's ability to promote central sympathetic stimulation and inhibition of neuronal catecholamine reuptake has brought upon its resurgence as an excellent sedation maintenance drug [7]. These effects favor hemodynamic stability. A prospective double-blind controlled study compared the use of ketamine vs. fentanyl for sedation in the ICU. It was observed that patients on ketamine had an increased MAP and a decreased incidence of shock. This characteristic is what makes it an excellent choice for induction of anesthesia for potentially unstable cardiac patients, especially when combined with midazolam. This benefit was observed in patients with septic cardiomyopathy [8].

In addition, clinicians have adapted 'ketofol,' a combination of ketamine and propofol especially for sedation cases. Propofol when used alone can cause myocardial depression and systemic vasodilation that both lead to hypotension, especially in a fasting patient. When propofol was used alone, it causesd a 20% reduction in systolic blood pressure in the first 5 and 10 minutes compare to 'ketofol' [10].

In addition, Ketamine tends to relax bronchiole smooth muscles. Thus, it can protect asymptomatic patients with asthma from developing bronchospasm and it can also effectively relieve bronchospasm in patients who already have respiratory problems before anesthesia. In addition, it has been used as an analgo-sedative in patients with status asthmaticus, not responding to the usual therapeutic options; as this can reduce the need for mechanical ventilation [8]. A review of prospective and observational studies showed a noticeable increase in chest wall dynamics in patients with status asthmaticus. They noticed that patients receiving ketamine continuous infusion also had reducible wheezing and even reduced bronchodilator requirement [7]. It should also be noted that unlike opioids, it does not increase histamine release; further reducing the possibility of bronchospasm [8].

These benefits extend to the pediatric population. Research has shown ketofol use as an induction agent as an alternative to propofol led to better laryngeal mask airway (LMA) insertion in children. In addition, during the LMA the use of ketofol showed faster induction time, lower injection pain, better jaw relaxation, better full mouth opening, and less incidence and duration of apnea when compared to using propofol alone [25]. Another study showed that induction with adjunctive use of ketamine and propofol, 1 mg/kg ketamine at induction and 5 mg/kg/h propofol infusion for maintenance for MRI sedation in children resulted in better induction quality, lower propofol infusion rate for maintenance, and faster time to full recovery [26]. Ketofol seems to have an effect that is dependent on the ratio of propofol to ketamine. In a clinical trial performed, it was determined that a 10:1 propofol ketamine ratio seems to have the greatest benefit during surgery due to better hemodynamic stability maintenance and faster recovery time [27].

5. Ketamine and opioid free anesthesia

With the opioid epidemic in recent years, clinicians are exploring options to provide pain relief with reduced or no opioid administration. Although opioids provide excellent analgesia, they can also produce unpleasant adverse effects such as nausea, vomiting, tolerance, pruritis, hyperalgesia, urinary retention, constipation, respiratory depression and have an extremely high potential for abuse. Approximately 2 million Americans use opioids for recreational purposes. According to the United State National Institute of Drug Abuse, overdose deaths involving prescription opioids rose from 3442 in 1999 to 17029 in 2017. Studies have shown that patients who consume high doses of opioids in the inpatient setting have a higher probability of report of increase opioid use after discharge. This is especially true for patients who leave the hospital with a prescription for opioids [28].

With regards to cancer pain control, the role of opioids has come into question in recent years as new data emerges about opioids, such as Morphine having pro tumor effects. Morphine may stimulate proliferation, facilitate metastasis, and promote angiogenesis leading to increased tumor burden. However, generalizations about these effects should not be extended to all opioids as research is still ongoing on this topic [29].

In recent years, clinicians are fast adopting Early Recovery After Surgery (ERAS) protocols that have an increased focus on a multimodal approach to pain control to reduce the consumption or even exposure to opioids. In the preoperative setting drugs such as celecoxib, acetaminophen and gabapentin are being utilized to begin pain control even before surgical incision is made. In the operating room Ketamine, among others such as Dexmedetomidine, Intravenous Lidocaine, Intravenous Magnesium, are some of the drugs on the forefront to achieve opioid free or opioid reduced pain relief.

In 2019 a study to evaluate the effect of Opioid Free Anesthesia (OFA) on post-operative morphine consumption and the post-operative course was initiated. Ketamine was used in both arms of OFA and Opioid Anesthesia (OA) for induction. A statistically significant result of reduced supplemental opioid consumption in the OFA group was observed (0.001). It should be noted, however, that ketamine was used in conjunction with lidocaine and dextromethorphan in the OFA group. In addition, the reduction in opioids used may also be due to reduced opioid tolerance. It was noted that postoperative pain scores did not differ between groups, indicating that OA and OFA provided comparable analgesia [30].

Multiple studies on the role of NMDA receptor antagonists in preventive analgesia have been reviewed. Preventive analgesia a concept in which the administration of a drug at any point in the perioperative period and the presumed associated reduction in central sensitization may reduce pain, analgesic consumption, or both beyond the clinical activity of the target drug. Their systemic review showed that ketamine and dextromethorphan produced significant preventive analgesic benefit in 58% and 67% of studies, respectively. In addition, a direct analgesic benefit of the drug occurred in the early postoperative period [5]. It can then be inferred that if pain is controlled early in surgery, then there may be reduced need for additional analgesic medications, including opioids.

A randomized, prospective, double blinded placebo- controlled study investigating the efficacy of preemptive ketamine infusions in patients with chronic pain undergoing elective back surgery was conducted. These patients had a history of at least 6 weeks (about 1 and a half months) of opiate use. They demonstrated that intraoperative preventative ketamine reduced opiate consumption in the acute postoperative period by 37% in these patients. In addition, it seemed that these patients who received ketamine infusions had a reduced pain sensation in the PACU (post anesthesia care unit) and even 6 weeks in the post operative period, leading to a reduction in morphine consumption [31]. As previously discussed, this reduction in pain sensation is due to reduction central sensitization *via* NMDA receptor antagonism, reduction in opiate tolerance, and some impact on the balance of neurotransmitters. This concept of preemptive analgesia was further explored by studying the effects of preemptive doses of ketamine before laparoscopic cholecystectomies at three doses; 1 mg.kg, 0.5 mg/kg and 0.25 mg/kg. In addition, researchers evaluated their effects on cardiovascular hemodynamics and hallucinations. There was a definitive role in reducing postoperative pain and analgesic requirement in patients. A low dose of 0.5 mg/kg was devoid of hemodynamic changes and hallucinations, making it the optimal dose for patients undergoing laparoscopic cholecystectomy [32].

Ketamine is being favored in bariatric surgery as obese patients tend to have obstructive sleep apnea and obesity hypoventilation syndrome that can be difficult to manage during induction and emergence of anesthesia. Due to its favorable stability on the cardiovascular system, respiratory system and gastrointestinal systems as detailed above. While only in a single case study, an opioid free anesthetic delivered to an obese lady with BMI of 50.1. She received an initial bolus of ketamine 5 $mg{\cdot}kg^{-1}$ was followed by a continuous infusion at 5 $\mu g{\cdot}kg^{-1}\ min^{-1.}$ She underwent surgery without complication, rapidly met all extubation criteria, was never hypoxic, and was ambulating unassisted after 90 minutes in the recovery room without pain. She received ketorolac and IV Acetaminophen as the multimodal regimen. No opioids were used [33]. This case study lays the foundation for an excellent randomized double blinded study to improve outcomes in bariatric surgery. Furthermore TIVA with propofol, ketamine and dexmedetomidine (59 patients) vs. opioids and volatile anesthetics (60 patients) and their effects on post-operative nausea and vomiting (PONV) has been studied. Patients in both groups had similar clinical characteristics, surgical procedure, and PONV risk scores and required similar amounts of postoperative opioid. 37.3% in the Opioid group compared to only 20% group reported PONV with a statistically difference (0.02). It was concluded that opioid-free TIVA is associated with a significant reduction in relative risk of PONV compared with balanced anesthesia [34].

Overall, OFA has gained in popularity to enhance early recovery and so spare opioids for the postoperative period. Pain is an extremely complex interaction of biological, cognitive, behavioral, cultural and environmental factors. Whether it is possible to deliver a safe and stable anesthesia without intraoperative opioids to many patients undergoing various surgical procedures. OFA still raises questions. Accurate monitoring to measure intraoperative nociception and guide the use of adjuvants is not available. Also, there is a need for procedure specific strategies as well as indications and contraindications to the technique. OFA does not seem to reduce the amounts of opioids prescribed at discharge which needs to be addressed and thought about by health care professionals.

6. Conclusion

Ketamine has made a strong resurgence as a versatile drug in the field of anesthesia. We reviewed the history of anesthesia from its discovery to its application as an anesthetic. In addition, we aimed to demonstrate how ketamine has favorable properties with regards to hemodynamics, its neuroprotective properties, psychomodulator effects, and anti-inflammatory effects. These favorable properties have made it one of the drugs on the forefront of the opioid free anesthesia concept discussed in this chapter. We remain excited about the ongoing research on Ketamine's role in treatment of patient with Post Traumatic Stress Disorder and various other applications in the field of Anesthesia.

Acknowledgements

We want to acknowledge Dr. Alex Bekker, MD, PhD, Chairman of Department of Anesthesiology for the encouragement and support.

Conflict of interest

The authors declare no conflict of interest.

Author details

Shridevi Pandya Shah*, Devanshi Patel and Antony Irungu
New Jersey Medical School, Newark, USA

*Address all correspondence to: pandyas1@njms.rutgers.edu

References

[1] Domino EF, Warner DS. Taming the ketamine tiger. Anesthesiology. 2010;113:678-684. doi: https://doi.org/10.1097/ALN.0b013e3181ed09a2

[2] Li L, Vlisides PE. Ketamine: 50 years of modulating the mind. Front Hum Neurosci. 2016;10:612. doi: 10.3389/fnhum.2016.00612

[3] Mion G. History of anaesthesia: the ketamine story - past, present and future. European Journal of Anaesthesiology. 2017;34(9):571-575. doi:10.1097/EJA.0000000000000638

[4] Domino EF, Chodoff P, Corssen P. Pharmacologic effects of CI-581, a new dissociative anesthetic, in man. Clin Pharmacol Ther. 1965;6:279-291. doi: 10.1002/cpt196563279

[5] McCartney CJ, Sinha A, Katz J. A qualitative systematic review of the role of N-methyl-D-aspartate receptor antagonists in preventive analgesia. Anesthesia and analgesia. 2004;98(5). doi: 10.1213/01.ane.0000108501.57073.38

[6] Lavender E, Hirasawa-Fujita M, Domino EF. Ketamine's dose related multiple mechanisms of actions: dissociative anesthetic to rapid antidepressant. Behav Brain Res. 2020;390:112631. doi: 10.1016/j.bbr.2020.112631

[7] Miller AC, Jamin CT, Elamin EM. Continuous intravenous infusion of ketamine for maintenance sedation. 2011;77(8):812-820

[8] Trimmel H et al. S(+)-ketamine: current trends in emergency and intensive care medicine. Wein Klin Wochenschr. 2018;130(9-10):356-366. doi: 10.1007/s00508-017-1299-3

[9] Merelman AH, Perlmutter MC, Strayer RJ. Alternatives to rapid sequence intubation: contemporary airway management with ketamine. West J Emerg Med. 2019;20(3):466-471. doi: 10.5811/westjem.2019.4.42753

[10] Stein MB, Simon NM. Ketamine for ptsd: Well, isn't that special. American Journal of Psychiatry. 2021;178(2):116-118. https://doi.org/10.1176/appi.ajp.2020.20121677

[11] Bittner EA et al. Acute and perioperative care of the burn-injured patient. Anesthesiology. 2015; 122:448-464. doi: https://doi.org/10.1097/ALN.0000000000000559

[12] Dale O et al. Does intraoperative ketamine attenuate inflammatory reactivity following surgery? A systematic review and meta-analysis. Anesthesia and analgesia. 2012;115(4):934-943. doi: 10.1213/ANE.0b013e3182662e30

[13] Hofbauer R et al. Ketamine significantly reduces the migration of leukocytes through endothelial cell monolayers. Crit Care Med. 1998;26(9):1545-1549. Doi: 10.1097/00003246-199809000-00022

[14] Weigand MA et al. Ketamine modulates the stimulated adhesion molecule expression on human neutrophils in vitro. Anesthesia and analgesia. 2000;90(1):206-212. Doi: 10.1097/00000539-200001000-00041

[15] Zanos, P., Moaddel, R., Morris, P. J., Riggs, L. M., Highland, J. N., Georgiou, P., Pereira, E. F., Albuquerque, E. X., Thomas, C. J., Zarate, C. A., & Gould, T. D. (2018). Ketamine and KETAMINE METABOLITE Pharmacology: Insights into therapeutic mechanisms. Pharmacological Reviews, *70*(3), 621-660. https://doi.org/10.1124/pr.117.015198

[16] Ackerman RS et al. The effects of anesthetics and perioperative

medications on immune function: a narrative review. Anesthesia and analgesia. 2021. Doi: 10.1213/ANE.0000000000005607

[17] Khoshraftar E et al. Antioxidant effects of propofol vs ketamine in humans undergoing surgery. Arch Iran Med. 2014;17(7):486-489

[18] Li D, Mashour GA. Cortical dynamics during psychedelic and anesthetized states induced by ketamine. Neuroimage. 2019;196:32-40. doi: 10.1016/j.neuroimage.2019.03.076

[19] Wang DS et al. Ketamine increases the function of gaba-aminobutyric acid type A receptors in hippocampal and cortical neurons. Anesthesiology. 2017;126:666-667. doi: https://doi.org/10.1097/ALN.0000000000001483

[20] Sun L et al. Pharmacodynamic elucidation of glutamate & dopamine in ketamine-induced anaesthesia. Chemic-Biological Interactions. 2020;326:109164. doi: https://doi.org/10.1016/j.cbi.2020.109164

[21] Garcia P, Sleigh J. Ketamine: a drug at war with itself. Anesthesiology. 2017;126:371-372. doi: https://doi.org/10.1097/ALN.0000000000001513

[22] Lahti AC et al. Subanesthetic doses of ketamine stimulate psychosis in schizophrenia. Neuropsychopharmacology. 1995;13: 9-19. https://doi.org/10.1016/0893-133x(94)00131-i

[23] Gitlin J et al. Dissociative and analgesic properties of ketamine are independent. Anesthesiology. 2020;133:1021-1028. https://doi.org/10.1097/ALN.0000000000003529

[24] Bar-Joseph, G., Guilburd, Y., Tamir, A., & Guilburd, J. N. Effectiveness of ketamine in decreasing intracranial pressure in children with intracranial hypertension. Journal of Neurosurgery: Pediatrics. 2009;4(1):40-46. https://doi.org/10.3171/2009.1.peds08319

[25] Yousef GT, Elsayed KM. A clinical comparison of ketofol (ketamine and propofol admixture) versus propofol as an induction agent on quality of laryngeal mask airway insertion and hemodynamic stability in children. Anesth Essays Res. 2013;7(2):194-199. doi:10.4103/0259-1162.118957

[26] Schmitz A et al. Sedation for magnetic resonance imaging using propofol with or without ketamine at induction in pediatrics - a prospective randomized double-blinded study. Paediatr Anaesth. 2018;28(3);264-274

[27] Cillo JE. Analysis of propofol and low-dose ketamine admixtures for adult outpatient dentoalveolar surgery: a prospective, randomized, positive-controlled clinical trial. 2012;70(3):537-546. doi: 10.1016/j.joms.2011.08.036

[28] Baboli, K. M., Liu, H., & Poggio, J. L. Opioid-free postoperative analgesia: Is it feasible? Current Problems in Surgery. 2020;57(7), 100794. https://doi.org/10.1016/j.cpsurg.2020.100794

[29] Amaram-Davila, J., Davis, M., & Reddy, A. Opioids and cancer mortality. Current Treatment Options in Oncology. 2020;21(3). https://doi.org/10.1007/s11864-020-0713-7

[30] Guinot, P.-G., Spitz, A., Berthoud, V., Ellouze, O., Missaoui, A., Constandache, T., Grosjean, S., Radhouani, M., Anciaux, J.-B., Parthiot, J.-P., Merle, J.-P., Nowobilski, N., Nguyen, M., & Bouhemad, B. (2019). Effect of opioid-free anaesthesia on post-operative period in cardiac surgery: A retrospective matched case-control study. BMC Anesthesiology, *19*(1). https://doi.org/10.1186/s12871-019-0802-y

[31] Loftus, R. W., Yeager, M. P., Clark, J. A., Brown, J. R., Abdu, W. A., Sengupta,

D. K., & Beach, M. L. Intraoperative ketamine Reduces Perioperative opiate consumption in Opiate-dependent patients with chronic back Pain Undergoing back surgery. Anesthesiology, 2010;113(3):639-646. https://doi.org/10.1097/aln.0b013e3181e90914

[32] Smischney NJ et al. Ketamine/propofol admixture (ketofol) is associated with improved hemodynamics as an induction agent: a randomized controlled trial. J Trauma Acute Care Surg. 2012;73(1):94-101. doi: 10.1097/TA.0b013e318250cdb8

[33] Aronsohn, J., Orner, G., Palleschi, G., & Gerasimov, M. Opioid-free total intravenous anesthesia with ketamine as part of an enhanced recovery protocol for bariatric surgery patients with sleep disordered breathing. Journal of Clinical Anesthesia. 2019;52:65-66. https://doi.org/10.1016/j.jclinane.2018.09.014

[34] Ziemann-Gimmel P et al. Opioid-free total intravenous aneasthesia reduces postoperative nausea and vomiting in bariatric surgery beyond triple prophylaxis. British Journal of Anaesthesia. 2014;112(5):906-911. https://doi.org/10.1093/bja/aet551

Chapter 5

Role of Ketamine as Part of the Anti-Hyperalgesic Approach in Opioid-Free Anesthesia (OFA) and Postoperative Analgesia (OFAA)

Carlos Ramírez-Paesano, Claudia Rodiera Clarens, José Carlos Torres Mandujano, Milen Bonev Bonev, Karen Salazar Loaiza, Florencia Borghetti, María Martínez Alberici, Josep Rodiera Olive and Jesus Santaliestra Fierro

Abstract

There is increasing evidence of the close relationship between persistent activation of the glutaminergic pathway, central sensitization, hyperalgesia and chronic pain. Opioids have long been the standard analgesics used in the perioperative. However, their side effects, namely opioid-induced hyperalgesia, opioid tolerance and post-operative dependence in patients with chronic pain that are to undergo aggressive surgeries have motivated anesthesiologists to develop alternative anesthetic techniques. They include analgesic and anti-inflammatory drugs that act by modulating the nociceptive pathways with an opioid-sparing effect and even opioid-free anesthesia (OFA). In OFA plus postoperative analgesia (OFAA) techniques, ketamine plays a fundamental role as an analgesic with its antagonist action on the N-Methyl-D-Aspartate-receptors (NMDAr). However, ketamine is limited to use at sub-anesthetic doses ("low-doses") due to its dose-dependent side effects. Consequently, other analgesic drugs with anti-NMDAr effects like magnesium sulfate and other non-opioid analgesics such as lidocaine and alpha-2-adrenergic agonists are often used in OFAA techniques. The aim of this text is to present a summary of the importance of the use of ketamine in OFA based on nociceptive pathophysiology. Additionally, the perioperative protocol (OFAA) with the anti-hyperalgesic approach of ketamine, lidocaine and dexmedetomidine co-administration in our center will be described. Some of the main indications for the OFAA protocol will be mentioned.

Keywords: Opioid-free anesthesia, OFA, Opioid-free anesthesia and analgesia, OFAA, minimizing-opioid-use, NMDA-receptors antagonists, ketamine-magnesium-lidocaine-dexmedetomidine-methadone, anti-hyperalgesia, central sensitization, opioid intolerance, opioid-induced hyperalgesia, craneocervical/thoracic fixation, complex spine surgery

IntechOpen

1. Introduction

Nociceptive phenomena associated with surgical trauma involve local and systemic inflammatory processes, activation of cellular and humoral immune mechanisms, and adrenergic and neuroendocrine activation. The activation of the glutaminergic pathway plays a determining role in secondary sensitization at the level of the central nervous system, which is responsible for nociceptive amplification, persistence of postoperative pain, and hyperalgesia.

Strategies to reduce perioperative opioid consumption and its consequent side effects have been based on the use of multimodal analgesia schemes. The development of opioid-free anesthesia (OFA) techniques, indicated for particular patient populations in which opioids may be harmful, requires the use of drug mixtures in which NMDA receptors (NMDAr) antagonists are integral. The most clinically used NMDAr inhibitors in anesthesia are ketamine and magnesium sulfate. Their co-administration in OFA techniques has synergistic analgesic effects. The concomitant use of intravenous lidocaine and dexmedetomidine provides additional benefits to the use of NMDAr antagonists to reduce the central sensitization phenomenon (SC), hyperalgesia and opioid-induced hyperalgesia (OIH).

2. NMDAr are involved in nociception even from the beginning of tissue trauma: peripheral hyperalgesia is an event modulated by a glutamatergic system in the dorsal root ganglia (DRG)

The nociceptive pathway undergoes important functional changes and modulation under surgical trauma (tissue damage and inflammation). This plasticity is mediated by many mechanisms, including peripheral and central sensitization. The paramount element for these modificationsis the result of release of many chemical mediators peripherally as well as neurotransmitters in the spinal cord and the brain [1].

Peripheral sensitization contributes to increased afferent stimulation of the spinal cord. It is mediated by many processes in which nerve tissues and immune cells act under a complex barrage of pain-mediating substances. The nociceptive impulse generated by an inflammatory event in peripheral tissue is regulated in the dorsal root ganglia (DRG) by a system that involves satellite glial cells and glutamatergic NMDA receptors (NMDAr) [2].

Mechanical inflammatory nociceptor sensitization is dependent on glutamate release in the DRG and subsequent NMDAr activation in satellite glial cells. That fact supports the idea that peripheral hyperalgesia is an event modulated by a glutamatergic system in the DRG. Moreover, retrograde sensitization of the primary sensory neuron has been proposed as an essential mechanism for induction and maintenance of peripheral inflammatory hyperalgesia. It has been suggested that this phenomenon is due to the release of glutamate in the spinal cord, which acts retrogradely on NMDARs present at the presynaptic terminals of the primary sensory neuron [3–5].

In summary, numerous receptors and ion channels are involved. Continued increased input to the spinal cord results in further central sensitizing changes.

3. What is the importance of glutaminergic pathway in the nociceptive process and secondary sensitization during surgical trauma?

The glutamate receptor NMDAr is the starting pointof secondary sensitization and the amplification of pain. Hence, the NMDAr may be a potential target for analgesic therapy in the context of opioid-free anesthesia and postoperative analgesia (OFAA).

The primary sensitization resulting from local inflammation of the tissue under surgical trauma activates the "asleep afferent" thereby increasing the total nociceptive afferent signals to the spinal cord, which is the beginning of the development of the central sensitization. The excitatory amino acid glutamate plays a central role both via the α-amino-3-hydroxy-5- methyl-4-isoxazolepropionate (AMPA) ion-channel linked receptor in acute pain transmission and via the N-methyl-d-aspartate (NMDA) receptor to mediate sensitizing effects. In the acute state, the NMDAr are limited by a voltage-dependent magnesium ion block of the channel. Increased afferent input from primary sensitization releases the magnesium ions and activates theNMDA receptors. NMDAr activation increases intracellular calcium flux and enhances the activation of the second-order neuron. The increase in intracellular calcium also stimulates cyclooxygenase, lipoxygenase and protein-kinases [2, 6].

Surgical stimulus activates C fibers and generatesa progressive build-up in the amplitude of response in dorsal horn neurons andbrings onthe Wind-up phenomenon, which is a specific initiator of central sensitization [1].

4. How does the glutaminergic pathway mediate the persistence of pain after surgery and chronic pain?

Neuropeptides like substance P and the calcitonin gene-related peptide (CGRP), released from primary afferent neurons, contribute to the activation of the NMDAr in pain states. Neuropeptides such as neurokinin A and B act on NK receptors and activate the NMDAr directly by inducing decreased potassium ion conductance and phosphorylation-induced increases of intracellular calcium, facilitating central sensitization and hyperalgesia. Brain-derived neurotrophic factor (BDNF) is produced by nerve growth factor (NGF)-dependent nociceptors and increases the glial inflammation. Moreover, BDNF augments spinal neuron excitability by phosphorylation-mediated stimulation of the NMDAr.

Finally, longer-term changes of central sensitization may be explained by transcriptional changes.

Hence, the significance ofthe spinal cord as a location for an anti-hyperalgesic approach leads us consider the important role the NMDA receptors have in central sensitization and their potential usefulness as a focus of analgesic therapeutics [7, 8].

Ketamine and magnesium sulfate are the most frequently used NMDAr antagonist drugs in anesthesia. Ketamine in association with lidocaine and dexmedetomidine infusions have led to the development of opioid-free anesthetic techniques (OFA). Moreover, the combination of low doses of ketamine with these adjuvant medications have shown an important opioid-sparing effect on postoperative pain control and has an additional anti-hyperalgesic effect [8].

5. Why should opioid use be minimized during the perioperative period?

Intravenous opioids are the commonly used analgesics during general anesthesia along with hypnotic drugs. Opioids provide potent analgesia, attenuate the neuroendocrine response triggered by surgery, and provide hemodynamic stability. However, these drugs have side effects like nausea, vomiting, decreased intestinal peristalsis, respiratory depression, histamine release and opioid-induced hyperalgesia mediated by NMDAr stimulation [6].

Multimodal postoperative analgesia has been the gold standard for more than 20 years. It makes for opioid-sparing and better outcomes than with drugs like morphine that are administered as a sole analgesic agent after surgery. OFA is based on the association of drugs and/or techniques that makes for good quality general anesthesia with no need for opioids. The association can combine NMDAr antagonists (ketamine, lidocaine, magnesium sulfate), sodium channel blockers (local anesthetics), anti-inflammatory drugs (NSAID, dexamethasone, lidocaine) and alpha-2 agonists (dexmedetomidine, clonidine) [9].

There is a group of patients in whom opioid use is relatively contraindicated. It is comprised of those with gastrointestinal intolerance susceptible to developing intestinal ileus, functional bladder disorders, a history of severe nausea and vomiting, sleep apnea syndrome, morbid obese, patients with mast cell activation syndrome (MCAS), autonomic symptoms like postural orthostatic tachycardia syndrome (POTS), patients with chronic pain, chronic fatigue syndrome and myalgic encephalomyelitis, patients with high-dose opioid use, opioid tolerance, opioid-induced hyperalgesia (OIH) and patients who are prone to drug dependence [9–13].

The above patients benefit from OFAA techniques. When feasible, the use of regional anesthesia is helpful. Then again, the substitution of opioids for analgesic drugs with different mechanisms of action is desirable when general anesthesia is indicated [14, 15].

6. Ketamine, magnesium, lidocaine and dexmedetomidine: an anti-hyperalgesic combination

Ketamine plays a fundamental role in OFA techniques since it is a potent NMDAr inhibitor that provides an excellent analgesic effect at sub-anesthetic doses. Since ketamine can cause dose-dependent side effects (cardiovascular excitation, hallucinations, psychomimetic events, nausea and vomiting as well as hyper-salivation), it is advisable to associate it with other NMDAr antagonists like magnesium sulfate or dextromethorphan to enhance its analgesic effect with lower doses.

Ketamine and magnesium have been widely described as improving postopera-pain control. The literature has consistently reported that both drugs provide effective postoperative analgesia and a reduction in opioid consumption. A meta-analysis that aggregated data from 2482 patients showed that intravenous ketamine reduces postoperative opioid use by 40% [16]. Similar results have been shown with the administration of intravenous magnesium [17–19].

Furthermore, experiments on the association of ketamine and magnesium may give us an important clue as to the useful of the association. In fact, pretreatment with ketamine has been demonstrated to improve the anti-nociceptive effect of magnesium [20]. Interestingly, myocardial and endothelial cells express NMDA receptor. Thus, a synergistic effect can be expected on the NMDA receptor in the cardiovascular system with the resulting cardiovascular stability by the competitive blocking actions of drugs [21, 22].

On the other hand, there are many publications that describe the use of intravenous lidocaine as a systemic analgesic with particular attenuating effects on the intraoperative inflammatory reaction at multiple levels (i.e., reduction of inflammatory biomarkers by direct action on cell membrane of monocytes, neutrophils and mast cell, PKC-mediated reduction of Ca^{++} intracellular influx and K^{+}_{A}-channels, action over cholinergic, adrenergic, GABAergic, NMDAr, and NK-1r pathways, etc.). Lidocaine has a non-relevant analgesic effect mediated by Na^{+}-channel blocks at therapeutic plasmatic concentrations [10, 23, 24].

Additionally, lidocaine modulates the immune response to surgical trauma with benefits in term of cancer recurrence. So, it is advisable to associate the intravenous infusion of lidocaine along with dexamethasone plus non-steroidal anti-inflammatory drugs (NSAIDs) to complement the analgesic effect of NMDA antagonists through the reduction of inflammation due to surgical trauma. Moreover, it has been shown that the intravenous lidocaine reduces the requirements for hypnotic drugs (propofol or sevoflurane) and has a dose-dependent anti-NMDAr effect [25–31].

Dexmedetomidine is an alpha-2 adrenergic agonist which acts at different levels of the nociceptive pathway like on the peripheral nerves, pre-synaptic receptors at the dorsal horn of the spinal cord and at the supraspinal level (Locus Coeruleus). The association of dexmedetomidine with OFA may provide additional benefits. They encompass the attenuation of the sympathetic nervous system, a reduction in intraoperative catecholamines release, a decrease in the requirements for hypnotics (propofol or inhalation anesthetics) due to its sedative effects, decreases in the post-operative psychomimetic side-effects of ketamine, the prevention of postoperative delirium and shivering [32, 33].

Meta-analyses have shown that clonidine and dexmedetomidine provide analgesia with an added opioid-sparing effect and PONV reduction [34, 35].

The authors has been using the OFAA protocol on patients with a medical history of postoperative nausea and vomiting, ERAS protocols in complex laparoscopic surgery that include bariatric surgery and patients with chronic pain, opioid treatment and OIH who are to undergo extensive/complex spinal surgery. The outcomes of our patients have undergone complex gastro-intestinal surgery have been consistent with the published literature. An important reduction in nausea and vomiting (20%), a faster recovery from intestinal peristalsis, adecrease in ileus and acute gastric remnant dilatation, and a reduction in the post-operative use of opioid rescue (30%) have been recorded in our case-series [36–38].

7. Is it feasible to provide a perioperative management focusing on anti-hyperalgesia and central sensitization for patient with chronic pain who are to undergo major spinal surgery?

Patients with severe spinal deformities like scoliosis, and cranio-cervical-thoracic instability due to connective tissue defects and Joint Hypermobility Syndrome often suffer from widespread chronic pain and hyperalgesia. In patients with Joint Hypermobility Syndrome (JHS) who developed cranio-cervical instability (CCI), both severe craniocervical pain and widespread pain (i.e., somatic/neuropathic/visceral), have multi-factorial causes, that are strongly related to chronic nociceptive neuro-inflammation, glial activation and neuronal plasticity in the spinal cordas well as in the brainstem and brain that lead to a common final pathway, which is the Central Sensitization phenomena (CS) [7, 10].

Furthermore, many patients with CCI, JHS, chronic fatigue and severe chronic pain receive different types of opioids, which further complicates pain due to OIH. Sometimes, these patients may suffer from a category of pain known as central intractable pain. It is a painful condition that does not respond to opioids and their use may even be detrimental to the patient [6, 7].

Therefore, considering the probable mechanisms of the chronic pain (CS and OIH) that affect patients with JHS and CCI as well as their frequent association with MCAS and POTS, the use of opioids in total intravenous anesthesia (TIVA) during occipitocervical~thoracic fixation (OCF) was halted in our practice. Intra-operative opioid-based analgesia has been replaced by infusions of lidocaine, ketamine, magnesium, dexmedetomidine and propofol as hypnotic [10, 39]. As stated before, they are coadjuvants with known anti-hyperalgesic properties. This OFAA protocol aims at improving postoperative pain control, minimizing postoperative opioid rescues and reducing preoperative opioid doses in those patients who have been prescribed those drugs over a long period (**Figure 1**).

Infusions of lidocaine, ketamine and dexmedetomidine are continued at lower doses during the post-operative period (for a maximum of one week) as part of a multimodal analgesia plan [10, 39]. The continued perioperative use of a lidocaine, ketamine and dexmedetomidine infusion and the gradual reduction of the doses over one week might overcome the peak of the inflammatory surgical-response. Therefore, its effect on pain and Central Sensitizationis to minimize opioid exposure and result in a reduction of VAS [8, 39–43].

In a case-series study of 42 patients with JHS that have undergone OCF [39], the authors found a lower VAS in the OFA group in the postoperative time ($p < 0.001$). The reduction in the VAS was more significanton the 1st postoperative day in the OFA group 5.35 (4.83–5.86) vs. the Opioid group (OP) 7.89 (7.56–8.23) ($p < 0.001$), meaning up to 32% decrease in the VAS of the OFA group. TheVAS at hospital-discharge was lower in the OFA group: 4.96 (4.54–5.37) vs. OP group: 6.39 (6.07–6.71) ($p < 0.001$). The methadone requirement was lower in the OFAgroup ($p < 0.001$). No methadone rescue was needed with 78% (IC 95%)of patients in OFA group. On the contrary, 95% (IC95%) in the OP group needed methadone rescue at high doses. The OFA group showed decreased ileus, nausea and vomiting ($p < 0.001$). Compared with preoperative values, there were decreased opioid

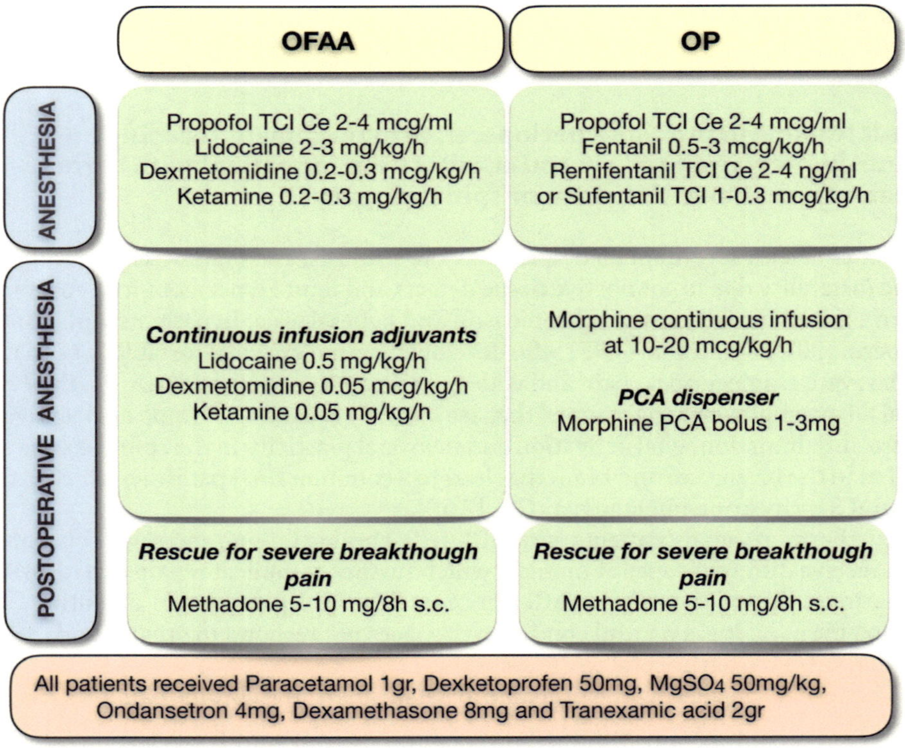

Figure 1.
Opioid-free anesthesia and analgesia (OFAA) vs. opioid based anesthesia and analgesia (OP) protocols for patients with joint hypermobility syndrome undergoing craneo-cervical fixation. Adapted from Ramírez-Paesano C., et al. [39].

requirements for 60.9% in the OFA group at hospital-discharge. A 77% reduction of anxiolytics requirements was also seen. In the OFA group, 17.4% (n = 4) of patients had visual hallucinations. Haloperidol was used in two patients [39].

The doses of lidocaine, ketamine, magnesium and dexmedetomidine proposed in the author's protocol seems to be a combination with balanced anti-nociceptive synergism. It coincides with recent publications that describe lidocaine, ketamine, dexmedetomidine and MgSO4 as the best options in both obese patients and complex spine surgery [23, 44].

According to the literature, there is more consensus on the benefits of OFA use in bariatric surgery or complex laparoscopy surgery. In term of the reduction of postoperative opioid requirements and a better recovery, the controversies that surround the benefits of OFA in major spinal surgery may be due to the diversity of surgical-procedures, the varying degrees of complexity of the cases and the exceptionally varied use of coadjuvants for post-operative multi-modal analgesia. However, there is strong evidence that opioid-inclusive anesthesia does not reduce postoperative pain but is associated with more side effects in comparison with the opioid minimizing approach. OFA management should be evaluated on a case-by-case basis.

With the current evidence, OFA management could not be confirmed as an independent factor in reducing postoperative pain in all the surgical settings in which it has been used. However, OFA management plus postoperative use of lidocaine, ketamine, and dexmedetomidine infusions (OFAA) as part of robust multimodal analgesia may explain the results seen in patients with extensive chronic pain, hyperalgesia and Central Sensitization phenomena [10, 39, 45, 46].

8. Is it possible to use some opioid as postoperative rescue in OFAA?

Many times patients undergoing extensive surgery require postoperative opioids as rescue for breakthrough pain control. The OFAA protocol used in our hospital includes methadone as rescue for severe postoperative pain [10, 39]. We believe that methadone is the most suitable opioid to use as rescue analgesic for severe pain due to its anti-MNDAr effect. Methadone decreases OIH and attenuates the central sensitization phenomenon. It also has a reducing effect on the reuptake of serotonin and norepinephrine. All these mechanisms of action make methadone a suitable opioid for use in OFAA protocols. In addition, the use of methadone with ketamine (both anti-NMDAr) shows a "boosting" and synergistic effect that enhances the opioid-sparing effect [47].

Recent publications have recommended the use of methadone (0.15–0.2 mg/kg bolus) at the start of anesthetic induction in complex spinal surgery [48]. Methadone has been shown to provide a postoperative opioid-sparing effect and improved pain control. These benefits appear to persist for months after surgery compared to other opioids such as morphine or hydromorphone [49].

A recent meta-analysis confirms the benefits of methadone use at the onset of anesthesia in extensive and painful surgeries [50, 51].

9. Are there some contraindications to the use of OFAA?

We should be noted that OFAA is no applicable to all patients. OFAA is relatively contraindicated in patients with node blocks, autonomous nervous system disfunctions including orthostatic hypotension as seen in patients with multiple systemic atrophy disease. Furthermore, OFAA should not be administered to patients with coronary stenosis or acute coronary isquemia as well as patients with hemodynamic instability, increased intracranial pressure or polytrauma. The peripheral vasodilation caused by

OFAA which could limit the perfusion of vital organs [52]. Finally, OFAA should not be administered to patients who have known allergies to some of its components.

10. What can be found in the literature on the risks and benefits of OFAA?

There is uncertainty in the literature on the balance between OFA benefits and risks. Some systematic reviews have shown an improvement in the incidence of postoperative pain, nausea and vomiting [53]. However, alpha-2-receptor agonists such as Dexmedetomidine or clonidine may be responsible of some side effects such as hypotension, bradycardia and sedation. Therefore, the safety of OFAA has been questioned [53–55]. The authors have not observed the aforementioned complications with the use of dexmedetomidine, probably because we did not administer starting boluses, and the maintenance doses used were limited to 0.2–0.3 mcg/kg/h.

A Meta-Analysis of randomized controlled trials including 2209 participants comparing OFAA to opioid based anesthesia (OBA) found no clinically significant effect of OFA on acute pain and opioid use after surgery in a large sample of studies. However, it found clinically important reductions in postoperative nausea, vomiting, shivering and sedation incidence showing a beneficial impact on postoperative patient comfort [56]. Definitive evidence-based conclusions related to the use of OFAA are still lacking. For this reason, it is important to continue exploring how to prevent its side effects as well as possible alternatives.

11. Conclusion

The activation of the glutaminergic pathway plays a determining role in secondary sensitization at the level of the central nervous system, which is responsible for nociceptive amplification, persistence of postoperative pain, and hyperalgesia.

The development of opioid-free anesthesia techniques, indicated for particular patient populations in which opioids may be harmful, requires the use of drug mixtures in which NMDAr antagonists are essential.

The most clinically used NMDA receptor inhibitors in anesthesia are ketamine and magnesium sulfate. They are the cornerstone to reduce or avoid the SC phenomenon, hyperalgesia and OIH in the surgical setting. Their co-administration in OFA techniques has synergistic analgesic and anti-hyperalgesic effects. The concomitant use of intravenous lidocaine and dexmedetomidine provides additional benefits to the use of NMDAr antagonists.

The authors consider that OFA has precise indications. However, the use of regional anesthetic techniques (whenever possible) or the use of intravenous mixtures with anti-hyperalgesic and opioid-sparing effects should be used, ifpossible, in patients with a history of chronic pain or with central sensitization phenomena and hyperalgesia who are to undergo extensive and very painful surgeries. Finally, methadone is a suitable opioid for use in modified OFAA protocols because its anti-NMDAr action and opioid-sparing effect.

Acknowledgements

The authorsthanks bariatric and spinal surgeons at Centro MedicoTeknon for their support in developing our OFAA protocol. We are also grateful tothe anesthesia/analgesia nursing team of "Anestalia", without them our OFAA protocol could not have been implemented.

Conflict of interest

The authors declare no conflict of interest and no funding.

Author details

Carlos Ramírez-Paesano*, Claudia Rodiera Clarens, José Carlos Torres Mandujano, Milen Bonev Bonev, Karen Salazar Loaiza, Florencia Borghetti, María Martínez Alberici, Josep Rodiera Olive and Jesus Santaliestra Fierro
Anesthesiology Department (Anestalia), Centro Médico Teknon (Quironsalud Group), Barcelona, Spain

*Address all correspondence to: cramirez@anestalia.com

References

[1] Farquhar-Smith Paul W. Anatomy, physiology and pharmacology of pain. Anaesth and Intensive Care Med. 2007; 9:1.

[2] Ferrari LF, Lotufo CM, Araldi D, Marcos A. Rodrigues MA. et al. Inflammatory sensitization of nociceptors depends on activation of NMDA receptors in DRG satellite cells. PNAS. 2014; 111(51): 18365. www.pnas.org/cgi/doi/10.1073/pnas.1420601111

[3] Ferreira SH, Lorenzetti BB. Glutamate spinal retrograde sensitization of primary sensory neurons associated with nociception. Neuropharmacology. 1994;33(11):1479-1485.

[4] Parada CA, Vivancos GG, Tambeli CH, Cunha FQ, Ferreira SH. Activation of presynaptic NMDA receptors coupled to NaV1.8-resistant sodium channel C-fibers causes retrograde mechanical nociceptor sensitization. Proc Natl Acad Sci USA. 2003; 100(5): 2923-2928.

[5] Ferreira SH, Lorenzetti BB. Intrathecal administration of prostaglandin E2 causes sensitization of the primary afferent neuron via the spinal release of glutamate. Inflamm Res. 1996; 45(10):499-502.

[6] Lee M, Silverman S, Hansen H, et al. A comprehensive review of opiod-induced hyperalgesia. Pain Physician. 2011; 14: 145-161.

[7] Ji R-R, Nackley A, Huh Y, et al. Neuroinflammation and Central Sensitization in Chronic and Widespread Pain. Anesthesiology. 2018; 129: 343-366.

[8] Bolyanatz P. A new paradigm: Prevention of central sensitization in pain management through minimizing opioid exposure. 2019. DOI:10.5772/intechopen.85192

[9] Beloeil H. Opioid-free anesthesia. BestPract Res Clin Anaesth. 2019;33(3):353-360. https://doi.org/10.1016/j.bpa.2019.09.002

[10] Ramirez-Paesano CR, Juanola G.A, Gilete G.V., et al. Opioid-Free Anesthesia Plus Postoperative Management Focused on Anti-Hyperalgesia Approach in Patients with Joint Hypermobility Syndrome Undergoing Occipital-Cervical Fixation: A Narrative Review and Authors' Perspective. Neurol Res Surg. 2020; 3(1): 1-11. doi:10.33425/2641-4333.1030

[11] Kharasch ED, Brunt LM. Perioperative opioids and public health. Anesthesiology 2016; 124:960-965.

[12] Steyaert A, Lavand'homme P. Prevention and treatment of chronic postsurgical pain: a narrative review. Drugs 2018; 78:339-354.

[13] Miclescu A. Chronic pain patient and anaesthesia. Rom J Anaesth Int Care. 2019; 26: 59-66.

[14] Mulier J, Dekock M. Opioid-free general anesthesia, a new paradigm? Best Pract Res Clin Anaesthesiol 2017; 31:441-443.

[15] Lavand'hommea P, Estebea JP. Opioid-free anesthesia: A different regard to anesthesia practice. CurrOpinAnesthesiol. 2018; 31: 556-561.

[16] Jouguelet-Lacoste J, La Colla L, Schilling D, et al. The use of intravenous infusion or single dose of low-dose ketamine for postoperative analgesia: a review of the current literature. Pain Med 2015 Feb;16(2):383e403.

[17] Jouguelet-Lacoste J, La Colla L, Schilling D, et al. The use of intravenous infusion or single dose of low-dose ketamine for postoperative analgesia: a review of the current literature. Pain Med 2015 Feb;16(2):383e403.

[18] Guo BL, Lin Y, Hu W, et al. Effects of systemic magnesium on post-operative analgesia: is the current evidence strong enough? Pain Phys 2015;18(5):405e18.

[19] De Oliveira Jr GS, Castro-Alves LJ, Khan JH, et al. Perioperative systemic magnesium to minimize postoperative pain: a meta-analysis of randomized controlled trials. Anesthesiology 2013;119 (1):178e90.

[20] Savic Vujovic KR, Vuckovic S, Srebro D, et al. A synergistic interaction between magnesium sulphate and ketamine on the inhibition of acute nociception in rats. Eur Rev Med Pharmacol Sci 2015;19(13):2503e9.

[21] Makhro A, Tian Q, Kaestner L, et al. Cardiac N-methyl D-aspartate receptors as a pharmacological target. J Cardiovasc Pharmacol 2016 Nov;68(5):356e73.

[22] Chen JT, Chen TG, Chang YC, et al. Roles of NMDARs in maintenance of the mouse cerebrovascular endothelial cell constructed tight junction barrier. Toxicol 2016 Jan 2;339:40e50.

[23] Farag E, Ghobrial M, Sessler DI, et al. Effect of perioperative intravenous lidocaine administration on pain, opioid consumption, and quality of life after complex spine surgery. Anesthesiology. 2013; 119: 932-940.

[24] Eipe N, Gupta S, Penning J. Intravenous lidocaine for acute pain: an evidence-based clinical update. BJA Education. 2016; 16: 292-298.

[25] Hans G.A., LauwickS.M., Kaba A., et al. Intravenous lidocaine infusion reduces bispectral index-guided requirements of propofol only during surgical stimulation.Br J Anaesth. 2010; 105: 471-479.

[26] Dunn L.K, Durieux M.E. Perioperative use of intravenous lidocaine Anesthesiology. 2017; 126: 729-737.

[27] Altermatt F.R., Bugedo D.A., Delfino A.E. et al. Evaluation of the effect of intravenous lidocaine on propofol requirements during total intravenous anaesthesia as measured by bispectral index.Br J Anaesth. 2012; 108: 979-983.

[28] Forster C, Vanhaudenhuyse A, Gast P, et al. Intravenous infusion of lidocaine significantly reduces propofol dose for colonoscopy: a randomised placebo-controlled study.Br J Anaesth. 2018;121(5):1059-1064. doi: 10.1016/j.bja.2018.06.019. Epub 2018 Aug 1.

[29] Nishizawa N, Shirasaki T, Nakao S, et al. The Inhibition of the N-Methyl-D-Aspartate Receptor Channel by Local Anesthetics in Mouse CA1 Pyramidal Neurons. AnesthAnalg 2002; 94:325-330.

[30] Nagy I, Woolf CJ. Lignocaine selectivity reduces C fibre evoked neuronal activity in rat spinal cord in vitro by decreasing N-methyl-D-aspartate and neurokinin receptor-mediated postsynaptic depolarizations; implications for the development of novel centrally acting analgesics. Pain. 1996; 64:59-70.

[31] Kim Ryungsa. Effects of surgery and anesthetic choice on immunosuppression and cancer recurrence. J Transl Med 2018;16: 8.https://doi.org/10.1186/s12967-018-1389-7

[32] Singh PM, Panwar R, Borle A, et al. Perioperative analgesic profile of dexmedetomidine infusions in morbidly obese undergoing bariatric surgery: a metaanalysis and trial sequential analysis. Surg Obes Relat Dis 2017; 13:1434-1446.

[33] Tsaousi GG, Pourzitaki C, Aloisi S, et al. Dexmedetomidine as a sedative

and analgesic adjuvant in spine surgery: a systematic review and meta-analysis of randomized controlled trials. Eur J Clin Pharmacol 2018; 74: 1377-1389.

[34] Blaudszun G, Lysakowski C, Elia N, et al. Effect of perioperative systemic alpha2 agonists on postoperative morphine consumption and pain intensity: systematic review and meta-analysis of randomized controlled trials. Anesthesiology 2012;116:1312-1322.

[35] Schnabel A, Meyer-Friessem CH, Reichl SU, et al. Is intraoperative dexmedetomidine a new option for postoperative pain treatment? A meta-analysis of randomized controlled trials. Pain 2013;154: 1140-1149.

[36] Ziemann-Gimmel P, Goldfarb AA, Koppman J, Marema RT. Opioid-free total intravenous anaesthesia reduces postoperative nausea and vomiting in bariatric surgery beyond triple prophylaxis. Br J Anaesth 2014; 112: 906-911. https://doi.org/10.1093/bja/aet551

[37] Mulier JP, Dillemans B. Anaesthetic factors affecting outcome after bariatric surgery, a retrospective levelled regression analysis. Obes Surg 2019; 29: 1841-1850. https://doi. org/10.1007/s11695-019-03763-1

[38] Malo-Manso A., Díaz-Crespo J., Escalona-Belmonte JJ., Romero-Molina S., et al. Impact of opioid free anaesthesia in bariatric surgery. An. Sist. Sanit. Navar. 2020; 43 (1): 51-56. https://doi.org/10.23938/ASSN.0757(in spanish)

[39] Ramirez-Paesano C, Juanola Galceran A, Rodiera Clarens C, et al. Opioid-free anesthesia for patients with joint hypermobility syndrome undergoing craneo-cervical fixation: a case-series study focused on anti-hyperalgesic approach. Orphanet J Rare Dis 2021;16:172. https://doi.org/10.1186/s13023-021-01795-4

[40] Mitra R, Prabhakar H, Rath GP, et al. A comparative study between intraoperative low-dose ketamine and dexmedetomidine, as an anaesthetic adjuvant in lumbar spine instrumentation surgery for the post-operative analgesic requirement. J Neuroanaesthesiol Crit Care. 2017;4:91-98.

[41] Cassuto J, Sinclair R, Bonderovick M. Anti-inflamatory of local anesthesia and their present and potential clinical indications. Acta Anaesthesiol Scand. 2006;50:265-282.

[42] Feizerfan A. Transition from acute to chronic pain. ContEducAnaesth Crit Care Pain. 2015;15(2):98-102. https://doi. org/10.1093/bjaceaccp/mku044

[43] Meiler S, Monk T, Mayfield JB, Head A. Can we alter long-term outcome? The role of inflammation and immunity in the perioperative period (Part II). APSF Newsletter. Spring. 2004;19(1):1-16.

[44] Baek S Y, Kim J W, Kim T W, Han W, et al. Opioid-free anesthesia with a mixture of dexmedetomidine, ketamine, and lidocaine in one syringe for surgery in obese patients. J Int Med Res. 2020; 48(10) 1-8. DOI: 10.1177/0300060520967830

[45] Frauenknecht J, Kirkham KR, Albrech A,E. Analgesic impact of intra-operative opioids vs. opioid-free anaesthesia: a systematic review and meta-analysis. Anaesthesia. 2019; 75:651-662.

[46] Maheshwari K, Avitsian R, Sessler DI, Makarova N, et al. Multimodal analgesic regimen for spine surgery: a randomized placebo-controlled trial. Anesthesiology. 2020;132: 992-1002.

[47] Kharasch E D, Clark JD. Methadone and Ketamine: Boosting Benefits and StillMore to Learn. Anesthesiology 2021;

134:676-679.DOI: 10.1097/ ALN.0000000000003752

[48] Glenn S. Murphy G S, Avram M J, Greenberg S B, et al. Perioperative Methadoneand Ketamine for Postoperative Pain Control in Spinal Surgical Patients A Randomized, Double-blind, Placebo-controlled Trial.Anesthesiology 2021; 134:697-708.

[49] Murphy G S, Avram M J, Greenberg S B, Shear T D, Mark A, Deshur M A, et al. Postoperative Pain and Analgesic Requirements in the First Year after Intraoperative Methadone for Complex Spine and Cardiac Surgery. Anesthesiology 2020; 132:330-342.

[50] Machado F C, Vieira J E, de Orange F A et al. Intraoperative Methadone Reduces Pain and Opioid Consumption in Acute Postoperative Pain: A Systematic Review and Meta-analysis. AnesthAnalg. 2019;129:1723-1732.

[51] Murphy G S, Wu Ch L, Mascha E J. Methadone: New Indications for an Old Drug? Anesth Analg. 2019;129(6):1456-1458.DOI:10.1213/ ANE.0000000000004472

[52] Mulier J. Opioid free general anesthesia: A paradigm shift? Revista Española de Anestesiología y Reanimación. 2017; 64 (8):427-430. DOI: 10.1016/j.redar.2017.03.004 (in Spanish)

[53] Frauenknecht J, Kirkham K R, Jacot-Guillarmod A, Albrecht E. Analgesic impact of intra-operative opioids vs. opioid-free anaesthesia: A systematic review and meta-analysis. Anaesthesia 2019; 74: 651-662.

[54] Grape S, Kirkham K.R., Frauenknecht J, Albrecht E. Intra-operative analgesia with remifentanil vs. dexmedetomidine: A systematic review and meta-analysis with trial sequential analysis. Anaesthesia 2019; 74: 793-800.

[55] Demiri, M, Antunes T, Fletcher D, Martinez V. Perioperative adverse events attributed to alpha2-adrenoceptor agonists in patients not at risk of cardiovascular events: Systematic review and meta-analysis. Br. J. Anaesth. 2019; 123: 795-807.

[56] Arthur S, Hakim H, Dominique F, Martínez V. Opioid free anesthesia Benefit-Risk Balance: A Sytematic review and Meta-Analysis of Randomized Controlled Trials. J. Clin Med. 2021, 10, 2069. http://doi.org/10.3390/jcm10102069

Chapter 6

Low-Dose Ketamine for Acute Postoperative Pain Treatment

Arunas Gelmanas, Migle Vitartaite, Ramunas Tamosiunas and Andrius Macas

Abstract

Treatment of acute postoperative pain is an essential part of perioperative care and if left untreated could complicate the healing period. Ketamine blocks nociceptive pain and pain arising from inflammation. Therefore, it is potentially beneficial in the postoperative period. After systematic review using "MEDLINE/PubMed (NLM)" database, we analyzed 18 studies published during 2011–2020 and found that 0.5 mg/kg/h ketamine bolus and 0.1–0.25 mg/kg/h ketamine infusion to be the most effective dose to alleviate postoperative acute pain. Ketamine, when compared with a placebo, did not have any impact on patients' satisfaction with postoperative pain management and overall well-being. Only three studies revealed more frequent adverse reactions to ketamine after surgery suggesting that ketamine did not have any impact on patients' postoperational rehabilitation. So, it is the option to recommend low-dose ketamine to be part of multimodal analgesia in acute severe postoperative pain treatment. It can be used in both opioid-dependent and opioid-tolerant patients. Ketamine bolus should be ≤0.35 mg/kg and infusion ≤1 mg/kg/h. One should avoid the use of ketamine in pregnant women, people with cardiovascular diseases, acute psychosis, impaired liver function, increased intracranial, and intraocular pressure. Intranasal ketamine may be considered for children during procedures outside of the operation room.

Keywords: low dose, ketamine, acute pain management

1. Introduction

Treatment of acute postoperative pain is an important part of perioperative care. Insufficient analgesia is related to adverse outcomes such as immunosuppression, hyperglycemia, aggravated early rehabilitation, deterioration in patients' quality of life, more common postoperative complications, a longer period of recovery after surgery, and progress from acute to chronic pain [1, 2].

Ketamine, a *N*-methyl-D-aspartate (NMDA) receptor antagonist, is a cheap and potentially opioid-sparing effect having drug, which in recent years attains more recognition for multimodal pain management [1, 3, 4]. NMDA receptors are related to nociceptive pain and pain arising from inflammation [5]. Blocking those receptors may contribute to the effectiveness of opioids and lower the prevalence of chronic pain syndrome [1, 4]. An adverse side effect of ketamine is dose-dependent and could be avoided by using anxiolytics for premedication, selecting patients more carefully before the operation, using antihypertensive drugs together with ketamine infusion [3].

U.S. Food and Drug Administration indications for the usage of ketamine are adjuvant to general anesthesia, induction agent for general anesthesia, sedation for short-time procedures [6]. This means that usage of ketamine for acute postoperative pain treatment is not based on official indications, because there is a lack of researches on this topic.

In recent years, there has been considerable interest in ketamine efficiency in treating acute postoperative pain. Guidelines published in 2018 indicate that a regimen of low-dose ketamine can be described as following—ketamine bolus lower than 0.35 mg/kg, infusion—lower than 1 mg/kg/h [5]. In 2015, Jouguelet-Lacoste with colleagues published a literature review that included five meta-analyses studying intravenous ketamine impact on postoperative pain inhibition. They revealed that ketamine lowers pain points and additional opioid consumption. Four out of five researches revealed that pain scores in the first 24 hours after operation lowered 87.5, 59, 54.5, and 25% compared to placebo [7]. In 2018, Cochrane systematic review included 130 pieces of research to find if low-dose ketamine effectively alleviates acute postoperative pain. Consumption of opioids in the first 24 hours was 8 mg less and the first 48 hours 13 mg less when compared with placebo. Pain at rest lowered 5/100 mm of visual analog scale (VAS), during movement 6/100 mm VAS in the first 48 hours [8].

Unfortunately, there were no guidelines on what dosage, which patient group, and in what way ketamine should be used. In 2018, the American Society of Regional Anesthesia and Pain Medicine together with the American Academy of Pain Medicine and the American Society of Anesthesiologists published guidelines on intravenous usage of ketamine for managing acute pain. They indicated the most suitable group of patients for using ketamine, its dosage, indications, contraindications, and trials supporting this evidence. The authors of these guidelines also pointed out that more trials should be done to determine the accurate and effective doses of ketamine for effective acute pain management [6].

2. Methods

The design of this systematic review of the literature is followed by the Preferred Reporting Items for Systematic Reviews and Meta-Analyses (PRISMA) statement guidelines. Data were identified from searches of MEDLINE (PubMed) database. The combination of keywords included terms "low" and "dose" and "ketamine" and "pain" and "postoperative" in PubMed Advanced Search Builder in all fields accordance with the PICO criteria: "Participants" were limited to 18 years and older, "interventions" covered were randomized controlled clinical trials on low-dose intravenous ketamine, "comparator"—comparing ketamine with placebo and/or a different dose of ketamine, and "outcomes" discovered after a thorough analysis of researches and classified according to the trial type and most common findings. Records were screened by the title, abstract, and full text. Inclusion criteria were as follows: (1) full-text articles published in English; (2) not older than 2011; (3) double- or triple-blinded randomized prospective trials of different ketamine intravenous dosage and/or placebo; (4) American Society of Anesthesiologists (ASA) I–III class; (5) age over 18 years; (6) VAS or Numeric Pain Scale (NPS) used for evaluation of acute postoperative pain. However, review or meta-analysis or systematic review articles, commentaries, abstract-only publications, guidelines, case reports, not randomized trials, ketamine given intramuscularly/orally/subcutaneous, ketamine given in the emergency department were excluded. The detailed search flowchart is presented in **Figure 1**.

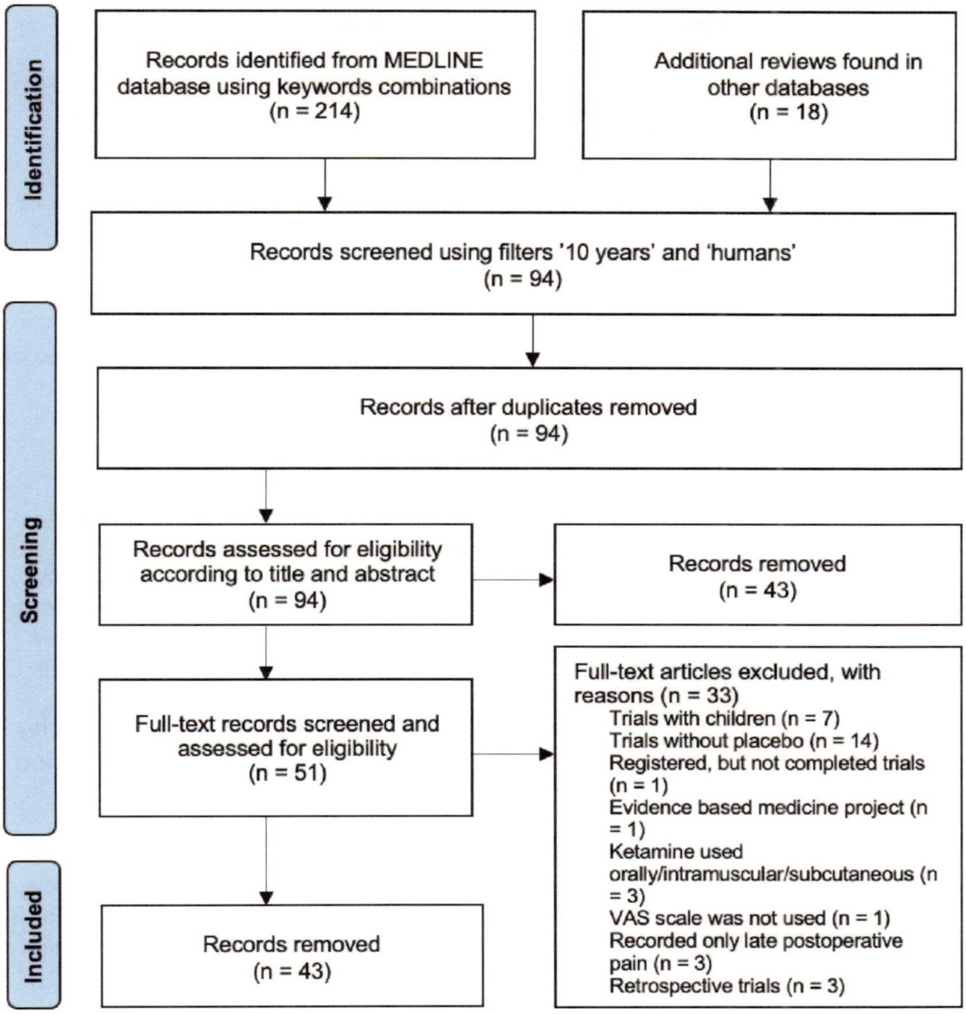

Figure 1.
Flowchart.

3. Results

3.1 Study selection process

The research yielded 214 results, extracted from one database. All duplicates were removed, and 94 articles were checked manually for relevance by screening their titles and abstracts. About 51 results met the inclusion criteria, but only 18 were included after a full-text review. Only full-text articles were selected because the information given in the abstract was not sufficient for the thorough analysis. The randomized trials, conducted in 2011–2020 and which compared different doses of ketamine and placebo given for patients during various surgeries to investigate the effect of the drug on the management of acute postoperative pain, were analyzed. About 33 publications were excluded for reasons explained in **Figure 1**.

3.2 Characteristics of included studies

Those 18 selected trials could be divided into several groups—those who investigate ketamine bolus dose (six trials), those who investigate different infusion dose peri- and postoperation (two trials), those who investigate both only during operation (six trials), and those who investigate bolus and infusion, which is continued during and after the operation (four trials). A summary of the results of 18 analyzed studies is provided in **Table 1**.

3.3 Synthesis of results

All 18 trials (bolus/infusion/both) included in this systematic review were investigated and compared in three categories—pain, overall satisfaction, and adverse reactions (AR). The summarized results can be seen in **Table 2**.

Subramaniam and colleagues [9] conducted a trial wanting to find out ketamine impact on pain management after laminectomy. Pain scores remained high despite analgesic therapy with ketamine, epidural bupivacaine, PCA with hydromorphone, and other adjuvants. No adverse reactions in the ketamine group were observed. Meanwhile, Kim with fellow authors [19] conducted a similar trial, but in PCA, they used fentanyl. Their research revealed that 0.5 mg/kg ketamine bolus and 2 μg/kg/min ketamine infusion statistically significantly lower fentanyl doses in the first 48 hours after surgery without more frequent adverse reactions. In both trials, pain evaluation in points did not differ.

Chumbley with colleagues' [24] trial revealed that 0.1 mg/kg IV ketamine bolus and 0.1 mg/kg/h infusion, started 10 min before thoracotomy, lowers consumption of opioids and pain scores at 48 h after surgery.

Yazigi with co-authors [18] injected IV 0.1 mg/kg ketamine bolus before the surgery and IV ketamine infusion of 0.05 mg/kg was continued for 72 hours after lobectomy during thoracotomy, same as bupivacaine that was injected through the intercostal catheter for 72 hours. Ketamine did not have any significant difference in pain scores, additional morphine consumption, sedation, and other adverse psychomimetic effects.

Parikh with other scientists [10] aimed to find out the efficiency of pain management by using ketamine for patients after open renal surgery. They favored the use of ketamine, as its bolus and infusion started after anesthesia induction which reduced pain scores in the first 12 hours, reduced or delayed the use of additional postoperative morphine, and does not cause a more frequent adverse reaction.

Kaur and colleagues [22] discovered that ketamine bolus and infusion were given only during surgery lowered pain scores in the first 6 hours, reduced opioid consumption, and did not have an adverse effect on patients after cholecystectomy.

Nielsen with co-authors [14] investigated opioid-dependent patients' pain management with ketamine bolus and infusion after back surgery. They did not find any difference in pain scores during 2–24 hours after surgery, but morphine consumption in the PCA in the first 24 hours was significantly lower in the research group. No statistical significance was observed on patients' overall satisfaction and adverse reaction rate.

Haliloglu with colleagues [23] researched ketamine bolus and infusion during C-section. Their trial revealed that ketamine reduced postoperative PCA morphine consumption in the first 24 hours, but it did not reduce pain scores in the research group in all hours except for the first 15 min after surgery.

Ates with others [26] injected ketamine bolus and infusion during septorhinoplasty and discovered that it reduces pain scores at every hour and lowers additional

DOI: http://dx.doi.org/10.5772/intechopen.100415

Author	Year of publishing, country	Surgery type	Number of patients	Type of anesthesia	Inclusion criteria	Pain and satisfaction evaluation
Subramaniam [9]	2011, USA	Lumbar/thoracic laminectomy	30	General anesthesia	Age 18 and older, ASA 1–3 class	VAS (0–10 cm) at 0, 1, 2, 4, 8, 12, 18, 24, 36, 48 h after surgery. Satisfaction on pain management at 48 h (1 p. bad, 10 p. good)
Parikh [10]	2011, India	Open renal surgery	60	General anesthesia	Age 18–70, ASA 1–2 class	VAS (0–10 cm) every 15 min at the first hour, and then at 4, 8, 12, 16, and 24 h after surgery
Bilgen [11]	2012, Turkey	C-section	140	General anesthesia	ASA 1–2 class, primiparas with an indication for C-section	NPS (0–10 p.) at 2, 6, 18, 24, 48 h after surgery
Mendola [12]	2012, Italy	Muscle-sparing posterolateral thoracotomy	62	General and epidural anesthesia	ASA 1–3 class	NPS (0–10 p.) at 1, 2, 4, 12, 18, 24 h and every 6 h following 3 days after surgery and 2 times a day until discharge
Song [13]	2013, Korea	1–2 level posterior lumbar fusion	50	General anesthesia	ASA 1–2 class, non-smoking women, age 20–65, with a risk for postoperative nausea and vomiting	VAS (0–100 mm) at 30 min, 6, 12, 24, 36, 48 h after surgery at rest and movement
Nielsen [14]	2017, Denmark	1–2 level middle lumbar fusion	147	General anesthesia	Chronic back pain for >3 months, age 18–85, ASA 1–3 class, BMI 18–40 kg/m^2, opioid usage for >6 months	VAS (0–100 mm) at 2, 6, 12, 18, 25 h after surgery at rest ant movement
Honarmand [15]	2011, Iran	Appendectomy	90	General anesthesia	ASA 1–2 class, age 18–60, no abscess or perforation	VAS (0–10 cm) at 0, 10, 20, 30 min, 6–12–18–24 h after surgery.
Menkiti [16]	2012, Nigeria	C-section	56	General anesthesia	ASA 1–2 class, age 18–60, no abscess or perforation	VAS (0–10 cm) at 0, 10, 20, 30 min, 6–12–18–24 h after surgery.
Nesek-Adam [17]	2012, Croatia	Laparoscopic cholecystectomy	80	General anesthesia	ASA 1–2 class, age 18–70	VAS (0–10 cm) and numeric pain scale (0–4 p.) 0, 1, 2, 4, 6, 12, 24 h after the surgery. Overall satisfaction evaluated after 24 h (1–5 p.)

Author	Year of publishing, country	Surgery type	Number of patients	Type of anesthesia	Inclusion criteria	Pain and satisfaction evaluation
Yazigi [18]	2012, Lebanon	Lobectomy during posterior dorsal thoracotomy, while having lung cancer	60	General anesthesia and intercostal nerve block	ASA 2–3 class	VAS (0–100 mm) 1, 6 12, 18, 24, 30, 36, 42, 48, 54, 60, 66, 72 h after the surgery. Ramsav sedation scale (1–6 p.)
Kim [19]	2013, Korea	Posterior decompression and posterior lumbar spinal cord surgery	60	General anesthesia	ASA 1–2 class	VAS (0–100 mm) 1, 6, 24, 48 h after the surgery and movement. Overall satisfaction evaluated after 48 h (1–5 p.)
Han [20]	2013, Korea	C-section	36	Spinal anesthesia	ASA 1–2 class, between 37 and 42 weeks of pregnancy	VAS (0–10) 2, 6, 24, 48 h after the surgery at a rest and while coughing Overall satisfaction evaluated after 48 h (1–5 p.)
Rahmanian [21]	2015, Iran	C-section	160	Spinal anesthesia	Singleton pregnancy	Numeric pain scale (0–10 p.) 1, 2, 6, 12 h after the surgery
Kaur [22]	2015, India	Open cholecystectomy	80	General anesthesia	ASA 1–2 class	VAS (0–100 mm) 0, 2, 4, 6, 12, 24 h after the surgery. Overall satisfaction evaluated after 24 h (1–5 p.) Nausea and sedation evaluation (0–3 p.)
Haliloglu [23]	2016, Turkey	C-section	52	General anesthesia	ASA 1–2 class	Numeric pain scale (0–10 p.) 15 min, 2, 6, 12, 18, 24 h after the surgery
Chumbley [24]	2019, UK	Thoracotomy	70	Not specified	≥18 years, able to read English	Numeric pain scale (0–10 p.) 24, 48 h after the surgery at a rest and while coughing
Boenigk [25]	2019, USA	Two or more levels of lumbar spinal cord surgery	124	General anesthesia	ASA 1–3 class	Numeric pain scale (0–10 p.) 0, 30 min. 1, 1. 5, 2, 4, 6, 8, 10, 12, 14, 16, 18, 20, 22, 24 h after the surgery
Ates [26]	2020, Turkey	Septorhinoplasty	48	General anesthesia	ASA 1–2 class	VAS (0–10 cm) 0, 1, 2, 4, 8, 12, 24 h after the surgery. Overall satisfaction is evaluated (1–5 p.)

Table 1.
Descriptive characteristics of the different trials which researched ketamine's bolus, infusion, or both.

Author	Research group (RG)	Control/other group (CG)	Postoperative pain management	Results			
				Pain	Overall satisfaction	Adverse reaction	Overall
Bolus and infusion during and after surgery							
Subramaniam	Intravenous (IV) ketamine bolus 0.15 mg/kg for induction and continuous infusion at 2 μg/kg/min during and after surgery for 24 h	Same scheme, but instead of ketamine IV NaCl 0.9%	Patient-controlled analgesia (PCA)—hydromorphone 0.125 boluses every 5 min (max 1.25 mg/h). Epidural block with bupivacaine. Nausea and vomiting—IV ondansetron 4 mg.	Not statistically significant	Not statistically significant	Not statistically significant, the control group experienced nausea and AR-related to central nervous system (CNS) more often	—
Kim	RG1—IV 1 μg/kg/min ketamine infusion started before incision and continued for 48 h and 0.5 mg/kg ketamine bolus/// RG2—same scheme, but infusion at 2 μg/kg/min and bolus 0.5 mg/kg	Same scheme, but instead of ketamine—IV NaCl 0.9%	PCA with fentanyl—15 μg bolus max every 5 min. Nausea or vomiting—IV 10 mg metoclopramide/4 mg ondansetron.	RG2 used less fentanyl than CG and RG1 ($p < 0.05$). VAS—not statistically significant	Same results among the group	No one had hallucinations or nightmares. Other things—not statistically significant	+
Chumbley	IV 0.1 mg/kg ketamine bolus 10 min before surgery and IV 0.1 μg/kg/h ketamine infusion for 96 h	Same scheme, but instead of ketamine—unknown placebo	Differ—thoracic epidural infusion/PCA ± paravertebral infusion of a local anesthetic	NPC 48 h after surgery lower in RG ($p = 0.03$). RG consumed less opioids at 24 and 48 h	Not examined	RG had vivid dreams and felt weaker than CG ($p = 0.001$ and $p = 0.02$). Nausea, vomiting, rash, and sedation did not differ.	+

Author	Research group (RG)	Control/other group (CG)	Postoperative pain management	Results			
				Pain	Overall satisfaction	Adverse reaction	Overall
Yazigi	Before the incision IV 0.1 mg/kg ketamine bolus IV 0.05 mg/kg/h ketamine infusion for 72 h	Same scheme, but instead of ketamine—IV NaCl 0.9%	72 h after the surgery—1 mg/mL 0.1 mL/kg/h bupivacaine through intercostal catheter. Also IV 1 g paracetamol, 50 mg ketoprofen every 6 h. If VAS > 40 mm—morphine sulfate titrated 2 mg bolus max every 5 min, max dose 0.1 mg/kg/h	No statistical difference—while coughing ($p = 0.7$), while at rest ($p = 0.75$)	Not examined	Not statistically significant for sedation, dizziness, nausea, or vomiting. For two patients in RG had hallucinations, impaired vision, or nightmares.	—
Bolus and infusion only during surgery							
Parikh	After the induction IV 10 mL (1 mg/mL–0.15 mg/kg) ketamine bolus and 50 mL (1 mg/mL–0.12 mL/kg/h-2 μg/kg/min) infusion until the end of the surgery	Same scheme, but instead of ketamine—IV NaCl 0.9%	When VAS > 40 - > morphine 1 mg	In the first 12 h after the surgery VAS was lower in the RG. In RG 5 patients needed an additional analgesic, in CG all patients needed it so morphine consumption at RG was lower than in the KG.	Not examined	Four patients in RG felt nausea or vomiting.	+
Nielsen	IV 0.5 mg/kg S-ketamine bolus after the induction and IV 0.25 mg/kg ketamine infusion until the last stich	Same scheme, but instead of ketamine—IV NaCl 0.9%	For everyone in the first 24 h—1 g paracetamol, orally every 6 h started from the 2nd h. PCA with 2.5 mg morphine boluses max every 5 min. For nausea or vomiting IV 4 mg ondansetron - > if not effective—droperidol	No statistical difference—when moving ($p = 0.63$) and at the rest ($p = 0.62$) at 2–24 h. RG used less morphine ($p < 0.001$).	Not statistically significant	Not statistically significant, but vomiting less frequent in the RG at 0–24 h.	+

DOI: http://dx.doi.org/10.5772/intechopen.100415

Author	Research group (RG)	Control/other group (CG)	Postoperative pain management	Results			
				Pain	Overall satisfaction	Adverse reaction	Overall
Haliloglu	At induction IV 0.5 mg/kg ketamine bolus and infusion 0.25 mg/kg/h until the end of operation	Same scheme, but instead of ketamine—IV NaCl 0.9%	NPS >4 in the recovery room - > 0.05 mg/kg morphine. PCA 0.5 mg/kg morphine at 1 mg boluses max every 10 min. If PCA not efficient—IV 75 mg diclofenac.	15 min after the surgery NPS lower in the RG (p = 0.001) at 2, 6, 12, 18, 24 h—did not differ (p > 0.05). Consumption of morphine 0–24 h was lower in the RG (p = 0.001)	Not examined	Spontaneous, involuntary eye movement, hallucinations, and dual vision did not occur to anyone. Most patients experienced nausea, vomiting, and itching, but no statistical difference (p > 0.05).	+
Kaur	IV 0.2 mg/kg ketamine bolus and infusion 0.1 mg/kg/h until the end of operation	Same scheme, but instead of ketamine—IV NaCl 0.9%	VAS >30 mm—IV 0.05 mg/kg morphine bolus. Medium and strong nausea–IV 0.1 mg/kg ondansetron	During the first 6 h, VAS was lower in the RG (p < 0.05), but not different at 12 and 24 h. RG patients needed less additional analgesic (p = 0.001). The usage of morphine was lower in the RG (p = 0.001).	Not statistically significant	No one experienced hallucinations, sedation, headache, dizziness, breathing disorder. Nausea and vomiting were similar, but statistically not different.	+
Ates	At induction IV 0.5 mg/kg ketamine bolus and 0.25 mg/kg/h infusion continued during operation	Same scheme, but instead of ketamine—IV NaCl 0.9%	For everyone at 12 and 24 h after the surgery—50 mg dexketoprofen. If VAS ≥ 4–1 mg/kg tramadol.	VAS was greater in the CG at 30 min. 1, 2, 4, 8, 12, 24 h (p < 0.05). CG needed more additional analgesics than RG (p = 0.022)	Higher in the RG (p = 0.003)	Nausea was more intense in the CG, but not statistically. RG did not experience hallucinations, arrhythmias, or vomiting.	+
Han	IV 0.5 mg/kg ketamine bolus and infusion 0.25 mg/kg/h during surgery	Same scheme, but instead of ketamine—IV NaCl 0.9%	PCA with 25 μg/mL fentanyl—as needed, max every 15 min. If VAS ≥ 5 or patient request—intramuscular 30 mg ketorolac.	At 2 h RG used less fentanyl (p = 0.033), but there was no difference at 6, 24, 48 h. VAS—not statistically significant.	Not statistically significant.	No one experienced hallucinations or nightmares.	—

Author	Research group (RG)	Control/other group (CG)	Postoperative pain management	Results			
				Pain	Overall satisfaction	Adverse reaction	Overall
Bolus							
Bilgen	Before the induction IV: RG1—ketamine 0.25 mg/kg; RG2—ketamine 0.5 mg/kg; RG3—ketamine 1 mg/kg bolus.	Same scheme, but instead of ketamine—IV NaCl 0.9%	PCA for 48 h after the surgery - > morphine chloride 0.5 mg/mL - > 1 mg bolus every 10 min. If needed—IV 75 mg diclofenac every 12 h. If NPS > 4, additional IV morphine 0.005 mg/kg.	No statistical difference (p = 0.2–0.9)	Not examined	No statistical difference (p = 0.3–0.7). In RG1—2 felt nausea, in RG2—3 felt nausea, 1 vomited and 1 experienced hallucination, in RG3—4 had spontaneous, involuntary eye movement, 1 vomited and had an occurrence of dual sight, in the CG—1 felt nausea and 1 experienced spontaneous, involuntary eye movement.	—
Song	After induction IV 0.3 mg/kg ketamine bolus + PCA (fentanyl 20 μg/kg, ondansetron 9 mg, ketamine 3 mg/kg)	Same scheme, but instead of ketamine—IV NaCl 0.9%	PCA and 25 mg meperidine, when VAS > 40 mm or if the patient asks. When nausea >6 points (in the system of 10 points, 0—no nausea, 10 strong and unbearable nausea) or if a patient asks—IV 4 mg ondansetron	No statistical difference—when moving or at the rest. RG used less fentanyl 48 h after the surgery (p = 0.035, 773 and 957 μg)	Not examined	RG felt nausea more common than CG at 0–6 h (p = 0.016). RG experienced dizziness in the first 48 h (p = 0.047). Three patients experienced hallucination/nightmares and dysphoria in the RG.	+

Author	Research group (RG)	Control/other group (CG)	Postoperative pain management	Results			
				Pain	Overall satisfaction	Adverse reaction	Overall
Honarmandt	IV 0.5 mg/kg 3 mL ketamine 15 min before the incision	Subcutaneous 0.5 mg/kg 3 mL ketamine/// subcutaneous infiltration of NaCl 0.9% 3 mL 15 min before the incision	If VAS > 4 cm—IV 0.4 mg/kg meperidine - > if it does not help in 10 min - > 0.2 mg/kg. Do not exceed 2 mg/kg in 4 h. Nausea >10 min. –0.1 mg/kg metroclopramide IV - > if needed, repeat after 1 h.	VAS scores were lower at 10, 20, 30 min in ketamine groups ($p < 0.05$) but did not differ between them. When comparing CG and RG groups at 6, 12, 18, 24 h VAS were lower in RG ($p < 0.05$). At 12, 18, 24 h VAS were lower in RG when compared with subcutaneous ketamine ($p < 0.05$)	Not examined	Sedation did not differ. AR did not differ, no one had delirium, hallucinations, or nightmares.	+
Menkiti	IV 0.15 mg/kg 2 mL ketamine bolus after spinal anesthesia	Same scheme, but instead of ketamine—IV NaCl 0.9%	If VAS >3 IV 75 mg diclofenac. If it does not help - > 30 mg pentazocine 0, every 4 h and 75 mg diclofenac every 8 h if needed.	CG VAS was bigger at 60, 90, 120 min. Statistically significant VAS > 3 p. differed at 90, 120, 150 min. RG received less analgesic after the surgery ($p < 0.001$)	Not examined	No significant difference, usually hypotension, trembling.	+

Author	Research group (RG)	Control/other group (CG)	Postoperative pain management	Results			
				Pain	Overall satisfaction	Adverse reaction	Overall
Adam	IV 100 mL NaCl 0.9% 20 min. Before anesthesia and 0.15 mg/kg 5 mL IV ketamine before incision///IV 1 mg/kg diclofenac in 100 mL NaCl 0.9% 20 min before anesthesia and 5 mL IV NaCl 0.9% before incision///IV 1 mg/kg diclofenac in 100 mL NaCl 0.9% 20 min before anesthesia and IV 0.15 mg/kg 5 mL ketamine before incision	IV 100 mL NaCl 0.9% 20 min before anesthesia and 5 mL IV NaCl 0.9% before incision	If VAS > 4—diclofenac IV. If no effect—IV 1.25 g metamizole and IV 100 mg tramadol in 100 mL 0.9% NaCl per 20 min.	VAS max 1 h after surgery. Ketamine and diclofenac group pain scores lower than CG at 1, 2, 4, 6 h and lower than ketamine group at 1, 2 h. During the first 6 h, pain scores were higher in CG rather than the ketamine and diclofenac group. During the first 4 h, ketamine and diclofenac are better than only ketamine. Diclofenac is better than CG or ketamine group at 2.6 h and 2.4 h, respectively.	Not statistically significant	Not statistically significant	—
Rahmaniam	5 min after delivery—IV 0.25 mg/kg ketamine bolus	Same scheme, but instead of ketamine IV NaCl 0.9%	If asked—100 mg rectal diclofenac suppository max every 6 h, max 4 times in 24 h. If NPS ≥5—intramuscular 50 mg petidine, max 2 times in 24 h.	CG VAS bigger that RG at 1, 2, 6, 12 h ($p < 0.001$). RG time until first analgesic longer than in the CG ($p < 0.001$). Total dose of petidine and diclofenac lower in the RG ($p < 0.001$).	Not examined	Vomiting is more common in CG ($p = 0.020$). Hallucinations are more common in the RG ($p = 0.032$).	+
Infusion during and after surgery							
Mendola	Before first incision IV 0.1 mg/kg/h ketamine infusion for 60 h	Same scheme, but instead of ketamine—IV NaCl 0.9%	If VAS > 3 p.— > PCA 5 mL max every 60 min. If not—1) IV paracetamol 45 mg/kg, 2) IV ketorolac 1.5 mg/kg, 3) morphine	Not statistically significant between NPS. 0.1 day after surgery RG needed more analgesics ($p = 0.0016$)	Not examined	Not statistically significant. RG 32, 5 vs. CG 25% experienced nausea, vomiting, hypotension, neurological symptoms.	+

Author	Research group (RG)	Control/other group (CG)	Postoperative pain management	Results			
				Pain	Overall satisfaction	Adverse reaction	Overall
Boenigk	IV 0.12 mg/kg ketamine infusion for 24 h and 0.2 mg/kg ketamine bolus during the first 30 min into Recovery Room	Same scheme, but instead of ketamine—IV NaCl 0.9% and same ketamine bolus	PCA with hydromorphone—0.2 mg max every 6 min, max 2 mg/h for 24 h in the Recovery Room. If NPS > 4—IV 0.2–0.3 mg hydromorphone.	Not statistically significant between NPS. Opioid-tolerant in RG consumed more hydromorphone than opioid-tolerant in CG ($p = 0.007$)	Not examined	Not statistically significant	+

Table 2.
Results of studies included in a systematic review.

consumption of opioids, the adverse reaction occurred less frequently, and overall satisfaction on pain management was better.

Different from other trials, Han with colleagues [20] did not find any statistically significant difference in reducing pain scores, overall satisfaction, and adverse reactions.

Bilgen with other researches [11] evaluated three different IV ketamine bolus doses (0.25, 0.5, 0.1 mg/kg) in patients after C-section. No differences were observed.

Menkiti with colleagues [16] found that VAS > 3 points were significantly more often assessed in the control group at 90, 120, 150 min. Also, the first analgesic was appointed for patients for a short amount of time in the research group.

Rahmaniam with colleagues [21] researched IV ketamine bolus after C-section. In the ketamine group, pain scores were lower in the 1, 2, 6, and 12 hours after surgery. Time until first analgesic and amount of them was lower in the ketamine group. Unfortunately, nausea and hallucinations occurred more frequently in the ketamine group.

Song and fellow co-authors [23] researched IV ketamine bolus (which was also given in the PCA) impacts on pain management after spinal cord surgery. At 48 hours, patients with PCA ketamine used less additional fentanyl than the control group. Also, research group participants experienced nausea at 0–6 hours and felt dizziness for 48 hours.

Honarmand and colleagues [15] discovered that 0.5 mg/kg IV ketamine bolus before appendectomy alleviates pain at 12, 18, and 24 hours better than the same dose given s/c or placebo.

Adam with other researchers [17] researched ketamine and diclofenac effects after laparoscopic cholecystectomy. It showed that ketamine without diclofenac has no significant difference.

Mendola and co-authors [12] were determined to find IV ketamine infusion, continued for 60 hours after surgery, impact on pain management. For 48 hours, the control group required more analgesics than the research group. Adverse reactions were not more common in the ketamine group.

Boenigk and colleagues [25] researched 0.2 mg/kg IV ketamine bolus and 0.12 mg/kg ketamine infusion on patients with and without opioid addiction. Those in the control group who have an addiction used more opioids for postoperative pain management than those who did not have an addiction.

4. Discussion

Multimodal analgesia is a key component for adequate and fulfilling postoperative pain management. Ketamine, together with adjuncts such as magnesium, lidocaine, dexamethasone, α2 agonists, incisional infiltration, acetaminophen, nonsteroidal anti-inflammatory drugs, or COX-2 selective given during surgery, is known to lessen the pain postoperatively by preventing neural sensitization that may lead to persistent pain as their primary purpose is to target the pain during various pathways in the central nervous system. Ketamine prescribed intravenously after the surgery may decrease overall opioid use, and it is a good analgesic for patients who develop tolerance to the analgesic properties of opioids [27].

The results of all these researches can be explained in several ways. Firstly, according to the type of surgery, Subramaniam [9] and Kim [19] investigated patients after spinal cord surgery, but Subramaniam [17] used IV ketamine 0.15 mg/kg and Kim [19] used a much bigger dose—0.5 mg/kg IV ketamine bolus. Ketamine was infused at the same speed at 24 and 48 hours, respectively. These reasons may have contributed to better outcomes of the Kim [19] trial, as patients used less postoperative analgesics when compared to the control group. Differently from these trials, Chumbley [24] and Yazigi [18] trial results cannot be explained like that, because IV ketamine bolus dose is the same, but Chumbley [24] used 0.1 mg/kg/h infusion for 48 hours (more common adverse reactions—vivid dreams, poor well-being) and Yazigi [18] used 0.5 mg/kg/h for 78 hours, but the results were favorable to Chumbley [24] where patients needed less additional analgesics. As in Chumbley [24], trial patients felt adverse reactions more frequently the prospects of early rehabilitation of these people would have been weaker.

As for ketamine bolus and infusion only during surgery, we can state that carrying out open renal surgery [10] and cholecystectomy [22], IV ketamine bolus (0.15 mg/kg and 0.2 mg/kg), and infusion (2 μg/kg/min and 2 μg/kg/min) alleviates pain better in the first 12 and 6 hours accordingly, reducing the postoperative amount of analgesics and not causing adverse reactions. Nielsen [14] trial (0.5 mg/kg ketamine bolus and 0.25 mg/kg infusion) showed that patients who used opioids before surgery consume less morphine. Haliloglu [23] and Han's [20] trials compared IV ketamine bolus 0.5 mg/kg and infusion 0.25 mg/kg—in the first one morphine consumption was lower in the research group for 24 hours, in the second one, no difference was observed. Best results were written in the Ates [26] trial (0.5 IV ketamine bolus and 0.25 mg/kg/h infusion)—pain scores, the demand of postoperative analgesics, and adverse reactions were lower in the ketamine group. Satisfaction of pain management was better in the ketamine group in only this trial.

Three trials compare the ketamine bolus effect on postoperative pain after C-section. In the first one [11], 0.25 mg/kg, 0.5 mg/kg, 1 mg/kg ketamine boluses did not have any impact on any factor. In the second one [16], 0.15 mg/kg ketamine bolus was determined to shorten the time of additional analgesia. In the third one [21], 0.25 mg/kg ketamine bolus revealed the best results—lower pain scores, longer time without analgesics and its dose, but nausea and hallucinations appeared more frequently. During spinal cord surgery [13], 0.3 mg/kg IV ketamine bolus triggered nausea and dizziness but lowered the number of additional analgesics. What is interesting, 0.5 mg/kg IV ketamine bolus caused fewer adverse reactions after appendectomy but also alleviated pain effectively in the first 24 hours after surgery [15]. A dose of 0.15 mg/kg IV ketamine bolus during laparoscopic cholecystectomy did not show any better results than a placebo. In only one trial, researchers investigated overall satisfaction which did not differ between the ketamine and placebo groups [17].

Comparing trials that investigated only ketamine infusion efficiency, we can summarize them into few fields—pain scores were not lower neither 0.1 mg/kg/h nor 0.12 mg/kg/h IV ketamine infusion. In the first research [12], the ketamine group required fewer postoperative analgesics. The same results were shown in the second trial, where patients before surgery used opioids [25]. Adverse reactions did not differ in any trial.

5. Conclusions

1. Pain intensity evaluated while using ketamine:

    a. Bolus and infusion (during and after surgery)—IV combination of 0.5 mg/kg ketamine bolus and 1 μg/kg/min infusion successfully lowered the necessity of postoperative analgesics,

    b. Bolus and infusion (during surgery)—IV combination of 0.5 mg/kg ketamine bolus and 0.25 mg/kg/h infusion successfully reduced postoperative pain and

IV 0.2–0.5 mg/kg bolus and 0.1–0.25 mg/kg/h infusion meaningfully diminished consumption of postoperative analgesics,

c. Infusion (during and after surgery)—IV 0.1 mg/kg/h ketamine bolus reduced consumption of postoperative analgesics,

d. Bolus—less analgesics were used when IV bolus dose were 0.25–0.3 mg/kg and IV 0.5 mg/kg bolus eased pain better for the first 24 h, 0.25 mg/kg for 12 h, 0.15 mg/kg for 3 hours.

2. In 17 trials, overall well-being and satisfaction of pain management did not differ between ketamine and placebo and in one trial, 0.5 mg/kg ketamine bolus and 0.25 mg/kg/h infusion were associated with better results.

3. Adverse reactions were more common in three pieces of research—the first being IV 0.1 mg/kg ketamine bolus and 0.1 mg/kg/infusion; second—IV 0.25 mg/kg ketamine bolus; and third—IV 0.3 mg/kg ketamine bolus, thus meaning that the early rehabilitation of patients in the rest of the trials would have been good.

6. Practical recommendations

These recommendations are prepared in accordance with guidelines issued in 2018 [6]:

1. Subanesthetic ketamine infusions should be considered for patients undergoing painful surgery (upper and lower abdominal, thoracic, and orthopedic (limbs and spine)).

2. Ketamine should be considered for both opioid-tolerant and opioid-dependent patient groups.

3. Ketamine bolus should not exceed 0.35 mg/kg, infusion 1 mg/kg/g dose, but it should always be considered according to a patient's factors.

4. Patients with cardiovascular disease, pregnant women, patients with active psychosis, hepatic dysfunction, elevated intracranial, and intraocular pressure should avoid using ketamine.

5. Intranasal ketamine should be considered using for children during short-time procedures and for whom intravenous ketamine is difficult to inject. Intranasal ketamine is effective for acute pain management and for amnesia and sedation during the procedure.

6. Evidence for the benefit of IV-PCA: Delivered ketamine as the only analgesic for acute pain is limited and there is moderate evidence for the benefit of the addition of ketamine to an opioid-based IV-PCA for acute and perioperative pain management.

Conflict of interest

The authors declare no conflict of interest.

Author details

Arunas Gelmanas[1*], Migle Vitartaite[2], Ramunas Tamosiunas[1] and Andrius Macas[1]

1 Department of Anaesthesiology, Lithuanian University of Health Sciences, Kaunas, Lithuania

2 Faculty of Medicine, Medical Academy, Lithuanian University of Health Sciences, Kaunas, Lithuania

*Address all correspondence to: arunas.gelmanas@kaunoklinikos.lt

References

[1] Laskowski K, Stirling A, McKay WP, Lim HJ. A systematic review of intravenous ketamine for postoperative analgesia. Canadian Journal of Anesthesia. 2011;**58**:911-923. DOI: 10.1007/s12630-011-9560-0

[2] Kehlet H, Jensen TS, Woolf CJ. Persistent postsurgical pain: Risk factors and prevention. The Lancet. 2006;**367**(9522):1618-1635. DOI: 10.1016/S0140-6736(06)68700-X

[3] Allen CA, Ivester JR. Low-dose ketamine for postoperative pain management. Journal of Perianesthesia Nursing. 2018;**33**(4):389-398. DOI: 10.1016/j.jopan.2016.12.009

[4] Niesters M, Martini C, Dahan A. Ketamine for chronic pain: Risks and benefits. British Journal of Clinical Pharmacology. 2014;**77**(2):357-367. DOI: 10.1111/bcp.12094

[5] Weinbroum AA. Non-opioid IV adjuvants in the perioperative period: Pharmacological and clinical aspects of ketamine and gabapentinoids. Pharmacological Research 2012;65(4):411-429. DOI:10.1016/j.phrs.2012.01.002

[6] Schwenk ES, Viscusi ER, Buvanendran A, Hurley RW, Wasan AD, Narouze S, et al. Consensus guidelines on the use of intravenous ketamine infusions for acute pain management from the American Society of Regional Anesthesia and Pain Medicine, the American Academy of Pain Medicine, and the American Society of Anesthesiologists. Regional Anesthesia and Pain Medicine. 2018;**43**(5):456-466. DOI: 10.1097/AAP.0000000000000806

[7] Jouguelet-Lacoste J, La Colla L, Schilling D, Chelly JE. The use of intravenous infusion or single dose of low-dose ketamine for postoperative analgesia: A review of the current literature. Pain Medicine. 2015;**16**(2):383-403. DOI: 10.1111/pme.12619

[8] Brinck EC, Tiippana E, Heesen M, Bell RF, Straube S, Moore RA, et al. Perioperative intravenous ketamine for acute postoperative pain in adults. Cochrane Database of Systematic Reviews. 2018;**12**(12):CD012033. DOI: 10.1002/14651858.CD012033.pub4

[9] Subramaniam K, Akhouri V, Glazer PA, Rachlin J, Kunze L, Cronin M, et al. Intra- and postoperative very low dose intravenous ketamine infusion does not increase pain relief after major spine surgery in patients with preoperative narcotic analgesic intake. Pain Medicine. 2011;**12**(8): 1276-1283. DOI: 10.1111/j.1526-4637.2011.01144.x

[10] Parikh B, Maliwad J, Shah VR. Preventive analgesia: Effect of small dose of ketamine on morphine requirement after renal surgery. Journal of Anaesthesiology Clinical Pharmacology. 2011;**27**(4):485-488. DOI: 10.4103/0970-9185.86592

[11] Bilgen S, Köner O, Türe H, Menda F, Fiçicioğlu C, Aykaç B. Effect of three different doses of ketamine prior to general anaesthesia on postoperative pain following Caesarean delivery: A prospective randomized study. Minerva Anestesiologica. 2012;**78**(4):442-449

[12] Mendola C, Cammarota G, Netto R, Cecci G, Pisterna A, Ferrante D, et al. S(+)-ketamine for control of perioperative pain and prevention of post thoracotomy pain syndrome: A randomized, double-blind study. Minerva Anestesiologica. 2012;**78**(7):757-766

[13] Song JW, Shim JK, Song Y, Yang SY, Park SJ, Kwak YL. Effect of ketamine as an adjunct to intravenous

patient-controlled analgesia, in patients at high risk of postoperative nausea and vomiting undergoing lumbar spinal surgery. British Journal of Anaesthesia. 2013;**111**(4):630-635. DOI: 10.1093/bja/aet192

[14] Nielsen RV, Fomsgaard JS, Siegel H, Martusevicius R, Nikolajsen L, Dahl JB, et al. Intraoperative ketamine reduces immediate postoperative opioid consumption after spinal fusion surgery in chronic pain patients with opioid dependency: A randomized, blinded trial. Pain. 2017;**158**(3):463-470. DOI: 10.1097/j.pain.0000000000000782

[15] Honarmand A, Safavi M, Karaky H. Preincisional administration of intravenous or subcutaneous infiltration of low-dose ketamine suppresses postoperative pain after appendectomy. Journal of Pain Research. 2012;**5**:1-6. DOI: 10.2147/JPR.S26476

[16] Menkiti ID, Desalu I, Kushimo OT. Low-dose intravenous ketamine improves postoperative analgesia after caesarean delivery with spinal bupivacaine in African parturients. International Journal of Obstetric Anesthesia. 2012;**21**(3):217-221. DOI: 10.1016/j.ijoa.2012.04.004

[17] Nesek-Adam V, Grizelj-Stojčić E, Mršić V, Rašić Z, Schwarz D. Preemptive use of diclofenac in combination with ketamine in patients undergoing laparoscopic cholecystectomy: A randomized, double-blind, placebo-controlled study. Surgical Laparoscopy, Endoscopy & Percutaneous Techniques. 2012;**22**(3):232-238. DOI: 10.1097/SLE.0b013e31824f8ae4

[18] Yazigi A, Abou-Zeid H, Srouji T, Madi-Jebara S, Haddad F, Jabbour K. The effect of low-dose intravenous ketamine on continuous intercostal analgesia following thoracotomy. Annals of Cardiac Anaesthesia. 2012;**15**(1):32-38. DOI: 10.4103/0971-9784.91479

[19] Kim SH, Kim SI, Ok SY, Park SY, Kim MG, Lee SJ, et al. Opioid sparing effect of low dose ketamine in patients with intravenous patient-controlled analgesia using fentanyl after lumbar spinal fusion surgery. Korean Journal of Anesthesiology. 2013;**64**(6):524-528. DOI: 10.4097/kjae.2013.64.6.524

[20] Han SY, Jin HC, Yang WD, Lee JH, Cho SH, Chae WS, et al. The effect of low-dose ketamine on post-caesarean delivery analgesia after spinal anesthesia. The Korean Journal of Pain. 2013;**26**(3):270-276. DOI: 10.3344/kjp.2013.26.3.270

[21] Rahmanian M, Leysi M, Hemmati AA, Mirmohammadkhani M. The effect of low-dose intravenous ketamine on postoperative pain following cesarean section with spinal anesthesia: A randomized clinical trial. Oman Medical Journal. 2015;**30**(1): 11-16. DOI: 10.5001/omj.2015.03

[22] Kaur S, Saroa R, Aggarwal S. Effect of intraoperative infusion of low-dose ketamine on management of postoperative analgesia. Journal of Natural Science, Biology and Medicine. 2015;**6**(2):378-382. DOI: 10.4103/0976-9668.160012

[23] Haliloglu M, Ozdemir M, Uzture N, Cenksoy PO, Bakan N. Perioperative low-dose ketamine improves postoperative analgesia following Cesarean delivery with general anesthesia. The Journal of Maternal-Fetal & Neonatal Medicine. 2016;**29**(6):962-966. DOI: 10.3109/14767058.2015.1027190

[24] Chumbley GM, Thompson L, Swatman JE, Urch C. Ketamine infusion for 96 hr after thoracotomy: Effects on acute and persistent pain. European Journal of Pain. 2019;**23**(5):985-993. DOI: 10.1002/ejp.1366

[25] Boenigk K, Echevarria GC, Nisimov E, von Bergen Granell AE,

Cuff GE, Wang J, et al. Low-dose ketamine infusion reduces postoperative hydromorphone requirements in opioid-tolerant patients following spinal fusion: A randomised controlled trial. European Journal of Anaesthesiology. 2019;**36**(1):8-15. DOI: 10.1097/EJA.0000000000000877

[26] Ates I, Aydin ME, Celik EC, Gozeler MS, Ahiskalioglu A. Perioperative intravenous low-dose ketamine infusion to minimize pain for septorhinoplasty: A prospective, randomized, double-blind study. Ear, Nose, & Throat Journal. 2021;**100**(4):254-259. DOI: 10.1177/0145561320974860

[27] Gritsenko K, Khelemsky Y, Kaye AD, Vadivelu N, Urman RD. Multimodal therapy in perioperative analgesia. Best Practice & Research. Clinical Anaesthesiology. 2014;**28**(1): 59-79. DOI: 10.1016/j.bpa.2014.03.001

Chapter 7

Ketamine for Chronic Pain

Cigdem Yildirim Guclu

Abstract

The treatment of chronic pain is a chronic problem for many specialities. It is generally based on an approach with antidepressants, anti-epileptics and opioids as drugs of first choice. It has been worked by many different protocols. Ketamine, which is known as a good anaesthetic, has been used for chronic pain. When the pain has a neuropathic component, ketamine is a promising treatment for pain management. Ketamine: by inhibiting the *N*-methyl-D-aspartate receptor and having some other effects like enhancement of descending inhibition and anti-inflammatory effects at central sites, takes part in chronic pain management. Besides having analgesic effects, there are some concerns about the side effects of ketamine. Some psychedelic symptoms as hallucinations, memory defects, panic attacks, nausea and vomiting, somnolence, cardiovascular stimulation and sometimes hepatoxicity may be seen in patients. Ketamine is generally well-tolerated in clinical settings. Close monitoring of patients receiving ketamine should be mandatory in order to be aware of central nervous system, haemodynamic, renal and hepatic symptoms as well as abuse.

Keywords: ketamine, neuropathic pain, chronic pain, pain management, NMDA receptors

1. Introduction

Chronic pain is classified as pain that lasts longer than three to 6 months. Besides medical treatment, it consists of many other issues, such as social, economic and psychological. The treatment of chronic pain is a chronic problem for many specialities; it is generally based on an approach with antidepressants, anti-epileptics and opioids as drugs of first choice. Still, there is no right choice for these patients and 60–70% remains untreated [1, 2].

Chronic pain management is arguably at its most effective when a multidisciplinary approach is used. Ketamine can optimise other (non-opioid) medications by reducing opioid requirements [3].

The socioeconomic burden due to chronic pain is another problematic issue and cannot be overestimated. In Europe, the reported burden of chronic pain is nearly equally steep, with the point prevalence estimated to be 25–30% [4].

Ketamine has been on the market as an alternative to phencyclidine since 1960s. In 1965, it is used as an anaesthetic. Ketamine produces dissociative anaesthesia as well as analgesia and amnesia. Because of its side effects like, the induction of a psychedelic state causing agitation, hallucinations and panic attacks, ketamine has limited use in contemporary anaesthesia.

Ketamine is a phenylpiperidine derivative structurally related to phencyclidine with 2(2-chlorophenyl)-2-(methylamino)-cyclohexanone as its chemical structure.

There are two different forms of ketamine: the racemic mixture (Ketalar®, Pfizer Inc., available in the US since 1966) and the S(+) enantiomer (S-ketamine or Ketanest-S®, Pfizer Inc.).

Ketamine is a potent N-Methyl-D-aspartate (NMDA) antagonist and is generally used in the treatment of acute and chronic pain, sedation, induction and maintenance of anaesthesia and ICU sedation [5]. It exerts its NMDA antagonism by binding to the phencyclidine receptor site when the channel is open. Its property to inhibit these receptors, it is postulated that ketamine can help treat chronic neuropathic pain [6]. Also, ketamine can be used as an antidepressant, making it useful in the concomitant treatment of pain and depression [7].

Ketamine is known to prevent central sensitization, so infusions of ketamine started intraoperatively and continued into the early postoperative period might prevent chronic postoperative pain, which is a problem impacting approximately 20% of surgical patients [8]. Ketamine, by inhibition of the N-Methyl-D-aspartate receptor (NMDAR), causes strong analgesia in neuropathic pain. Also, NMDAR is involved in the process of chronification of pain [9].

Ketamine also interacts with other receptors such as opioidergic, muscarinic and mono aminergic receptors. But still, little is known about the contributions of these receptor systems to the various effects of ketamine [10].

There are many routes that ketamine can be given; IV, IM, SC, oral, rectal, nasal, transdermal, epidural, or intrathecal [11]. Orally administered ketamine undergoes extensive first-pass metabolism, primarily via N-demethylation, resulting in small ketamine concentrations and large nor-ketamine concentrations in blood and tissue [12].

One of the challenging concepts about chronic pain patients should be treated in an inpatient setting. When outpatient treatment is planned, other issues must be considered like lack of monitoring, increased risk of toxicity and abuse. Smart dosing regimens, patient (and doctor) training, frequent contact and close monitoring of drug are needed for home treatment of ketamine [13].

The multimodal approach is the most effective treatment of chronic pain. Ketamine is often administered together with opioid analgesics, post-operatively and in the treatment of chronic cancer pain.

2. Central pain

Ketamine has been studied for central pain after spinal cord injury. Oral and parenteral ketamine was found to be effective. It reduced continuous and evoked pain in these patients, and it is related to only mild side effects [14]. Ketamine showed an analgesic effect in a case with neuropathic pain after cauda equina trauma [15]. Ketamine was found effective in a patient with central poststroke pain after subarachnoid haemorrhage, besides providing analgesia, ketamine also helped the opioids and anticonvulsants to be tapered and discontinued [16]. The authors used midazolam for premedication and used iv incremental dose. With 50 mg oral dosing nightly, increasing to 50 mg 3 times a day resulted in relief of allodynia and hyperalgesia.

3. Complex regional pain syndromes

Complex regional pain syndrome is a chronic pain condition having both autonomic and inflammatory features. It occurs acutely in about 7% of patients who have limb fractures, limb surgery, or other injuries. Only a small percentage of it turns into a chronic form. This transition is often paralleled by a change from 'warm complex regional pain syndrome,' with inflammatory characteristics dominant, to 'cold complex regional pain syndrome' in which autonomic features dominate. Many complex mechanisms take role in this period. This may include peripheral and central sensitization, autonomic changes and sympatho-afferent coupling, inflammatory and immune alterations, brain changes, and genetic and psychological factor. Effective management of the chronic form of the syndrome is often challenging. There are reports about epidural use of ketamine in patients with complex regional pain syndromes and refractory to other treatments [16, 17]. Dose for epidural ketamine suggested was 0.3 mg/kg followed by 25 mcg/kg/h with only transient side effects like headache and nausea.

4. Fibromyalgia

Fibromyalgia is a disorder characterised by widespread musculoskeletal pain accompanied by fatigue, sleep, memory and mood issues. Fibromyalgia is thought to amplify painful sensations by affecting the way your brain and spinal cord process painful and nonpainful signals. Symptoms usually appear after physical trauma, surgery, infection or significant psychological stress. In other cases, symptoms gradually accumulate over time with no single triggering event.

In patients with fibromyalgia, ketamine which is given 0.3 mg/kg iv, showed an increase in endurance and reduction in pain intensity, tenderness at trigger points, referred pain, temporal summation, muscular hyperalgesia, and muscle pain at rest. It is suggested that ketamine by reducing central sensitization, is effective in fibromyalgia.

5. Ischemic pain

Peripheral vascular disease is a common reason of limb pain-causing considerable suffering. In its early stages, it can present as intermittent claudication, but with multiple levels of occlusion rest pain can develop. Patients presenting with critical limb ischemia face a 13% risk of primary amputation. The pain often responds poorly to different treatment strategies including opioids.

As ischemic pain of arteriosclerosis may consist of both nociceptive and neuropathic components, it is generally poorly responsive to opioids. When compared with ketamine with a potent dose dependent analgesic effect (0.15, 0.3, 0.45 mg/kg iv) in clinical ischemic pain but with a narrow therapeutic window, ketamine may show better analgesia in these patients [18]. Also dose dependent side effect such as disturbed cognition and perception recorded for these patients.

6. Neuropathic pain

According to aetiology, neuropathic pain syndromes are heterogeneous; in clinical aspect, they have many similarities. Pain, dysesthesias and hyperalgesia are the main features of neuropathic pain syndromes. Unfortunately, standard pharmacologic therapies are generally insufficient.

Current interest in ketamine focuses on its ability to alleviate chronic pain, especially when chronic pain has a neuropathic component. Chronic neuropathic pain is the most widely investigated indication for IV ketamine. Different doses have been tried between 0.25 and 0.75 mg/kg iv. Most side effects are observed with high doses. Neuropathic pain results from lesions of the somatosensory nervous system causing alterations in structure and function so that pain occurs spontaneously and responses to noxious and innocuous stimuli are amplified [19].

Another condition that generally manifests with neuropathic pain is chronic diabetes. In mice, this can be modelled with high-dose injection of streptozotocin which selectively kills pancreatic beta cells through DNA alkalization. Ketamine when given systemic infusion at 20 mg/kg/day for 5 days showed to reduce heat and mechanical hyperalgesia for several weeks following treatment.

7. Acute on chronic neuropathic pain

Ketamine is frequently used for managing acute episodes of refractory neuropathic pain. In these situations, generally, large doses of opioids are used which leads to development of severe hyperalgesia. The mechanism of opioid induced hyperalgesia is not certain, one of the leading theories is overactivation and stimulation of the NMDA-receptor, so this proposed mechanism would explain why NMDA receptor modulators such as ketamine are effective in treating the condition. Ketamine with 10 mg/h iv suggested for opioid hyperalgesia. Also, subcutaneous administration can be a good alternative for these patients to get time for finding iv access.

8. Orofacial pain

Neuropathic pain related to 'nerve damage in the trigeminal region' is one of the chronic pain topics, which generally needs many interventions for pain relief. Ketamine can be an alternative for these kinds of pain issues. NMDA receptor inhibition by ketamine might change the sensitization, so ketamine causes pain relief even after ketamine has been eliminated from the body. The optimal dose suggested as 60 mg per oral, 6 times a day found [20]. Some side effects like dizziness and fatigue were well tolerated.

9. Phantom/stump pain

After amputation of a limb, most amputees suffer from stump and phantom limb pain. Many medical and surgical therapies have been tried, but only a few treatments have been found to be effective. Both peripheral and spinal mechanisms have been accused of underlying mechanism. Studies show that C-fibre input may induce a central hyperexcitability in dorsal horn neurons. There is evidence that this hyperexcitability in part is mediated by excitatory amino acids acting at NMDA receptor sites and that excitatory amino acid receptor antagonists may block this central hyperexcitability and its clinical manifestations.

Case series and case reports support ketamine use in stump and phantom pain. Ketamine showed a significant increase in pressure thresholds and reduced hyperpathia. Especially for patients who did not benefit from conventional treatments, iv ketamine was very effective. Doses such as 0.1 mg/kg iv over 5 min then infusion of 7 g/kg/min for 45 min and 0.125–0.3 mg/kg iv then continuous sc infusion 0.125–0.2 mg/kg/h for maintenance showed effective results. Also, other papers support the use of oral ketamine to control phantom pain (50 mg/6 hr) [21].

10. Postherpetic neuralgia

Nerve injury may lead to persistent pathological pain with hyperalgesia and pain evoked by non-noxious stimuli. Long-lasting hyperexcitability in nociceptive neurons initiated by increased activity in primary afferents may play a role in the pathogenesis of nerve injury pain. In particular, the N-methyl-o-aspartic acid receptors may be important for the development of long-lasting changes in neuronal excitability. NMDA receptor blockers inhibit the progressive increase in action potential discharge (wind-up) and neuronal hyperexcitability produced by repeated stimulation of small-diameter primary. NMDA receptor blockers also inhibit nociceptive behaviour in animals caused by nerve injury.

Ketamine is effective for pain relief in postherpetic neuralgia. Ketamine produces significant pain relief and also reduces allodynia and hyperpathia [22]. Relief of continuous pain was observed at the smallest dose but was most marked at the largest (0.05, 0.075, 0.1, 0.15 mg/kg/h. sc). The number and severity of spontaneous pain attacks are also reduced. Ketamine administration showed even complete resolution of ophthalmic postherpetic neuralgia [23].

11. Headache, backpain and others

Patients with refractory chronic migraine suffer from continuous pain and non-painful symptoms, substantial disability, and have generally failed treatments with multiple medications. Patients with severe pain have often failed typically inpatient or outpatient infusion treatment, so few options remain for them.

Ketamine use for headaches has demonstrated benefits. Subcutaneous ketamine of 80 μg/kg was associated with an approximately 50% reduction in acute migraine-related pain and an approximate 75% reduction in chronic migraine-related pain [24].

Unfortunately, there was weak or no evidence supporting ketamine infusions for immediate improvements in pain management of mixed neuropathic pain, PLP, PHN, fibromyalgia, cancer pain, ischemic pain, migraine headache and low-back pain. Evidence only supports ketamine infusions for intermediate or long-term improvements in pain management of CRPS [25].

Some reports suggest that ketamine decreases the rate of chronic postoperative pain when administered as a pre-incisional dose (0.15–1 mg/kg iv) followed by an intraoperative infusion, and intravenous ketamine has been shown to significantly reduce chronic pain incidence following certain types of surgeries [26].

Multimodal approach to chronic pain is found to be the most effective treatment. In general, ketamine is administered with opioids, post-operatively and in the treatment of chronic cancer pain. A Cochrane review showed that ketamine is effective in reducing morphine consumption, and is related to less pain and less nausea and vomiting [27]. Also, ketamine positively affect opioid treatment in cancer pain [28]. The ability of ketamine to reduce the incidence (and severity) of opioid side effects is important as side effects reduce patient compliance. So, an opioid-ketamine combination may be useful in non-neuropathic pain states (e.g., in the palliative setting) or in mixed nociceptive/neuropathic pain states (e.g., in cancer pain).

Studies show that ketamine has also anti-depressant effects [29]. In fact, clinical studies showed that a subanaesthetic dose of ketamine produces antidepressant effects Ketamine has a positive effect on depressive symptoms in otherwise therapy-resistant patients. Because depression and chronic pain share common mechanistic pathways, Most chronic pain patients face depression or depression-like symptoms.

In fact, the treatment of chronic pain may serve two purposes, treating the pain and ameliorating the depressive symptoms. When the pain is treated and the depression simultaneously resolves, or the reverse is true.

Some experimental reports conclude that ketamine has also anti-inflammatory, neuroprotective and anti-tumour effects [30].

12. Intravenous ketamine for chronic pain

Intravenous ketamine infusions have the advantages of avoiding first-pass metabolism and also controlling the way of administration. But this requires inpatient settings allowing the healthcare team to monitor for adverse conditions and track treatment efficacy.

A meta-analysis including seven different studies examining both neuropathic and non-neuropathic pain conditions showed a significant analgesic effect for intravenous ketamine infusions. The median ketamine dose of 0.35 mg/kg was reached after 5 h. In these studies, maximum analgesic effect was observed between 48 h and 2 weeks post-infusion. The studies showed no efficacy difference between ketamine as a sole agent or adjuvant therapy [31]. This meta-analysis reported that ketamine shows significant promise for the treatment of a wide variety of chronic pain conditions, including neuropathic and non-neuropathic. Due to the long-acting nature of ketamine's analgesia, outpatients treatments could be effective with visits required as frequently as infusions are needed.

Ketamine can be used as a third-line agent in intractable cancer pain. In a case study of cancer patients with intractable pain, ketamine infusions at a rate of 1.5 mg/kg/day reduced total daily morphine use by 50% after patients were sent home with ketamine/morphine pain pumps [32].

13. Oral and nasal ketamine for chronic pain

Oral and nasal formulations generally do not need are direct physician supervision in contrast to infusions, so oral and nasal formulations are more desirable for management of long-term pain conditions. Despite requiring higher doses due to extensive metabolism, oral administrations have also been found to be effective in providing analgesia.

A study with a daily dose of 2 mg/kg, ketamine showed reduction in pain in two-thirds of patients while one-half of patients reported some adverse event [33].

Intranasal ketamine, although now mostly taken part in the treatment of depression, has also been tried for management of cancer pain. Intranasal ketamine was found to be successful in 65% of breakthrough cancer pain patients and achieved a Numerical Pain Intensity Scale (NPIS) score that was at least 40% lower than pre-treatment levels [34].

14. Ketamine as a topical agent

Ketamine as a topical agent may be preferred for patients in whom systemic ketamine administration via oral or IV routes is not desirable administration. Topical application provides the benefit of keeping plasma concentrations and therefore potential side effects at a minimum.

Topical ketamine has been tried in chronic regional pain syndrome, studies reported effective reduction in pain measures, tactile allodynia and Visual Analog

Scale pain score. Besides being a good alternative in pain management, still, there is concern about the systemic levels of ketamine [35].

15. Concerns

Ketamine besides being an anaesthetic is used to treat various chronic pain syndromes, especially those that have a neuropathic component. Inhibition of the N-methyl-D-aspartate receptor and probably some other mechanisms like enhancement of descending inhibition and anti-inflammatory effects at central sites results in strong analgesia even with low doses.

The side effects of ketamine noted in clinical studies include psychedelic symptoms (hallucinations, memory defects, panic attacks), nausea/vomiting, somnolence, cardiovascular stimulation and hepatoxicity. There are also risks ranging from the bladder and renal complications to persistent psychological behaviour and memory defects by the increase in ketamine usage. Also, abuse is another problem.

Cognitive side effects of ketamine frequently limit its use. Since its discovery, ketamine was known to produce dissociative and psychomimetic effects. These effects are also responsible for the continued abuse of ketamine [36].

Studies showed that ketamine produces structural and physiological changes in the brain, even a decrease in grey and white matter volumes in the pre-frontal cortex and white matter degeneration in the left temporoparietal lobe has been reported [37].

Regardless of the mechanism of these cognitive disorders, many research has been done to find out what drugs may be able to prevent them. Several of these studies have demonstrated that benzodiazepines, specifically midazolam and haloperidol, reduced undesired psychotic side effects and nausea associated with ketamine administration [38].

Cystitis related to ketamine use is another problem, especially for long term users. The increase in neurotrophin in bladder tissue accused to cause the chronic inflammation of the bladder and urinary tract in ketamine cystitis [39].

Elevation of serum liver enzymes has been reported in patients receiving ketamine infusions, but these levels decreased back to baseline within 10–14 days following treatment [40].

Due to ketamine's central inhibition effect of norepinephrine reuptake in adrenergic nerves, an increase in cardiac output via elevations in heart rate, systolic blood pressure, and diastolic blood pressure can be observed. Also, ketamine acts as a sympathomimetic on the cardiovascular system [41].

Because of dissociative and hallucinogenic effects of ketamine, it has been abused. Even therapeutic doses are generally less than street-use doses, ketamine still maintains addictive potential.

In clinical settings, ketamine is generally well tolerated, especially when benzodiazepines are used to suppress the psychotropic side effects. Patients receiving ketamine should be monitored closely, especially for CNS, haemodynamic, renal and hepatic symptoms as well as abuse. Until definite proof is obtained ketamine administration should be restricted to patients with therapy-resistant severe neuropathic pain.

16. Conclusion

Ketamine as an analgesic can be used for several indications and in many ways. It may be used most effectively to reduce the symptoms of allodynia, hyperalgesia and hyperpathia rather than acting as a traditional analgesic. This could be consistent with NMDA receptor blockade limiting or reducing central sensitization, although the ability of ketamine to interact with such a wide variety of receptors means that this is currently only speculative.

There are various dose regimens for different application ways for ketamine. Most of the data is based on case reports. Still, there are also concerns about side effects and with different premedication like lorazepam or midazolam, most of the side effects may resolve.

The data provides encouraging suggestions about ketamine for chronic pain situations. To talk about pros of ketamine for chronic pain management:

- Ketamine is tried for many types of pain and found most useful
- Pain related to neuropathies can be relieved by ketamine
- Ketamine can be effective for pain where opioids are ineffective, and hyperalgesia occurred cause of opioids.
- Ketamine can be used during the perioperative period both for acute analgesia management and for preventing chronic pain.
- Ketamine can be applied by many routes; epidural, subcutaneous, intravenous.
- Ketamine has an antidepressant effect, which plays an important role in the management of chronic pain.

Author details

Cigdem Yildirim Guclu
Department of Anesthesiology and ICU, Ankara University Faculty of Medicine, Ibni-Sina Hospital, Ankara, Turkey

*Address all correspondence to: drcigdemyldrm@yahoo.com.tr

References

[1] Dworkin RH, O'Connor AB, Audette J, Baron R, Gourlay GK, Haanpää ML, et al. Recommendations for the pharmacological management of neuropathic pain: An overview and literature update. Mayo Clinic Proceedings. 2010;**85**:S3-S14

[2] Finnerup NB, Otto M, McQuay HJ, Jensen TS, Sindrup SH. Algorithm for neuropathic pain treatment: An evidence based proposal. Pain. 2005;**118**:289-305

[3] Clardk JD. Ketamine for chronic pain old drug new trick? Anesthesiology. 2020;**133**:13-15

[4] Leadley RM, Armstrong N, Lee YC, Allen A, Kleijnen J. Chronic diseases in the European Union: The prevalence and health cost implications of chronic pain. Journal of Pain & Palliative Care Pharmacotherapy. 2012;**26**:310-325

[5] Quibell R, Prommer EE, Mihalyo M, Twycross R, Wilcock A. Ketamine. Journal of Pain and Symptom Management. 2011;**41**(3):640-649

[6] O'Brien SL, Pangarkar S, Prager J. The use of ketamine in neuropathic pain. Current Physical Medicine and Rehabilitation Reports. 2014;**2**(2): 128-145

[7] Zhang K, Hashimoto K. An update on ketamine and its two enantiomers as rapid-acting antidepressants. Expert Review of Neurotherapeutics. 2019;**19**(1):83-92

[8] Correll D. Chronic postoperative pain: Recent findings in understanding and management. F1000Res. 2017;**6**:1054

[9] Petrenko AB, Yamakura T, Baba H, Shimoji K. The role of N-methyl-D-aspartate (NMDA) receptors in pain: A review. Anesthesia and Analgesia. 2003;**97**:1108-1116

[10] Wolff K, Winstock AR. Ketamine: From medicine to misuse. CNS Drugs. 2006;**20**:199-218

[11] Azevedo VM, Lauretti GR, Pereira NL, Reis MP. Transdermal ketamine as an adjuvant for postoperative analgesia after abdominal gynaecological surgery using lidocaine epidural blockade. Anesthesia and Analgesia. 2000;**91**:1479-1482

[12] Grant IS, Nimmo WS, Clements JA. Pharmacokinetics and analgesic effect of i. m. and oral ketamine. British Journal of Anaesthesia. 1981;**53**:805-810

[13] Niesters M, Martini C, Dahan A. Ketamine for chronic pain: Risks and benefits. British Journal of Clinical Pharmacology. 2014;**77**(2):357-367

[14] Eide PK, Stubhaug A, Stenehjem AE. Central dysesthesia pain after traumatic spinal cord injury is dependent on N-methyl-daspartate receptor activation. Neurosurgery. 1995;**37**:1080-1087

[15] Fisher K, Hagen NA. Analgesic effect of oral ketamine in chronic neuropathic pain of spinal origin: A case report. Journal of Pain and Symptom Management. 1999;**18**:61-66

[16] Takahashi H, Miyazaki M, Nanbu T, et al. The NMDA-receptor antagonist ketamine abolishes neuropathic pain after epidural administration in a clinical case. Pain. 1998;**75**:391-394

[17] Lin T-C, Wong C-S, Chen F-C, et al. Long-term epidural ketamine, morphine and bupivacaine attenuate reflex sympathetic dystrophy neuralgia. Canadian Journal of Anaesthesia. 1998;**45**:175-177

[18] Persson J, Hasselstrom J, Wiklund B, et al. The analgesic effect of racemic ketamine in patients with chronic

ischaemic pain due to lower extremity arteriosclerosis obliterans. Acta Anaesthesiologica Scandinavica. 1998;**42**:750-758

[19] Costigan M, Scholz J, Woolf CJ. Neuropathic pain: A maladaptive response of the nervous system to damage. Annual Review of Neuroscience. 2009;**32**:1-32

[20] Rabben T, Skjelbred P, Oye I. Prolonged effect of ketamine, an N-methyl-d-aspartate receptor inhibitor, in patients with chronic pain. The Journal of Pharmacology and Experimental Therapeutics. 1999;**289**:1060-1066

[21] Franks JF, Olesen AS, Mikkelsen SS, Borgbjerg FM. Ketamine in the management of intractable phantom pain. Ugeskrift for Laeger. 1995;**157**: 3481-3482

[22] Eide PK, Jorum E, Stubhaug A, et al. Relief of post-herpetic neuralgia with the N-methyl-d-aspartic acid receptor antagonist ketamine: A double-blind, cross-over comparison with morphine and placebo. Pain. 1994;**58**:347-354

[23] Hoffmann V, Coppejans H, Vercauteren M, Adriaensen H. Successful treatment of postherpetic neuralgia with oral ketamine. The Clinical Journal of Pain. 1994;**10**:240-242

[24] Nicolodi M, Sicuteri F. Exploration of NMDA receptors in migraine: Therapeutic and theoretic implications. International Journal of Clinical Pharmacology Research. 1995;**15**:181-189

[25] Cohen SP, Bhatia A, Buvanendran A, et al. Consensus guidelines on the use of intravenous ketamine infusions for chronic pain from the American Society of Regional Anesthesia & PainMedicine (ASRA), the American Academy of Pain Medicine (AAPM) and the American Society of Anesthesiologists (ASA). Regional Anesthesia and Pain Medicine. 2018;**43**:521-546

[26] Chaparro LE, Smith SA, Moore RA, Wiffen PJ, Gilron I. Pharmacotherapy for the prevention of chronic pain after surgery in adults. Cochrane Database of Systematic Reviews. 2013;**7**

[27] Bell RF, Dahl JB, Moore RA, Kalso E. Perioperative ketamine for acute postoperative pain. Cochrane Database of Systematic Reviews. 2006;**1**:CD004603

[28] Bell RF, Eccleston C, Kalso E. Ketamine as adjuvant to opioids for cancer pain. A qualitative systematic review. Journal of Pain and Symptom Management. 2003;**26**:867-875

[29] Berman RM, Cappiello A, Anand A, Oren DA, Heninger GR, Charney DS, et al. Antidepressant effects of ketamine in depressed patients. Biological Psychiatry. 2000;**47**:351-354

[30] Hirota K, Lambert DG. Ketamine: New uses for an old drug? British Journal of Anaesthesia. 2011;**107**: 123-126

[31] Orhurhu V, Orhurhu MS, Bhatia A, Cohen SP. Ketamine infusions for chronic pain: A systematic review and meta-analysis of randomized controlled trials. Anesthesia and Analgesia. 2019;**129**(1):241-254

[32] Lossignol DA, Obiols-Portis M, Body JJ. Successful use of ketamine for intractable cancer pain. Supportive Care in Cancer. 2005;**13**(3):188-193

[33] Marchetti F, Coutaux A, Bellanger A, Magneux C, Bourgeois P, Mion G. Efficacy and safety of oral ketamine for the relief of intractable chronic pain: A retrospective 5-year study of 51 patients. European Journal of Pain. 2014;**9**(7):984-993

[34] Carr DB, Goudas LC, Denman WT, Brookoff D, Staats PS, Brennen L, et al. Safety and efficacy of intranasal ketamine for the treatment of

breakthrough pain in patients with chronic pain: A randomized, double-blind, placebo-controlled, crossover study. Pain. 2004;**108**(1-2):17-27

[35] Finch PM, Knudsen L, Drummond PD. Reduction of allodynia in patients with complex regional pain syndrome: A double-blind placebo-controlled trial of topical ketamine. Pain. 2009;**146**(1-2):18-25

[36] Domino EF, Chodoff P, Corssen G. Pharmacologic effects of CI- 581, a new dissociative anesthetic, in man. Clinical Pharmacology and Therapeutics. 1965;**6**:279-291

[37] Liao Y, Tang J, Corlett PR, Wang X, Yang M, Chen H, et al. Reduced dorsal prefrontal gray matter after chronic ketamine use. Biological Psychiatry. 2011;**69**(1):42-48

[38] Mercadante S, Lodi F, Sapio M, Calligara M, Serretta R. Long- term ketamine subcutaneous continuous infusion in neuropathic cancer pain. Journal of Pain and Symptom Management. 1995;**10**(7):564-568

[39] Jhang JF, Hsu YH, Kuo HC. Possible pathophysiology of ketamine-related cystitis and associated treatment strategies. International Journal of Urology. 2015;**22**(9):816-825

[40] Kiefer RT, Rohr P, Ploppa A, Dieterich HJ, Grothusen J, Koffler S, et al. Efficacy of ketamine in anesthetic dosage for the treatment of refractory complex regional pain syndrome: An open-label phase II study. Pain Medicine. 2008;**9**(8):1173-1201

[41] Suleiman Z, Ik K, Bo B. Evaluation of the cardiovascular stimulation effects after induction of anaesthesia with ketamine. Journal of the Western African College of Surgeons. 2012;**2**(1):38-52

Chapter 8

Ketamine for Non-Neuropathic Pain

Subbulakshmi Sundaram and
Ashok Swaminathan Govindarajan

Abstract

Chronic pain is one of the leading causes of years lost to disability, as most of the time it is refractory to conventional treatment. Recent advances in understanding the pain mechanisms have favored the use of ketamine as a rescue agent in refractory chronic pain conditions, as it has potential modulating effect on both sensory-discriminative and affective motivational components of pain. Preclinical studies also suggested the antinociceptive effect of sub anesthetic dose of ketamine against central and peripheral neuropathic pain conditions and non-neuropathic pain conditions such as inflammatory and nociceptive pain states. Subanesthetic infusion of ketamine along with adjuvants such as midazolam and clonidine is found to reduce the psychomimetic and cardiovascular side effects of ketamine. Even though the consensus guidelines for intravenous use of ketamine for chronic pain advocate the use of ketamine only for complex regional pain syndrome, various other clinical studies suggested its role in other refractory painful conditions. Hence the present topic focuses specifically on the effect of ketamine on non-neuropathic pain conditions such as complex regional pain syndrome, fibromyalgia, headache, ischemic limb pain, etc. Many studies had shown that ketamine not only reduces the pain scores but also the analgesic medications, which further improves the well-being and quality of life.

Keywords: ketamine, non-neuropathic pain, nociplastic pain, refractory pain syndromes, NMDA receptor antagonist

1. Introduction

Chronic pain (CP) is one of the most leading causes of disabilities affecting more than 30% of people worldwide [1–3]. It is a disease in its own right [4]. Individuals with moderate to severe pain experience a marked decrease in the physical, psychological, and social well-being. It further affects the quality of life, reduces the ability to perform routine activities, and leads to work absenteeism. Economic costs associated with the management of chronic pain in United States include direct healthcare costs ranging from \$260 to \$330 billion and indirect cost ranging from \$300 to \$350 billion per annum [5]. The leading causes of year lost to disability worldwide in 2013 include low back pain, neck pain, migraine, and musculoskeletal disorders [6].

Management of CP is often based on trial-and-error approach with tricyclic antidepressants, anticonvulsants, and narcotics. Many studies have also suggested that combination of drugs is superior to single agent for CP management [7]. Recent advances in understanding the pain mechanism have favored the use of ketamine as a rescue agent in refractory chronic pain syndromes [8]. The most recent definition of neuropathic pain by International Association for the Study for Pain (IASP) excludes the pain states characterized by central sensitization in the absence of a discrete nerve injury such as CRPS-1 and fibromyalgia [8]. Further the new pain descriptor nociplastic pain includes the condition associated with altered processing of pain that does not fit into nociceptive category such as fibromyalgia, CRPS-1, nonspecific chronic back pain, irritable bowel syndrome, and other functional visceral pain disorders [9]. Drugs used to be effective for one type of pain have been shown in various studies to be effective for other type of pain also [10, 11]. Even though the preclinical studies supported the antinociceptive effect of ketamine against central and peripheral neuropathic pain states, there is growing evidence suggesting its analgesic effect in inflammatory and non-neuropathic pain conditions also [12–14]. Hence the present topic focuses specifically on the effect of ketamine on non-neuropathic pain conditions.

2. Newer concepts of pain

Pain can be classified as nociceptive, neuropathic, and nociplastic in origin. Nociceptive pain results from stimulation of primary nociceptive nerve endings by actual or threatened tissue damage, while integrity of nerve fibers is preserved. In contrast to nociceptive pain, neuropathic pain results from direct injury or disease affecting somatosensory nervous system. Recently defined nociplastic pain is the pain that arises from altered nociception despite no clear evidence of actual or threatened tissue damage causing the activation of peripheral nociceptors or evidence for disease or lesion of the somatosensory nervous system causing pain. Characterization of altered nociception is yet to be defined [15]. Another widely, used terminology is mixed pain. It is a complex overlap of various known pain types (nociceptive, neuropathic, and nociplastic) in any combination acting simultaneously and/or concurrently to cause pain in the same area [16].

2.1 Chronic pain

Acute pain is reduced with the removal of painful stimulus, while chronic pain persists beyond the useful limit of pain signal and often extends beyond 3–6 months after the initial tissue injury has healed. IASP along with World Health Organization (WHO) proposed a new chronic pain classification for the 11th edition of International Classification of Diseases (ICD) as chronic primary pain and chronic secondary pain. Chronic primary pain is defined as the pain in one or more anatomical region that persists or recurs for longer than 3 months; it is associated with significant emotional stress and functional disability, and the symptoms are not better accounted for by another diagnosis. Chronic secondary pain is considered as a symptom of another condition, whereas in chronic primary pain, the pain itself is considered as a disease. These conditions often exhibit central sensitization along with psychological distress and pain catastrophizing. For example, chronic widespread pain, fibromyalgia (CRPS 1) temporomandibular disorder, irritable bowel syndrome, most back pain, and neck pain syndromes [17].

Approximately 30% of world's population suffer from chronic pain, and it is more common in females and in old population [18, 19]. Other risk factors include low socioeconomic status, geographical and cultural factors, and psychological factors such as anxiety and depression. Increase in prevalence may negatively affect the global health status and overall economy of countries [20].

Even though the acute pain or traumatic injury may proceed the development of chronic pain, mechanism behind the chronic pain may differ from those implicated in acute pain [21]. In contrast to acute pain, the diagnosis of chronic pain is not often straightforward. It often involves biomedical and psychological factors. Standardized questionnaires such as LANSS, Pain DETECT, and DN_4 are used to evaluate pain along with functional abilities and emotional distress in chronic pain patients. Detailed history, clinical examination and confirmatory tests are often necessary for presumption of diagnosis. Several studies have reported the successful short-term management of chronic nonmalignant pain with ketamine infusion.

3. Ketamine

3.1 History

Ketamine initially labeled as CI-581 is a phencyclidine derivative prepared by Professor Calvin from Parke Davis. After experimental studies on animals, first human trial was conducted on prisoners on August 3, 1964 by Dr. Domino and Dr. Corssen. They found that ketamine could rapidly produce analgesia with unique state of altered consciousness, which was later named as "dissociative anesthesia" by Toni, wife of Dr. Domino. Because of its sympathomimetic effects and wide safety margin, ketamine was used as war anesthetic to American soldiers in Vietnam war [22].

3.2 Ketamine and its isomers

Ketamine [2-(2-chlorophenyl)-2-(methyalmino)-cyclohexanone ketamine] is a racemic mixture of two optical enantiomers [23]. S(+) ketamine is two times stronger than parent compound and four times stronger than R(−) ketamine. It has also anti-hyperalgesic effects [24]. R(−) ketamine has potent antidepressant effect [25]. Ketamine undergoes demethylation and hydroxylation and metabolites are conjugated and excreted in urine [26]. Nor ketamine is the main metabolite, and it is one-third to one-fifth as potent as its parent compound [27].

Ketamine can be safely administered through several routes with varying bioavailability: intravenous (100%), intramuscular (93%), oral (20%), nasal (50%), and rectal (20%) and even epidural [28]. FDA has approved the use of intranasal S (+) ketamine along with antidepressant in treatment-resistant depression [29].

3.3 N-Methyl-D-aspartate receptor

Discovery of N-methyl-D-aspartate (NMDA) receptor and its noncompetitive inhibition by ketamine has revolutionized the use of ketamine as a potent antihyperalgesic drug in various painful states.

NMDA receptors are important for learning, memory, and synaptic plasticity, and it is also involved in amplification of pain signals and opioid intolerance. Non-competitive antagonism of NMDA receptor by ketamine occurs by two different mechanisms. It decreases the frequency of channel opening by allosteric mechanism and reduces the time spent in the acute open state [30]. Ketamine equally binds to NMDA subtypes 2A to 2D and results in favorable effect compared with other subtype selective NMDA antagonists [31]. It inhibits NMDA-mediated responses both in spinal cord and thalamus. Its non-competitive antagonism allows the endogenous agonist glutamate to continue to binding to these sites. Ketamine at lower concentration blocks closed channels, while higher concentration blocks both open and closed channels [32]. Ketamine can also interact with NMDA receptors present at periphery [33].

3.4 Action on other receptors

Ketamine also binds to μ, κ, and δ receptors; however, this interaction is not responsible for its analgesic effect as their block is not antagonized by naloxone [34–36]. At high doses it also produces local anesthetic effect by blockade of sodium channel receptors [37].

Ketamine's interaction with monoaminergic system is significant with the stimulation of non-adrenergic neurons and inhibition of catecholamine uptake, and it provokes hyperadrenergic condition (norepinephrine, dopamine, serotonin) [38]. R(−) isomer inhibits only neuronal uptake while S(+) isomer inhibits extra neuronal uptake also [22]. Ketamine also has a direct inhibitory effect on nicotinic and muscarinic receptors [39].

Ketamine also acts on other non-NMDA pathways that play significant role in pain and mood regulation including the blockade of Na-K channel (hyperpolarization-activated cyclic nucleotide gated (HCN), activation of high affinity D_2 receptors and L-type voltage-gated calcium channels, facilitation of gamma aminobutyric acid A (GABA-A) signaling, and enhancement of descending inhibitory pathways [32, 40, 41].

Ketamine can also block large conductance Kca channels (BK channel) and preferentially suppresses spinal microglia hyperactivation after nerve injury, which may explain its potent effect against neuropathic pain [42]. Direct inhibition of nitric oxide synthase could also contribute to its analgesic and anesthetic properties [43].

4. Consensus guidelines of ketamine infusion for chronic pain

Over the past few years, the use of ketamine infusion for the management of CP had increased dramatically but with wide variation in dose, monitoring, and selection of patients. This has led to the creation of consensus Guidelines to start ketamine infusion for CP by American Society of Regional Anesthesia and Pain Medicine along with American Academy of Pain Medicine and American Society of Anesthesiologists [44].

1. Ideally treatment session should be carried out in inpatient settings under the care of anesthetists, nurse anesthetists, or emergency physicians experienced in ketamine administration and trained in advanced cardiac life support. Availability of personnel and equipment for resuscitation at all times is mandatory (Grade A recommendation).

2. There is a grade B recommendation for the use of ketamine infusion for (CRPS) and Grade D recommendation against fibromyalgia, ischemic limb pain, migraine headache, and low back pain.

3. There is moderate evidence to support the use of higher dosage of ketamine over longer periods for chronic pain conditions.

4. Prior to infusion of ketamine base line ECG should be considered for individuals at high risk of cardiovascular events. Baseline and post infusion liver function tests should be considered for individuals with baseline liver dysfunction

(alcohol abusers, chronic hepatitis) or for patients who also are expected to receive high doses of ketamine at frequent intervals (Grade C evidence).

5. Ketamine should not be used in patients with poorly controlled cardiovascular disease and poorly controlled psychosis (Grade B). It should be avoided in patients with severe hepatic impairment, but may be administered judiciously with proper monitoring in patients with moderate disease (Grade C). Basic monitoring such as hemodynamic and respiratory parameters, sedation levels using a validated scale same as individuals receiving ketamine in a non-chronic treatment regime irrespective of the dose and route of administration are essential.

6. There is limited direct evidence to support the preemptive use of benzodiazepines and α2 agonists, and there is no evidence to support antidepressant, antihistaminic, or anticholinergic medications prior to start of ketamine infusion at sub-anesthetic doses for CP treatment.

7. There is moderate evidence to support intranasal ketamine for breakthrough pain and low-level evidence for use of oral ketamine and other NMDA antagonists as follow-up therapy after infusion.

8. Given the refractory nature of patients who receive ketamine infusion, the positive outcome could be considered as 30% pain relief or greater in conjunction with patient satisfaction and/or more objective indicators of meaningful benefit such as 12.8% improvement in Oswestry disability index score in a patient with back pain or 20% or greater reduction in opioid use.

5. Ketamine in complex regional pain syndrome

Complex regional pain syndrome (CRPS) was recognized as a distinct pain condition during American civil war in 1864 by Mitchell [45], and it had been described by various names since that time.

It is a chronic pain condition characterized by autonomic and inflammatory features, and it is most often followed by fracture, soft tissue injury, or any surgical procedure, which is often disproportionate in magnitude or duration to the normal course of pain after similar tissue trauma. In 10% of the cases, no inciting cause can be identified [46].

CRPS is subdivided into type 1 and type 2 on the basis of absence or presence of major peripheral nerve injury. The diagnostic features are almost similar in both subtypes although there is difference in etiology, which contributes to uncertainty about the role of neuropathic mechanism [46].

Incidence is found to be greater in females compared with males, and many patients recover within a year, but smaller group may progress to CP. Possible contributing mechanisms include peripheral and central sensitization, autonomic changes and sympathetic afferent coupling, inflammatory and immune alterations in higher centers along with genetic and psychological factors [46]. So effective management of chronic form is often difficult. CRPS causes significant morbidity, and 80% of patients with CRPS are severely disabled [47]. So it needs multidisciplinary care aimed at attaining adequate pain relief, functional restoration, and psychological improvement. Many patients are poorly responsive to regular therapeutic approaches, and ketamine has been shown to decrease pain levels in refractory cases of CRPS in several studies.

5.1 Effect of topical application of ketamine

Various routes of application of ketamine for CRPS had been explained in several studies. Topical application of ketamine in inflammatory and neuropathic pain conditions resulted in reduction of pain by downregulation of NMDA, α-3-amino-3-hydroxy-5-methyl-4-isoxazole propionic acid (AMPA), and kainite receptors [48]. It had been evidenced that application of 10% ketamine cream reduced tactile allodynia and pain scores within 30 min in CRPS patients. Systemic level of ketamine remained undetectable in the study, which suggested the peripherally mediated effect [49]. Another study showed that topical application of ketamine (0.25–1.5%) to the affected areas of limbs relieved pain and swelling in the early dystrophic stage of CRPS 1. This could be due to the local analgesic effect or peripherally mediated NMDA antagonistic effect of ketamine [50, 51].

5.2 Effect of epidural ketamine

Similarly early stage of CRPS was treated with very low dose of epidural ketamine for 10 days in a patient to get prolonged pain relief up to 8 months, which suggested the role of ketamine on NMDA receptors on dorsal horn neurons [52].

5.3 Effect of sub-anesthetic infusion of ketamine

Kirkpatrick in his study found that patients with lower limb CRPS responded better than upper limb CRPS for graded dose of ketamine for 5 days [53]. However, the study on mouse model of CRPS showed that subcutaneous ketamine reduces the nociceptive sensitization better in chronic stage than in acute stage [54].

A randomized controlled trial on 60 CRPS1 patients had shown that duration of disease did not affect the response of ketamine in sub-anesthetic dose. The study group received a continuous sub-anesthetic titrated dose of S(+) ketamine ranging from (1.2–7.2% μg/kg/m) for 4.2 days. S(+) ketamine is 2–4 times more potent than racemic ketamine and required less dose for the same analgesic effects with minimal side effects. Recovery is also quicker with S(+) ketamine due to its rapid clearance compared with R(−) ketamine. Median duration of illness was 7.4 years (0.1–31.9 years). ketamine was found to produce significant reduction in pain scores for 10–12 weeks compared with placebo [55].

Pharmacokinetic-pharmacodynamic study on these patients had shown that concentration of ketamine reduced rapidly on the termination of infusion, but analgesic effect outlasts the treatment period by 10 weeks [56]. This is in contrast with the effect of S (+) ketamine in acute experimental pain where the analgesic effect correlates with its plasma concentration [57]. Prolonged effect of sub-anesthetic dose of ketamine could be due to the long-term desensitization of NMDA receptors in spinal cord or restoration of inhibitory sensory control in the brain [58].

Another low-dose ketamine (0.35 mg/kg/min not to exceed 25 mg/h) study on 19 out patients over 4 h for 10 days showed significant reduction (50%) in affective component of pain. Activity watch scores were significantly reduced. Low dose infusion can be done in outpatient basis and is cost-effective also. However, study was stopped halfway by stressing that higher ketamine dose provided much greater pain relief for prolonged period without any complication [59].

This was also suggested by Goldberg, who studied effect of ketamine infusion at two different doses for two different time periods. In his first study with low-dose ketamine for 10 days in 40 CRPS patients, he found significant reduction in pain scores, with increased ability to initiate movement and tendency to decreased autonomic regulation. A total of 36 patients had pain relief for 2 weeks, while eight patients had pain relief for 12 weeks similar to Sigterman's study [55], but here they have used racemic ketamine [60].

In his second study on 16 patients with moderate-dose ketamine for 5 days, he found significant reduction in pain scores compared with 10 days regime at the end of infusion (2.8 ± 0.65 *vs* 5.4 ± 0.91). Pain relief experienced on second day of infusion continued to increase over the fifth day of infusion and correlated well with the maximum plasma levels of ketamine and nor-ketamine. Author also suggested the possible role of downstream metabolites in prolonged analgesia. Similar to Sigterman's study, the pain relief extended up to 12 weeks, although in few cases it prolonged up to 6 m. Significant reduction of pain was reported in 10 out of 16 patients [61]. Another study demonstrated longer duration of pain relief after second treatment of ketamine infusion than the first one in CRPS patients [62]. The sustained effect could also be due to antagonistic effect of ketamine on other receptors. The presence and therapeutic significance of single nucleotide polymorphism of the NMDA receptor cannot be overlooked and opens new route for research [61].

5.4 Ketamine coma

In refractory and generalized CRPS patients, the anesthetic dose of ketamine in range of (3–7 mg/kg/h) produced significant reduction in pain. As ketamine's analgesic potency and duration of clinical effect are dose-dependent, author had evaluated anesthetic dose of ketamine in these refractory patients along with midazolam and clonidine. Significant pain relief was observed at 1, 3, 5, 6 months. Quality of life and ability to perform work are significantly improved in many of the patients at 3 and 6 months. Ten out of 20 patients were completely pain free for 5–11 years, and they had not taken any pain medication further [63]. On the first day of infusion, mobilization of neurogenic edema fluid occurs, later on third day, venous tone returns to the affected extremity [64]. Few patients experienced muscle weakness and weight loss. No neurocognitive adverse effects were observed at 6 weeks after anesthetic infusion of ketamine in another study. It could also be due to reduction in pain and pain medicine uptake [65]. However, in 20% of patients, nosocomial, urinary, and pulmonary complications have occurred. No long-term psychiatric impairments have been seen in any of these 20 CRPS patients [63].

6. Effect of ketamine in other pain conditions

Although there is a grade D recommendation for the use of ketamine in fibromyalgia, cancer pain, ischemic pain, and migraine headache [44], various studies have demonstrated its beneficial effects in alleviating pain in fibromyalgia, phantom limb pain, ischemic limb pain, and headache [66–69].

6.1 Effect of ketamine in fibromyalgia

Fibromyalgia, a functional pain syndrome, is characterized by widespread musculoskeletal pain, fatigue, sleep abnormality, and somatic hyperalgesia. Mean estimated global prevalence of fibromyalgia is 2.7% with female preponderance. Patients often experience pain from head to toe; cognitive dysfunction and memory deficit are common severe symptoms of fibromyalgia. Autonomic disturbances manifest in all areas of body, which correlate with severity of fibromyalgia. It is associated with many of the features of central sensitization including hyperalgesia, allodynia, and temporal summation [70].

Diffuse pain processing in the brain is altered, and it correlates with fibromyalgic nociplastic pain. Increased substance P in cerebrospinal fluid, decreased μ opioid receptor availability along with high level of opioids in cerebrospinal fluid, and reduced levels of noradrenaline, serotonin neurotransmitters are seen compared with healthy individuals [71–73]. It is often difficult to identify the cause of the nociplastic alteration as it may not be caused by single etiology. Evaluation should be holistic including all symptoms experienced by the patients along with aggravating factors and functional capabilities of the patients. Integrated multidisciplinary approach including patient education, fitness, medical management, and psychotherapy is often needed [70].

Sorenson had found that ketamine produced significant reduction in pain scores and increased endurance in fibromyalgia patients compared with morphine and lidocaine [66]. Graven-Nielsen had also demonstrated that ketamine reduced referred pain, temporal summation, and muscular hyperalgesia in fibromyalgia patients [11]. However, Noppers had reported only short-term benefits after (0.5 mg/kg) of S(+) ketamine corresponding to its plasma concentration in 24 fibromyalgia patients. It is in contrast with the prolonged benefits of long-term infusion of ketamine in CRPS patients, which suggested that duration of infusion is critical rather than the dose of ketamine [74]. Other studies had also proved that long-term infusion produces cascade of molecular changes both at spinal and supraspinal sites [58].

This large inter-patient variability in response to ketamine infusion may occur from a dosing effect, duration of treatment, individual differences in metabolic degradation, genetic variation of NMDA receptors [64]. This variability in response was also reported by Rabben in trigeminal neuropathic patients with 0.4 mg/kg of intramuscular ketamine [75]. Another possibility of varied response in patients could be heterogeneity in pathophysiology of fibromyalgia [71]. Guedj had demonstrated distinct brain function single- photo emission computed tomography (SPECT) pattern in responders and non-responders to ketamine [76].

6.2 Headache

In refractory cases of migraine, titrated doses of ketamine had reduced pain severity in acute states [69]. A randomized controlled trial has reported that 25 mg of intranasal ketamine reduced the severity of aura in migraine patients [77]. Combination of ketamine (0.5 mg/kg in 2 h) and magnesium sulfate (3000 mg in 30 min) had demonstrated immediate pain relief in two cluster headache patients. It also produced reduction in pain intensity and attack frequency for up to 6 weeks along with reduction in suicidal tendencies [78]. Previous studies on effectiveness of memantine against refractory migraine had further suggested the role of NMDA antagonists against headache [79].

6.3 Visceral pain syndrome

Preclinical studies on ketamine in rats have shown to reverse sensitization in visceral pain syndromes, which provides a good rationale for using ketamine in irritable bowel syndrome [80, 81]. Non-responding refractory pancreatic pain in a pediatric patient has shown reduction in pain scores and morphine requirement after sub-anesthetic infusion of ketamine [82].

6.4 Ischemic limb pain

Randomized controlled trial on 35 patients with ischemic limb pain had shown that combination of low dose ketamine and opioid produced significant pain relief compared with opioid alone [68]. Animal studies had shown that ischemia can produce hyperalgesia and allodynia, hence the addition of low-dose ketamine along with opioid produced enhanced analgesic effect in these patients [68]. Ketamine also tends to reduce the pain in vasoocclusive crisis in sickle cell anemia patients [83].

7. Adverse effects and adjuvants

Ketamine is associated with adverse psychomimetic, cardiovascular, and gastrointestinal effects resulting from its action on various receptors [84–86]. Double-blinded randomized controlled trial using midazolam and clonidine as premedication along with low-dose ketamine up to 5.2 μg/kg/min showed no psychomimetic and cardiovascular adverse effects [59]. However, another study calculated number needed to harm; "harm" defined as ketamine-induced psychomimetic adverse effects; where author found that number needed to harm for hallucination to be 21 when ketamine was used alone and number increased to 35 when used in combination with benzodiazepines suggesting that adjuvant may lessen but not eliminate psychomimetic effects [87]. Research is being conducted to develop wearable device to deliver low, non-dissociative dose of ketamine. Studies on animals and ketamine abusers raised the concern of hepatotoxicity and cystitis on prolonged use [88]. In humans, the incidence of hepatotoxicity and cystitis found to be increased with higher and frequent doses of ketamine; however, the liver enzyme levels were back to normal after withdrawing the drug [63].

8. Conclusion

Medicine is an art as well as science, and the evidence-based medicine not only relies on scientific literature but also the judgment of clinician and patient preferences and satisfaction. The use of ketamine infusion for chronic pain is an evolving treatment that shows great promise. Though the consensus guidelines for intravenous use of ketamine for chronic pain advocate the use of ketamine only for complex regional pain syndrome, various other clinical studies suggested its role in other chronic refractory painful conditions. Effect of ketamine on various receptors not only affects the sensory component but also the affective motivational component of pain. It decreases pain scores along with the reduction of analgesic medications, which further improves well-being and the quality of life. However, continuous refinement of treatment protocol is essential along with emphasis on both long-term safety and effectiveness.

Author details

Subbulakshmi Sundaram[1*] and Ashok Swaminathan Govindarajan[2]

1 Anaesthesiology, Rajah Muthiah Medical College and Hospital, Annamalai University, Annamalainagar, Tamil Nadu, India

2 Plastic Surgery, Rajah Muthiah Medical College and Hospital, Annamalai University, Annamalainagar, Tamil Nadu, India

*Address all correspondence to: subbulakshmisundaram76@gmail.com

References

[1] Cohen SP, Vase L, Hooten WM. Chronic pain: An update on burden, best practices, and new advances. The Lancet. 2021;**397**(10289):2082-2097

[2] Elzahaf RA, Tashani OA, Unsworth BA, Johnson MI. The prevalence of chronic pain with an analysis of countries with a human development index less than 0.9: A systematic review without meta-analysis. Current Medical Research and Opinion. 2012;**28**(7):1221-1229

[3] Souza JB, Grossmann E, Perissinotti DM, Oliveira Junior JO, Fonseca PR, Posso ID. Prevalence of chronic pain, treatments, perception, and interference on life activities: Brazilian population-based survey. Pain Research and Management. 2017;**2017**

[4] Taylor AM, Phillips K, Taylor JO, Singh JA, Conaghan PG, Choy EH, et al. Is chronic pain a disease in its own right? Discussions from a pre-OMERACT 2014 workshop on chronic pain. Journal of Rheumatology. 2015;**42**(10):1947-1953

[5] Gaskin DJ, Richard P. The economic costs of pain in the United States. The Journal of Pain. 2012;**13**(8):715-724

[6] Vos T, Barber RM, Bell B, Bertozzi-Villa A, Biryukov S, Bolliger I, et al. Global, regional, and national incidence, prevalence, and years lived with disability for 301 acute and chronic diseases and injuries in 188 countries, 1990-2013: A systematic analysis for the global burden of disease study 2013. The Lancet. 2015;**386**(9995):743-800

[7] Chaparro LE, Wiffen PJ, Moore RA, Gilron I. Combination pharmacotherapy for the treatment of neuropathic pain in adults. Cochrane Database of Systematic Reviews. 2012;7:CD008943

[8] Finnerup NB, Attal N, Haroutounian S, McNicol E, Baron R, Dworkin RH, et al. Pharmacotherapy for neuropathic pain in adults: A systematic review and meta-analysis. The Lancet Neurology. 2015;**14**(2): 162-173

[9] Kosek E, Cohen M, Baron R, Gebhart GF, Mico JA, Rice AS, et al. Do we need a third mechanistic descriptor for chronic pain states? Pain. 2016; **157**(7):1382-1386

[10] Cohen KL, Harris S. Efficacy and safety of nonsteroidal anti-inflammatory drugs in the therapy of diabetic neuropathy. Archives of Internal Medicine. 1987;**147**(8): 1442-1444

[11] Graven-Nielsen T, Kendall SA, Henriksson KG, Bengtsson M, Sörensen J, Johnson A, et al. Ketamine reduces muscle pain, temporal summation, and referred pain in fibromyalgia patients. Pain. 2000; **85**(3):483-491

[12] Le Roy C, Laboureyras E, Gavello-Baudy S, Chateauraynaud J, Laulin JP, Simonnet G. Endogenous opioids released during non-nociceptive environmental stress induce latent pain sensitization Via a NMDA-dependent process. The Journal of Pain. 2011; **12**(10):1069-1079

[13] Schwenk ES, Dayan AC, Rangavajjula A, Torjman MC, Hernandez MG, Lauritsen CG, et al. Ketamine for refractory headache: A retrospective analysis. Regional Anesthesia & Pain Medicine. 2018; **43**(8):875-879

[14] Orhurhu V, Orhurhu MS, Bhatia A, Cohen SP. Ketamine infusions for chronic pain: A systematic review and meta-analysis of randomized controlled trials. Anesthesia & Analgesia. 2019; **129**(1):241-254

[15] Trouvin AP, Perrot S. New concepts of pain. Best Practice & Research Clinical Rheumatology. 2019;**33**(3): 101415

[16] Freynhagen R, Parada HA, Calderon-Ospina CA, Chen J, RakhmawatiEmril D, Fernández-Villacorta FJ, et al. Current understanding of the mixed pain concept: A brief narrative review. Current Medical Research and Opinion. 2019;**35**(6):1011-1018

[17] Nicholas M, Vlaeyen JW, Rief W, Barke A, Aziz Q, Benoliel R, et al. The IASP classification of chronic pain for ICD-11: Chronic primary pain. Pain. 2019;**160**(1):28-37

[18] Saxena AK, Jain PN, Bhatnagar S. The prevalence of chronic pain among adults in India. Indian Journal of Palliative Care. 2018;**24**(4):472-477

[19] Greenspan JD, Craft RM, LeResche L, Arendt-Nielsen L, Berkley KJ, Fillingim RB, et al. Studying sex and gender differences in pain and analgesia: A consensus report. Pain. 2007;**132**:S26-S45

[20] Mills SE, Nicolson KP, Smith BH. Chronic pain: A review of its epidemiology and associated factors in population-based studies. British Journal of Anaesthesia. 2019;**123**(2): e273-e283

[21] Voscopoulos C, Lema M. When does acute pain become chronic? British Journal of Anaesthesia. 2010;**105** (Suppl. 1):i69-i85

[22] Mion G. History of anaesthesia: The ketamine story–past, present and future. European Journal of Anaesthesiology (EJA). 2017;**34**(9): 571-575

[23] Adams JD, Castagnoli N, Trevor AJ. Quantitative analysis of ketamine enantiomers. In: Proceedings of the Western Pharmacology Society. Vol. 21. 1978. pp. 471-472

[24] Lee SK. The use of ketamine for perioperative pain management. Korean Journal of Anesthesiology. 2012;**63**(1): 1-2

[25] Hashimoto K. The R-stereoisomer of ketamine as an alternative for ketamine for treatment-resistant major depression. Clinical Psycho pharmacology and Neuroscience. 2014;**12**(1):72-73

[26] Clements JA, Nimmo WS, Grant IS. Bioavailability, pharmacokinetics, and analgesic activity of ketamine in humans. Journal of Pharmaceutical Sciences. 1982;**71**(5):539-542

[27] Kurdi MS, Theerth KA, Deva RS. Ketamine: Current applications in anesthesia, pain, and critical care. Anesthesia, Essays and Researches. 2014;**8**(3):283-290

[28] Pai A, Heining M. Ketamine. Continuing Education in Anaesthesia, Critical Care & Pain. 2007;**7**(2):59-63

[29] Kryst J, Kawalec P, Pilc A. Efficacy and safety of intranasal esketamine for the treatment of major depressive disorder. Expert Opinion on Pharmacotherapy. 2020;**21**(1):9-20

[30] Orser BA, Pennefather PS, MacDonald JF. Multiple mechanisms of ketamine blockade of N-methyl-D-aspartate receptors. The Journal of the American Society of Anesthesiologists. 1997;**86**(4):903-917

[31] Collins S, Sigtermans MJ, Dahan A, Zuurmond WW, Perez RS. NMDA receptor antagonists for the treatment of neuropathic pain. Pain Medicine. 2010;**11**(11):1726-1742

[32] Vadivelu N, Schermer E, Kodumudi V, Belani K, Urman RD, Kaye AD. Role of ketamine for analgesia

in adults and children. Journal of Anaesthesiology, Clinical Pharmacology. 2016;**32**(3):298-306

[33] Culp C, Kim HK, Abdi S. Ketamine use for cancer and chronic pain management. Frontiers in Pharmacology. 2021;**11**:2360

[34] Smith DJ, Perrotti JM, Mansell AL, Monroe PJ. Ketamine analgesia is not related to an opiate action in the periaqueductal gray region of the rat brain. Pain. 1985;**21**(3):253-265

[35] Sleigh J, Harvey M, Voss L, Denny B. Ketamine–More mechanisms of action than just NMDA blockade. Trends in Anaesthesia and Critical Care. 2014; **4**(2-3):76-81

[36] Bansinath M, Warner W, Tang CK, Turndorf H, Puig MM. On the mechanism of the interaction of ketamine and halothane in vitro. General Pharmacology. 1992;**23**(6): 1183-1187

[37] Frenkel C, Urban BW. Molecular actions of racemic ketamine on human CNS sodium channels. British Journal of Anaesthesia. 1992;**69**(3):292-297

[38] Koizuka S, Obata H, Sasaki M, Saito S, Goto F. Systemic ketamine inhibits hypersensitivity after surgery via descending inhibitory pathways in rats. Canadian Journal of Anesthesia. 2005;**52**(5):498-505

[39] Durieux ME. Inhibition by ketamine of muscarinic acetylcholine receptor function. Anesthesia & Analgesia. 1995;**81**(1):57-62

[40] Hayashi Y, Kawaji K, Sun L, Zhang X, Koyano K, Yokoyama T, et al. Microglial Ca^{2+}-activated K^{+} channels are possible molecular targets for the analgesic effects of S-ketamine on neuropathic pain. Journal of Neuroscience. 2011;**31**(48):17370-17382

[41] Niesters M, Aarts LP, Sarton E, Dahan A. Influence of ketamine and morphine on descending pain modulation in chronic pain patients: A randomized placebo-controlled cross-over proof-of-concept study. British Journal of Anaesthesia. 2013;**110**(6): 1010-1016

[42] Chen X, Shu S, Bayliss DA. HCN1 channel subunits are a molecular substrate for hypnotic actions of ketamine. Journal of Neuroscience. 2009;**29**(3):600-609

[43] Gordh T, Karlsten R, Kristensen J. Intervention with spinal NMDA, adenosine, and NO systems for pain modulation. Annals of Medicine. 1995;**27**(2):229-234

[44] Cohen SP, Bhatia A, Buvanendran A, Schwenk ES, Wasan AD, Hurley RW, et al. Consensus guidelines on the use of intravenous ketamine infusions for chronic pain from the American Society of Regional Anesthesia and Pain Medicine, the American Academy of Pain Medicine, and the American Society of Anesthesiologists. Regional Anesthesia & Pain Medicine. 2018;**43**(5):521-546

[45] Lau FH, Chung KC. Silas Weir Mitchell, MD: The physician who discovered causalgia. The Journal of Hand Surgery. 2004;**29**(2):181-187

[46] Bruehl S, Warner DS. An update on the pathophysiology of complex regional pain syndrome. The Journal of the American Society of Anesthesiologists. 2010;**113**(3):713-725

[47] Zhao J, Wang Y, Wang D. The effect of ketamine infusion in the treatment of complex regional pain syndrome: A systemic review and meta-analysis. Current Pain and Headache Reports. 2018;**22**(2):1-8

[48] Coggeshall RE, Carlton SM. Ultrastructural analysis of NMDA,

AMPA, and kainate receptors on unmyelinated and myelinated axons in the periphery. Journal of Comparative Neurology. 1998;**391**(1):78-86

[49] Finch PM, Knudsen L, Drummond PD. Reduction of allodynia in patients with complex regional pain syndrome: A double-blind placebo-controlled trial of topical ketamine. Pain. 2009;**146**(1-2):18-25

[50] Ushida T, Tani T, Kanbara T, Zinchuk VS, Kawasaki M, Yamamoto H. Analgesic effects of ketamine ointment in patients with complex regional pain syndrome type 1. Regional Anesthesia & Pain Medicine. 2002;**27**(5):524-528

[51] Wagner LE, Gingrich KJ, Kulli JC, Yang J. Ketamine blockade of voltage-gated sodium channels: Evidence for a shared receptor site with local anesthetics. The Journal of the American Society of Anesthesiologists. 2001;**95**(6):1406-1413

[52] Takahashi H, Miyazaki M, Nanbu T, Yanagida H, Morita S. The NMDA-receptor antagonist ketamine abolishes neuropathic pain after epidural administration in a clinical case. Pain. 1998;**75**(2-3):391-394

[53] Kirkpatrick AF, Saghafi A, Yang K, Qiu P, Alexander J, Bavry E, et al. Optimizing the treatment of CRPS with ketamine. The Clinical Journal of Pain. 2020;**36**(7):516-523

[54] Tajerian M, Leu D, Yang P, Huang TT, Kingery WS, Clark JD. Differential efficacy of ketamine in the acute versus chronic stages of complex regional pain syndrome in mice. Anesthesiology. 2015;**123**(6): 1435-1447

[55] Sigtermans MJ, Van Hilten JJ, Bauer MC, Arbous MS, Marinus J, Sarton EY, Dahan A. Ketamine produces effective and long-term pain relief in patients with Complex Regional Pain Syndrome Type 1. Pain. 2009;**145**(3):304-311

[56] Dahan A, Olofsen E, Sigtermans M, Noppers I, Niesters M, Aarts L, et al. Population pharmacokinetic–pharmacodynamic modeling of ketamine-induced pain relief of chronic pain. European Journal of Pain. 2011; **15**(3):258-267

[57] Sigtermans M, Noppers I, Sarton E, Bauer M, Mooren R, Olofsen E, Dahan A. An observational study on the effect of S (+)-ketamine on chronic pain versus experimental acute pain in Complex Regional Pain Syndrome type 1 patients. European Journal of Pain. 2010;**14**(3):302-307

[58] Borsook D. Ketamine and chronic pain—Going the distance. Pain. 2009;**145**(3):271-272

[59] Schwartzman RJ, Alexander GM, Grothusen JR, Paylor T, Reichenberger E, Perreault M. Outpatient intravenous ketamine for the treatment of complex regional pain syndrome: A double-blind placebo controlled study. Pain. 2009;**147**(1-3): 107-115

[60] Goldberg ME, Domsky R, Scaringe D, et al. Multi-day low dose ketamine infusion for the treatment of complex regional pain syndrome. Pain Physician. 2005;**8**(2):175-179

[61] Goldberg ME, Torjman MC, Schwartzman RJ, Mager DE, Wainer I. Pharmacodynamic profiles of ketamine (R−) and (S+) with five day inpatient infusion for the treatment of complex regional pain syndrome. Pain Physician. 2010;**13**(4):379

[62] Correll GE, Maleki J, Gracely EJ, Muir JJ, Harbut RE. Subanesthetic ketamine infusion therapy: A retrospective analysis of a novel therapeutic approach to complex

regional pain syndrome. Pain Medicine. 2004;**5**(3):263-275

[63] Kiefer RT, Rohr P, Ploppa A, Dieterich HJ, Grothusen J, Koffler S, et al. Efficacy of ketamine in anesthetic dosage for the treatment of refractory complex regional pain syndrome: An open-label phase II study. Pain Medicine. 2008;**9**(8):1173-1201

[64] Schwartzman RJ, Alexander GM, Grothusen JR. The use of ketamine in complex regional pain syndrome: Possible mechanisms. Expert Review of Neurotherapeutics. 2011;**11**(5):719-734

[65] Koffler SP, Hampstead BM, Irani F, Tinker J, Kiefer RT, Rohr P, et al. The neurocognitive effects of 5 day anesthetic ketamine for the treatment of refractory complex regional pain syndrome. Archives of Clinical Neuropsychology. 2007;**22**(6):719-729

[66] Sörensen J, Bengtsso A, Bäckman E, Henriksson KG, Bengtsson M. Pain analysis in patients with fibromyalgia: Effects of intravenous morphine, lidocaine, and ketamine. Scandinavian Journal of Rheumatology. 1995;**24**(6): 360-365

[67] Stannard CF, Porter GE. Ketamine hydrochloride in the treatment of phantom limb pain. Pain. 1993;**54**(2): 227-230

[68] Mitchell AC, Fallon MT. A single infusion of intravenous ketamine improves pain relief in patients with critical limb ischaemia: Results of a double blind randomised controlled trial. Pain. 2002;**97**(3):275-281

[69] Pomeroy JL, Marmura MJ, Nahas SJ, Viscusi ER. Ketamine infusions for treatment refractory headache. Headache: The Journal of Head and Face Pain. 2017;**57**(2):276-282

[70] Sarzi-Puttini P, Giorgi V, Marotto D, Atzeni F. Fibromyalgia: An update on clinical characteristics, aetiopathogenesis and treatment. Nature Reviews Rheumatology. 2020;**16**(11):645-660

[71] Russell IJ, Orr MD, Littman B, Vipraio GA, Alboukrek D, Michalek JE, et al. Elevated cerebrospinal fluid levels of substance P in patients with the fibromyalgia syndrome. Arthritis & Rheumatism: Official Journal of the American College of Rheumatology. 1994;**37**(11):1593-1601

[72] Harris RE, Clauw DJ, Scott DJ, McLean SA, Gracely RH, Zubieta JK. Decreased central μ-opioid receptor availability in fibromyalgia. Journal of Neuroscience. 2007;**27**(37): 10000-10006

[73] Russell IJ, Vaeroy H, Javors M, Nyberg F. Cerebrospinal fluid biogenic amine metabolites in fibromyalgia/ fibrositis syndrome and rheumatoid arthritis. Arthritis & Rheumatism: Official Journal of the American College of Rheumatology. 1992;**35**(5):550-556

[74] Noppers I, Niesters M, Swartjes M, Bauer M, Aarts L, Geleijnse N, et al. Absence of long-term analgesic effect from a short-term S-ketamine infusion on fibromyalgia pain: A randomized, prospective, double blind, active placebo-controlled trial. European Journal of Pain. 2011;**15**(9):942-949

[75] Rabben T, Øye I. Interindividual differences in the analgesic response to ketamine in chronic orofacial pain. European Journal of Pain. 2001;**5**(3): 233-240

[76] Guedj E, Cammilleri S, Colavolpe C, Taieb D, de Laforte C, Niboyet J, et al. Predictive value of brain perfusion SPECT for ketamine response in hyperalgesic fibromyalgia. European Journal of Nuclear Medicine and Molecular Imaging. 2007;**34**(8): 1274-1279

[77] Afridi SK, Giffin NJ, Kaube H, Goadsby PJ. A randomized controlled trial of intranasal ketamine in migraine with prolonged aura. Neurology. 2013;**80**(7):642-647

[78] Moisset X, Clavelou P, Lauxerois M, Dallel R, Picard P. Ketamine infusion combined with magnesium as a therapy for intractable chronic cluster headache: Report of two cases. Headache: The Journal of Head and Face Pain. 2017; **57**(8):1261-1264

[79] Bigal M, Rapoport A, Sheftell F, Tepper D, Tepper S. Memantine in the preventive treatment of refractory migraine. Headache: The Journal of Head and Face Pain. 2008;**48**(9):1337-1342

[80] Olivar T, Laird JM. Differential effects of N-methyl-D-aspartate receptor blockade on nociceptive somatic and visceral reflexes. Pain. 1999;**79**(1):67-73

[81] Chizh BA. Low dose ketamine: A therapeutic and research tool to explore N-methyl-D-aspartate (NMDA) receptor-mediated plasticity in pain pathways. Journal of Psycho pharmacology. 2007;**21**(3):259-271

[82] Mulder DJ, Sherlock ME, Lysecki DL. NMDA-receptor antagonism in pediatric pancreatitis: Use of ketamine and methadone in a teenager with refractory pain. Journal of Pediatric Gastroenterology and Nutrition. 2018;**66**(5):e134-e136

[83] Uprety D, Baber A, Foy M. Ketamine infusion for sickle cell pain crisis refractory to opioids: A case report and review of literature. Annals of Hematology. 2014;**93**(5):769-771

[84] Laskowski K, Stirling A, Mckay WP, Lim HJ. A systematic review of intravenous ketamine for postoperative analgesia. Canadian Journal of Anesthesia/Journal canadiend'anesthésie. 2011;**58**(10): 911-923

[85] Waxman K, Shoemaker WC, Lippmann M. Cardiovascular effects of anesthetic induction with ketamine. Anesthesia and Analgesia. 1980;**59**(5): 355-358

[86] Niesters M, Martini C, Dahan A. Ketamine for chronic pain: Risks and benefits. British Journal of Clinical Pharmacology. 2014;**77**(2):357-367

[87] Elia N, Tramèr MR. Ketamine and postoperative pain—A quantitative systematic review of randomised trials. Pain. 2005;**113**(1-2):61-70

[88] Wai MS, Chan WM, Zhang AQ, Wu Y, Yew DT. Long-term ketamine and ketamine plus alcohol treatments produced damages in liver and kidney. Human & Experimental Toxicology. 2012;**31**(9):877-886

Section 4

Non-Anaesthetic Use of Ketamine

Chapter 9

Perspective Chapter: NMDA Treatments for CNS Disorders

Chih-Hung Lin, Po-Chang Shih and Guochuan Emil Tsai

Abstract

The N-methyl-D-aspartate receptor (NMDAR), a glutamate-gated ion channel, mediates various physiological functions, such as synaptic plasticity, learning, and memory. Any homeostatic dysregulation of NMDAR may cause central nervous system (CNS) disorders, such as Alzheimer's disease, depression, and schizophrenia. The involvement of NMDA dysfunction promotes advanced research on developing NMDAR pharmaceutics for treating CNS disorders. NMDAR enhancers, by direct or indirect potentiating NMDAR functions, have been used to recover NMDAR functions for treating schizophrenia. Interestingly, NMDAR blockers, by direct or indirect inhibiting NMDAR functions, have also been utilized for CNS disorders, such as Alzheimer's disease and depression. In this chapter, the current strategy of NMDAR modulation for CNS disorders are elaborated on to discern underlying neurophysiological mechanisms of how homeostatic regulation of NMDAR plays a vital role in the normal and pathological states, respectively.

Keywords: NMDAR, CNS pathology, agonism, antagonism, homeostasis

1. Introduction

Glutamatergic signaling plays a critical role in the CNS function under physiological and pathophysiological states via two major types of receptor: ionotropic glutamate receptors (iGluRs) and metabotropic glutamate receptors (mGluRs) [1]. mGluRs consist of three subgroups (Group I-III), while iGluRs comprise four subgroups (AMPARs, KARs, GluδS, and NMDARs). Among all GluRs, NMDARs play a crucial role in brain development, mediating the physiological functions, such as synaptic plasticity, learning, and memory. NMDARs are voltage-dependent glutamate- or aspartate-gated cation channels with two prerequisites for channel opening: 1) depolarization-induced unblockage of magnesium ions; 2). concomitant binding of glutamate (or aspartate) and glycine (or D-serine). When the NMDARs are either aberrantly enhanced or encumbered opening, various CNS symptoms/disorders may develop, such as depression, psychosis, and cognitive impairment.

CNS disorders still loom over many people's health with limited effective treatment. The role of NMDARs playing in CNS disorders has been gaining attention owing to the finding of ketamine as an antidepressant [2]. This new therapeutic mechanism promotes NMDARs as an emerging therapeutic target. Ketamine, a NMDAR antagonist, exerts rapid and robust antidepressant effects in depressed patients [3]. On the contrary, a NMDAR agonist, D-serine, could alleviate schizophrenic and depressive symptoms in the clinical trial [4]. These contrary modulations on NMDAR further support the importance of NMDAR homeostasis leveraged by NMDAR modulators [5].

NMDAR modulators, with positive or negative modulation, have been designed to alleviate various symptoms of CNS through distinct mechanisms. Positive NMDAR modulators elevate NMDARs via direct and indirect approaches. Direct NMDAR enhancers fit into the glutamate site or glycine site of NMDARs, or they bind the allosteric pockets of the glutamate/glycine sites. In contrast to direct enhancement, several NMDAR enhancers improve NMDAR functions by modulating indirect pathways, for example, by inhibiting glycine transporter or D-amino acid oxidase (DAAO). Negative NMDAR modulators, on the contrary, work as competitive antagonists to directly occupy the glycine site, or bind an allosteric site (known as non-competitive antagonists), or block NMDAR channel pore (known as uncompetitive antagonists) [6]. All above modulators have shown potential for clinical use in CNS disorders but without one-size-fits-all approach.

2. CNS disorders alleviated by NMDAR modulators

2.1 Neurological disorders

The excitatory neurotransmission of mammalian CNS is largely dictated through glutamate and its receptors, particularly NMDAR. Because its critical roles in mediating synaptic plasticity related to learning and memory formation, the dysfunction of the NMDAR-based signaling is implicated in the neurological disorders such as Alzheimer's disease (AD), Parkinson's disease (PD), and Huntington's disease (HD), as described below.

2.1.1 Alzheimer's disease

AD is the most common cause of dementia to induce not only cognitive impairments in memory and thought, but also behavioral and psychiatric symptoms [7]. Current understanding to AD relies on two main histopathological abnormalities: (1) amyloid plaques composed of amyloid ß (Aß) peptides cleaved from amyloid precursor proteins in the brain tissue, and (2) the formation of intraneuronal neurofibrillary tangles due to phosphorylated and aggregated tau proteins. Although Aß and tau serve as the most discussed mechanisms through which cause AD, no effective treatment was developed successfully. Coincidently, the neurotransmitter systems, including cholinergic, adrenergic and glutamatergic pathways are considered critical in AD progression and development [8]. In this chapter, we focus on the discussion of how NMDAR involves in AD.

NMDAR is the major regulator associated with long-term synaptic plasticity. Studies have reported that AD brains contain neurotoxins consisted of soluble Aß oligomers. The binding of Aß 42 oligomers to forebrain synaptosomes is associated with post-synaptic density complexes containing NMDAR subunits NR1 and NR2B [9]. Consistently, Aß oligomers were found to ablate long-term potentiation in hippocampal brain slices and the cortices of AD brains via overactivating extrasynaptic NMDAR containing NR2B [10]. The over-activation of extrasynaptic NMDAR linked to neurodegeneration in AD has also been supported by the pharmacotherapeutic use of NMDAR inhibitor memantine [11].

Indirect modulation of NMDAR via glutamate release or glycine transporter-1 (GlyT1) are considered feasible for AD. An escalated stimulation via glutamatergic signaling causes glutamate excitotoxicity that results in damaged nerve cells, and such neuronal toxicity is coined "excitotoxicity". In AD, glutamate uptake and recycling systems are severely impaired [12], which therefore increases glutamate availability, resulting in excessive NMDAR stimulation. Additionally, Aß peptides may increase glutamate availability by weakening glutamate uptake and recycling systems [13] that may contribute to AD pathology. On the other hand, at glutamatergic synapses, glycine is transported by GlyT1, a Na^{+}/Cl^{-}-dependent carrier protein playing a major role in maintaining glycine concentration below saturation at postsynaptic NMDAR, sculpturing GlyT1 as an intriguing target for NMDAR modulation.

Overall, direct and indirect NMDAR inhibition strategies through the discussed mechanisms to attenuate the overactivation of NMDA function have shown rationale for developing medicine for late-stage AD to attenuate the neuronal death.

2.1.2 Parkinson's disease

PD, the second most common neurodegenerative disease, is a progressive disorder with symptoms of onset gradually, motor disturbances and cognitive impairment. Due to the rapidly aging population worldwide, PD also receives increasing attention from communities [14]. The pathophysiology of PD is due to the degeneration of pigmented dopaminergic neurons, resulting in functional changes to the circuitry of basal ganglia nuclei. Accordingly, levo-dopa, a precursor of dopamine, and dopamine receptor agonists have been serving as the standard treatments for PD. However, long-term use of these standard therapies contribute to the loss of efficacy and development of disfiguring motor complications [15]. Novel PD treatments based on different mechanism is long awaited.

Regulating glutamatergic receptors, particularly NMDAR, has been found to be altered in the basal ganglia of PD where NMDAR is widely expressed. Specifically, NR2B-containing NMDARs may significantly influence the PD pathology while NR2B was found to be substantially distributed in the striatum and other basal ganglia areas. An increasing body of literature has reported that not only experimental PD models but also PD patients present substantially elevated NMDA-sensitive glutamate binding in the striatum [16]. In levo-dopa-treated rodent and primate, GluN2A and the ratio of GluN2A/GluN2B are increased. The findings are also reported in PD patients [17], suggesting that attenuated NMDAR activity may help halt the progression of PD.

Alternately, reshaping synaptic connections for PD patients via brief activation of NMDAR can increase axonal growth rate and axonal branching. The brief NMDAR activation can be achieved through inhibiting GlyT1 to increase levels of extracellular glycine [18]. In addition, activating NMDAR via weak NMDAR glycine binding agonists can also achieve similar effects. This hypothesis remains to be investigated.

2.1.3 Huntington's disease

HD is a progressive CNS disorder due to a single defective gene on chromosome 4 that encodes the protein huntingtin. The defect is hereditary and will eventually develop symptoms in lifetime. At the beginning of symptom onset, patients often have subtle abnormalities in mood, usually followed by a lack of coordination and unsteady gaits [19].

Since the altered function of huntingtin induces neuronal cell death, research focuses on mechanisms towards regulation of such cell death. It has been revealed that the formation of the nuclear protein aggregates, oxidative stress, and mitochondrial dysfunction are associated with neuronal cell death in HD [20]. NMDARs have also been found to regulate neuronal cell death of HD, and by modulating

NMDAR activity, psychotic symptoms of HD due to low NMDA function can be alleviated simultaneously. In this chapter, we focus on the discussion of NMDAR in HD.

Animal studies have shown that neuroexcitatory agonists kainic or quinolinic acids can induce lesions similar to those in HD, indicating that excitotoxicity from NMDAR over-activation could contribute to the progression of the disease [21]. Post-synaptic density protein 95 (PSD-95), a scaffolding protein, can bind huntingtin and the NR2 subunit of NMDAR. At the molecular level in HD, the presence of abnormal huntingtin protein causes the interruption of PSD-95 binding onto NMDAR. The unbinding of PSD-95 results in excitotoxicity and neuronal cell death consistent with HD [20]. Therefore, among the known mechanisms inducing HD progression, NMDAR remains a primary target to develop therapeutic intervention.

2.2 Psychiatric disorders

Existing high concentration of post-synaptic NMDAR in limbic structures [22] highlights the homeostasis of NMDAR activity as be of uttermost significance in behavioral regulation of the brain. The dysfunction of NMDAR can cause a variety of psychiatric disorders such as depression, schizophrenia, bipolar disorder (BD), and anxiety disorder [23].

2.2.1 Depression

Depression is a chronic mental disorder characterized by persistent low mood, loss of interest/pleasure, lack of appetite, sleep disturbance, low energy, and poor concentration. Depression can affect people irrespective of age, ethnicity, and gender. Major depressive disorder (MDD) is the most studied type of depression characterized by one or more major depressive events, that is, the presence of low mood and/or loss of interest for at least 14 days in company with depression symptoms. MDD leads to suicide that takes 2160 self-harm deaths per day in US [24]. Decades of research on depression have yielded several mechanisms that may explain its pathophysiology, including biogenic amine (e.g., monoamine) hypothesis, abnormal endocrine factors, genetic and environmental factors, neurogenesis, and the dysregulation of second messenger systems, which have been extensively reviewed elsewhere [25]. Among them, monoamine-based mechanisms were the most studied with successful development of antidepressants.

Although monoamine treatments are available for MDD, they have not been optimal. Currently, standard monoamine antidepressants require one month or more to exert antidepressant effects [26]. Such time lag has put MDD patients at risk of suicide and other self-harm acts. In recent decades, the NMDAR has emerged as a central player in MDD research, resulting in a paradigm shift from the monoamine-based to the NMDAR-based hypothesis. The NMDAR-based hypothesis of depression originated from early findings in the 1990's that NMDAR antagonists exerted quick antidepressant-like action [27]. Subsequently, many studies have reported abnormal glutamate levels in frontal and occipital cortices in MDD; however, these findings infer the complex role of NMDAR in the brain of MDD patients. The regionally decreased glutamate level in the brain demonstrates an association with the pathophysiology of MDD [28]; on the contrary, the elevated glutamate levels occurs in medication-free MDD patients during an active depressive episode, in remission, and in young people [29]. Since glutamate is a major excitatory neurotransmitter dictating the neural plasticity and process of learning and memory, the alteration to NMDAR causes region-specific maladaptive neurocircuitry in depression and decreases in cognitive controls over negative emotion.

At the molecular level, postmortem brain analyses from MDD patients show alterations in the NMDAR subunit profile, such as reduced GluN2A and GluN2B subunits in locus coeruleus, and decreased GluN1 and GluN2A expression levels but no changes to those of GluN2B, GluN2C and GluN2D subunits in dorsolateral prefrontal cortex of MDD subjects [30]. Further studies have found that biologically, the activation of NMDAR requires both the binding of glycine and glutamate onto their binding sites, and therefore, modulating the release of the two amino acids into synapses are considered feasible. At glutamatergic synapses, glycine is transported by GlyT1, maintaining glycine concentration below saturation at post-synaptic NMDAR. Accordingly, GlyT1 has become an intriguing target for NMDAR activity modulation [31]. Alternatively, inhibiting glutamate levels at synapses renders reduced glutamate binding to NMDAR [32]. In summary, the above findings provide a solid basis for developing chemotherapeutics for treating MDD via modulating NMDA.

2.2.2 Schizophrenia

Schizophrenia is a psychotic illness presenting symptoms with processing thoughts and contents, and develops positive, negative and/or cognitive symptoms. Concurrently, depression and suicidal thoughts and attempts happen often in people suffering from schizophrenia. Because schizophrenia patients require lifelong treatment, early intervention may improve the long-term outlook. Conventional therapies for schizophrenia are developed based on a dopamine hypothesis which has been prevailing to explain symptoms associated with the positive symptoms. However, these treatments have not been optimal and often induce substantial adverse side effects [33].

Glutamate hypofunction hypothesis of schizophrenia has been supported by several lines of studies. Low level of glutamate in cerebrospinal fluid was reported in patients with schizophrenia [34]. The worsening of schizophrenic symptoms was observed in patients treated with NMDAR inhibitors such as ketamine. Healthy people administered with similar inhibitors were reported to develop symptoms of schizophrenia [35]. Building on these data, upregulating NMDA function serves as a promising target for treating schizophrenia [36].

Although NMDAR is a focus for antipsychotic drug development for schizophrenia, direct activation of the NMDAR via targeting the glutamate site is reported to cause excitotoxicity. The finding suggests the demand for targeting the glycine site as an alternative, but direct approach. To reduce glycine site vacancy, a number of studies have synthesized amino-acid derivatives to occupy it [37]. Alternatively, enhancing the glycine levels through GlyT1 inhibition has also shown promise, which is used as an adjunct to conventional therapies [38].

2.2.3 Bipolar disorder

BD, as its name suggested, causes extremes of mood fluctuations that a person will be either in emotional highs (mania or hypomania) or lows (depression). BD is a lifelong disease that episodes of mood swings may occur infrequently or several times in a year. Typically, BD patients spend more time in depressive mood than mania or hypomania. Currently, treatments for BD are limited to symptom reduction and prevention of the occurrence of mood episodes [39].

Neuroimaging [40] and genetic findings [41] have revealed that glutamatergic abnormality is associated with the pathophysiology of BD, indicating NMDAR may play a role in the disease. The use of NMDAR inhibitor further evidences the role of NMDAR in the regulation of BD. Ketamine has shown to improve depressive symptom. One of possible mechanisms of ketamine in regulating BD symptoms is to increase presynaptic levels of glutamate which in turn binds to AMPAR instead of NMDAR. The increased ratio of AMPAR-to-NMDAR neurotransmission is implicated to induce the antidepressant effects of ketamine [42].

At the molecular level, postmortem findings suggest that BD is associated with a reduced expression of NR1 subunit in the prefrontal cortex [30]. The genetic polymorphisms in the 3'UTR region of GRIN2B gene that encodes for the NR2B subunit has been found to play a role in BD etiology, although its expression level is not significantly different from the control [43]. Together, these studies suggest NMDAR is associated with BD.

2.2.4 Anxiety disorder

Having occasional anxiety is a normal part of life. However, intense, excessive, and persistent worries and fear about specific situation would be in the category of anxiety disorder that needs intervention. Types of anxiety disorders include panic attack, generalized anxiety disorder, and separation anxiety disorder. An anxiety patient may experience one or more of them and can experience anxiety at very young age [44].

Benzodiazepine and selective serotonin reuptake inhibitors (SSRIs) or selective serotonin-norepinephrine reuptake inhibitors (SNRIs) are recommended as first line drug treatment, because of their more favorable profile than tricyclic antidepressants and monoamine oxidase inhibitors. Nevertheless, some SNRIs are also antagonists of metabolic enzyme cytochrome P450, therefore causing drug–drug interactions [45]. In addition, discontinuation of SSRIs or SNRIs may experience withdrawal reactions [46]. These unwanted outcomes suggest an essential for developing next generation anxiolytic treatments based on novel mechanisms.

Fear often occurs together and share similar stress responses with anxiety, and therefore, both are often put into the same context when discussing the underlying mechanisms. Currently, studies have found that the neuronal modulatory systems in brain areas contributing to fear and anxiety share a high degree of overlap [47]. In particular, regulating extinction learning of fear through NMDAR within amygdala, medial prefrontal cortex, and hippocampus is considered critical among the neuronal modulatory systems [48]. Hippocampus and amygdala of the medial temporal lobe situate at the interface between cognition and emotion, which is believed to be potential sites where NMDAR inhibitors exert anxiolytic effects [49]. NMDAR regulates emotionality and cognition, and its antagonists have shown promising effects on them. In contrast to NMDAR antagonism, partial activation of NMDAR facilitates fear extinction in rodents. In clinical setting, partial agonists used as an adjuvant increase psychotherapeutic effects in patients suffering fear-related disorders [50]. These finding suggest that a balanced modulation of NMDAR activity can bring benefits for the patients with anxiety disorder.

3. NMDAR modulators for CNS disorders

3.1 Positive NMDAR modulators

In this section, positive NMDAR modulators for CNS disorders will be discussed (**Figures 1** and **2**, **Table 1**). To enhance NMDAR function, two approaches could achieve: direct or indirect modulation. For direct modulation, three types of enhancers are categorized according to their binding sites: glutamate site, glycine site, and allosteric site of NMDAR.

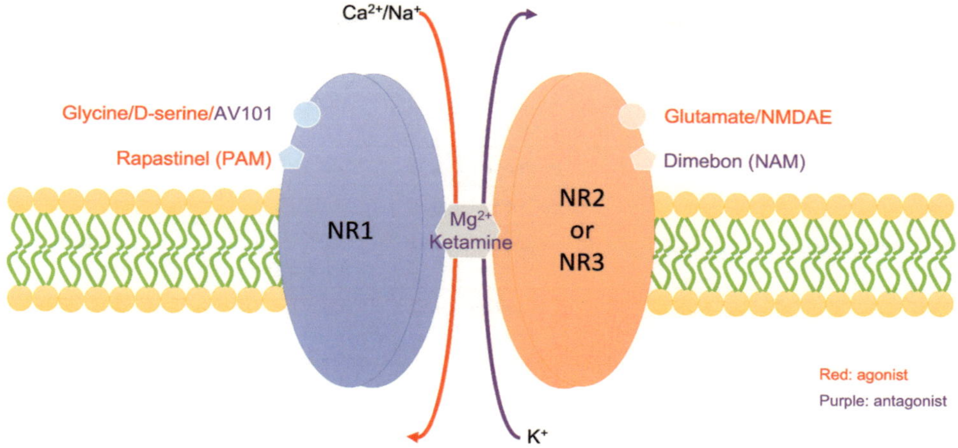

Figure 1.
Scheme of direct agonism/antagonism via various binding sites of NMDAR. NAM, negative allosteric modulators; PAM, positive allosteric modulators.

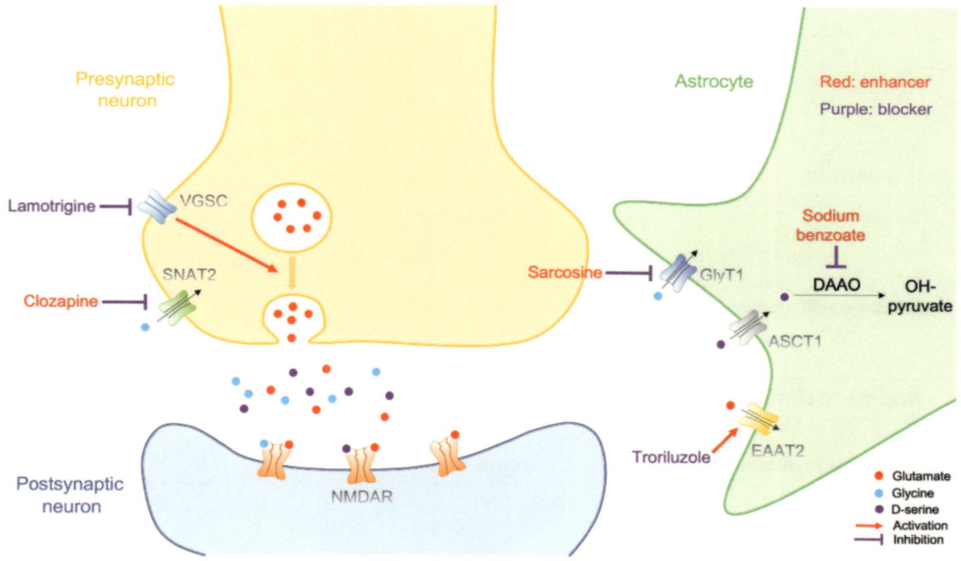

Figure 2.
Indirect NMDAR agonism/antagonism through activation or inhibition on diverse channels or transporters or enzymes. ASCT-1, alanine/serine/cysteine transporter-1; DAAO, D-amino acid oxidase; EAAT2, excitatory amino acid transporter-2; GlyT1, glycine transporter-1; NMDAR, N-methyl-D-aspartate receptor; SNAT2, sodium-coupled neutral amino-acid transporter-2; VGSC, voltage-gated sodium channel.

3.1.1 Direct NMDAR enhancers

3.1.1.1 NMDAR glutamate site agonists

Cognitive deficits occur often in elderly MDD patients, hardly to be relieved with the existing treatment. NMDA enhancement via the glutamate site has been proved to enhance cognitive functions in previous studies [81]. NMDA enhancer (NMDAE), binding the NMDAR glutamate site as an agonist, has been offered for the elderly (>55 years) and adults (18–55 years) with MDD. To testify the efficacy, safety, and the cognitive improvement of NMDAE in those patients, the NMDAE

Drug	Mechanism	Disease	Study
Positive NMDAR modulators			
NMDAE	glutamate site agonist	MDD	NCT03414931 NCT04637620
Glycine	glycine site agonist	Schizophrenia	[53]
D-alanine	glycine site agonist	Schizophrenia	[54]
D-serine	glycine site agonist	MDD Schizophrenia	NCT04721249 NCT00322023
D-cycloserine	glycine site partial agonist	AD MDD Schizophrenia BD Anxiety	[55] NCT00408031 [56] NCT01833897 NCT00515879
Rapastinel (GLYX-13/BV-102)	PAM	MDD	NCT01684163
Apimostinel (NRX-1074)	PAM	MDD	NCT02067793
Clozapine	Indirect enhancer (SNAT2 inhibitor)	PD MDD Schizophrenia BD	NCT00004826 [57] [58] [59]
BI 425809	Indirect enhancer (GlyT1 inhibitor)	AD Schizophrenia	NCT02788513 NCT02832037
Bitopertin (RO-4917838)	Indirect enhancer (GlyT1 inhibitor)	Schizophrenia	NCT01235585
Sarcosine	Indirect enhancer (GlyT1 inhibitor)	PD MDD Schizophrenia	NCT01785628 NCT00977353 [60]
D-Amino acid oxidase inhibitor	Indirect enhancer (D-serine retention)	AD MDD Schizophrenia	[61] [62] NCT01908192
Negative NMDAR modulators			
AV-101 (L-4-chlorokynurenine)	glycine site antagonist	PD MDD	NCT04147949 NCT02484456
Dimebon (Latrepirdine)	NAM	AD HD	NCT00377715 NCT00497159
Dextromethadone (D-methadone/ REL-1017)	NAM	MDD	NCT04688164
Rislenemdaz (CERC-301/MK-0657)	NAM	MDD	NCT01941043
Amantadine	Uncompetitive antagonist	PD HD	NCT00632762 [63]
Memantine	Uncompetitive antagonist	AD PD MDD Schizophrenia BD Anxiety	[64] [65] [66] [67] [68] [69]
Dextromethorphan	Uncompetitive antagonist	MDD BD	NCT04226352 [70]

Drug	Mechanism	Disease	Study
Nuedexta (Dextromethorphan+ Quinidine)	Uncompetitive antagonist	MDD BD	NCT01882829 [71]
AVP-786 (Dextromethorphan+ Quinidine + Deuterium)	Uncompetitive antagonist	AD MDD Schizophrenia	NCT03393520 NCT02153502 NCT03896945
AXS-05 (Axsome, Dextromethorphan+ Bupropion)	Uncompetitive antagonist	AD MDD	NCT04797715 NCT02741791
(R,S)-Ketamine	Uncompetitive antagonist	MDD BD Anxiety	[72] [73] [74]
(S)-Ketamine (Esketamine)	Uncompetitive antagonist	MDD BD	[75] NCT03965871
(R)-Ketamine (Arketamine)	Uncompetitive antagonist	MDD	NCT04108234
Neramexane	Uncompetitive antagonist	AD	[76]
Nitrous oxide (N_2O)	Uncompetitive antagonist	MDD Anxiety	[77] NCT02243826
Lamotrigine	Indirect blocker (glutamate release inhibitor)	MDD Schizophrenia BD	[78] [67] [78]
Riluzole (BHV-0223)	Indirect blocker (glutamate release inhibitor)	AD MDD BD Anxiety	[79] [52] [52] [80]
Troriluzole (BHV-4157)	Indirect blocker (glutamate uptake activator)	AD Anxiety	NCT03605667 NCT03829241

AD, Alzheimer's disease; BD, bipolar disorder; GlyT1, Glycine transporter-1; HD, Huntington's disease; MDD, major depressive disorder; NAM, negative allosteric modulators; PAM, positive allosteric modulators; PD, Parkinson's disease; SNAT2, sodium-coupled neutral amino-acid transporter-2.

Table 1.
NMDAR modulators for CNS disorders [6, 51, 52].

treatment results were compared with sertraline (SSRI) and placebo. The results of those clinical studies are not disclosed as of August 2021 (NCT03414931 and NCT04637620). The potential risk of this approach is the excitotoxicity caused by overactivation through the glutamate-binding site.

3.1.1.2 NMDAR glycine site agonists

Another ligand binding site on NMDAR is the glycine site, which can also be targeted to modulate the NMDAR activation for the treatments of psychiatric disorders [82]. Glycine, acting as an agonist via binding the glycine site, can ameliorate negative symptoms in schizophrenia patients [53]. This preliminary finding encourages the development of other endogenous co-agonists, such as D-alanine. D-alanine, working as an add-on antipsychotic medication, improved schizophrenic symptoms without significant side effects, which further supports that the pathophysiology of schizophrenia is due to the hypofunction of NMDA neurotransmission [54]. D-serine, an NMDAR co-agonist without psychotomimetic effects, emerges as a novel glutamatergic antidepressant as an adjuvant therapy in MDD patients (NCT04721249). On the other hand, the therapeutic effects of D-serine at low dose (30 mg/kg/d) in schizophrenic patients are inconsistent. Some clinical studies showed significant improvement in positive, negative, and cognitive symptoms [83], whereas others presented no significant improvement [84]. Interestingly, high doses of D-serine (≥60 mg/kg/d) could possess consistent significant improvement in negative symptoms, strongly suggesting a therapeutic dose–response of D-serine for the treatment of schizophrenia (NCT00322023).

D-cycloserine (DCS), a partial agonist of NMDAR with agonism at low doses but antagonism at high doses depending on the intrinsic tone of NMDA function [85], exhibits controversial therapeutic effects on CNS disorders. In some AD studies, a dose as high as 100 mg/d could improve the cognitive symptoms, while a low dose of 15 mg/d could improve memory deficits [55, 86]. However, other studies presented no cognitive improvement from low (10 mg/d) to high dose (500 mg/d) in AD patients [87].

When the high dose of DCS (≥ 500 mg/d) was employed in MDD patients, depressive symptoms could be improved (NCT00408031) [88]. These observations implied that NMDAR antagonism might be a potential target for the development of novel antidepressant. The clinical studies of DCS at a dose of 50 mg/d is argumentative, some claimed to possess significant clinical improvement [89], while the others found no clinical improvement [90]. In the dose finding phase, the dose of 100 mg/d of DCS seemed to be more effective than 50 or 250 mg/d in improving schizophrenic symptoms [56]. In combination with ketamine, DCS could ameliorate depression symptoms in BD (NCT01833897). Cognitive behavioral therapy with DCS also reduced social anxiety (NCT00515879) and PTSD [91]. Overall, the dose selection of DCS determines its agonistic vs. antagonistic effects on NMDAR, hence modulating its therapeutic efficacy for a variety of CNS disorders.

3.1.1.3 NMDAR allosteric site enhancers (positive allosteric modulators (PAM))

Rapastinel (GLYX-13/BV-102), an amidated tetrapeptide acting as a NMDA allosteric glycine site partial agonist, is administered intravenously to treat MDD in clinical trial (NCT01684163). Rapastinel infusion achieved antidepressant effects without psychotomimetic properties and serious adverse events, therefore acquiring FDA Fast-Track and Breakthrough Therapy designations for adjunctive treatment of MDD. However, rapastinel failed to meet primary and key secondary endpoints in three acute studies (RAP-MD-01, −02, −03 by Allergan).

Apimostinel (NRX-1074), a chemical structure like rapastinel with an additional benzyl group, is administered intravenously and orally under the studies of efficacy and safety evaluation for MDD patients and healthy individuals (NCT02067793 and NCT02366364). Benefiting from its molecular weight and orally stability, apimostinel is 100-fold more potent than rapastinel and is also well tolerated without psychotomimetic symptoms [92]. The findings of the studies are not available yet.

3.1.2 Indirect NMDAR enhancers

To enhance NMDAR function, "consolidating" amino acids (e.g., glycine or D-serine, glutamate, and aspartate) in the synaptic cleft could achieve that goal. With the use of inhibitors of amino acid transporters or degrading enzymes, the concentration of those specific amino acids could sustain in the synaptic cleft to boost NMDAR function [58]. Clozapine, a modest inhibitor of sodium-coupled neutral amino acid transporter-2 (SNAT2), indirectly activates NMDAR via augmenting synaptic glycine levels. Clozapine could also improve symptoms of psychosis, tremor, and dyskinesias in PD patients (NCT00004826) [58]. In addition to reducing the risk of hospital re-admission for MDD patients, clozapine administration also demonstrated higher efficacy than quetiapine by ameliorating depressive symptoms [57]. As approved by Food and Drug Administration (FDA) of the USA, clozapine is utilized to treat treatment-resistant schizophrenia and symptoms of self-harm in patients with schizophrenia. Clozapine is also more effective than other antipsychotics in improving treatment-resistant bipolar disorder [59]. However, clozapine can cause potentially lethal agranulocytosis.

Other than SNAT2 inhibitor, GlyT1 inhibitor could also increase synaptic glycine level by blocking the GlyT1 to enhance NMDAR function. BI 425809, a selective GlyT1 inhibitor, emerges as a potential treatment of cognitive impairment of AD and schizophrenia. Although BI 425809 failed to improve cognition in AD study (NCT02788513), it improved cognition in patients with schizophrenia (NCT02832037). Bitopertin (RO-4917838), a selective and potent GlyT1 inhibitor, modulates both glutamatergic and dopaminergic neurotransmission in animal models of schizophrenia [93]. In six active treatment arms across three clinical studies, only one of them proved improvement in symptoms of schizophrenia (NCT01235585) [94]. However, the magnitude of improvement was small. Because of its strong antagonism, bitopertin induces NMDAR internalization, counterproductive to improve the NMDA function.

Sarcosine, a potent endogenous non-selective GlyT1 inhibitor, was applied in cognitive- and mood-related clinical studies. In PD patients, sarcosine improved depression and neuropsychiatric symptoms, especially in patients with mild–moderate severity (NCT01785628). Both in animal models and in depressed patients, sarcosine improved depression-like behaviors, further strengthening GlyT1 inhibitor as a novel class of promising antidepressant (NCT00977353) [31]. In most clinical studies of sarcosine in patents with schizophrenia, improvement in schizophrenic symptoms were reported [60]. However, when being adjunctive with clozapine, sarcosine could not produce improvement in schizophrenic patients [95]. This phenomenon may be explained by the "ceiling effect": additional NMDAR activation may not be induced due to maximal NMDAR enhancement achieved by clozapine administration alone. In contrast, the combination therapy of sarcosine and sodium benzoate (a D-amino acid oxidase (DAAO) inhibitor) enhances the cognitive function of patients with schizophrenia [96].

DAAO, a flavoenzyme for D-amino acids (e.g., D-serine and D-alanine) degradation, could be strategically inhibited to increase endogenous D-serine levels at the synaptic cleft, resulting in strengthening NMDAR functions. In post-mortem studies, patients with schizophrenia possessed higher expression and activity of DAAO in the cortex and cerebellum [97]. Thus, DAAO inhibition provides a good rationale to be a novel therapeutic target for schizophrenia treatment. Sodium benzoate, a prototype competitive DAAO inhibitor, generated antipsychotic effects in the phencyclidine-induced model of schizophrenia [98]. In some clinical studies, sodium benzoate adjunctive therapy improved symptomatology of patients with schizophrenia [99], and a larger scale clinical trial is undergoing (NCT01908192). In patients with early-phase AD, sodium benzoate predominantly enhanced cognitive and universal functions [61]. Sodium benzoate may enlarge gray matter via synaptogenesis and neurogenesis in MDD treatment [62].

3.2 Negative NMDAR modulators

NMDAR antagonism has been a therapeutic strategy for a variety of CNS disorders [100]. To achieve NMDAR antagonism, several negative NMDAR modulators have been offered to treat patients with CNS disorders through distinct underlying mechanisms: direct blocking in competitive, non-competitive, and uncompetitive ways, and indirect blocking. All negative NMDAR modulators are introduced in this section (**Figures 1** and **2**, **Table 1**).

3.2.1 Direct NMDAR blockers

3.2.1.1 Competitive NMDAR glycine site antagonists

AV-101 (L-4-chlorokynurenine), a pro-drug of 7-Chlorokynurenic acid (7-CKA), is able to cross the blood–brain barrier and transform to 7-CKA in astrocytes [101]. 7-CKA is a potent and selective NMDAR glycine site antagonist [102]. In preclinical studies, AV-101 demonstrated dose-dependent antidepressant-like effects in animal models [103]. However, AV-101 monotherapy failed to produce the anti-depressant effects in the clinical study (NCT02484456) [104]. On the other hand, AV-101 treatment for patients with PD will be conducted (NCT04147949).

3.2.1.2 Non-competitive NMDAR antagonists (negative allosteric modulators (NAM))

Dimebon (Latrepirdine), an NAM at the polyamine-binding site of NMDARs, was originally used as an antihistamine [51]. Assessed in clinical trials, dimebon significantly improved the neuropsychiatric symptoms of patients with mild-to-moderate AD (NCT00377715) [105]. In patients with HD, short-term administration of dimebon is beneficial for cognitive improvement (NCT00497159) [106]. Dextromethadone (D-methadone/REL-1017), a non-competitive NMDAR antagonist, provided antidepressant activity via mTORC1-mediated synaptic plasticity in the mPFC in animal models [107]. As dextromethadone performs as a rapid-acting treatment for depression in clinical studies (NCT03051256), it gained FDA Fast-Track designation as an adjunctive treatment for MDD. A phase III clinical trial of dextromethadone is currently ongoing (NCT04688164). Rislenemdaz (CERC-301/MK-0657), a NMDAR NR2B-selective antagonist, induced antidepressant properties in patients with treatment-resistant MDD [108]. Nevertheless, in a phase II study, no obvious antidepressant effects were produced by rislenemdaz (NCT01941043).

3.2.1.3 Uncompetitive NMDAR antagonists (NMDAR channel blockers)

Amantadine, a low-affinity uncompetitive NMDAR antagonist with rapid blocking channel kinetics, could ameliorate several clinical symptoms in PD, and the long-term efficacy of chronic treatment with amantadine might improve apathy and fatigue in PD patients (NCT00632762) [109]. For Huntington chorea, amantadine treatment delivered no beneficial effects but brought subjectively better feelings to patients [63]. Memantine, an adamantane derivative like amantadine, is an uncompetitive, moderate affinity, open-channel NMDAR blocker with strong voltage dependency and rapid blocking and unblocking kinetics [110]. Despite being approved by the US FDA for treating moderate-to-severe AD with safe and well tolerated profile, the efficacy of memantine is inconsistent at best. Some studies proved the clinical improvement of memantine in patients with moderate to severe AD [64], while other studies showed little clinical benefits of memantine towards AD treatment [111]. Several clinical results of memantine treatment in PD were also contradictive [65]. In MDD and BD clinical studies, memantine failed to show antidepressant effects in patients [66, 68]. As treatment for schizophrenic symptoms, adjunct memantine uncovered a beneficial effect in ten studies, but no effects in two studies [67]. One study of memantine revealed minimal improvement in seven patients with anxiety [69].

Dextromethorphan, an uncompetitive NMDA receptor antagonist, is used as a cough suppressant with sedative and dissociative effects. In recent research, dextromethorphan and dextromethorphan-based compounds are considered as potential rapid-acting antidepressants, and therefore its therapeutic effect in MDD is evaluated in the clinical study (NCT04226352). In a BD study, dextromethorphan had no significant antidepressant effects compared with placebo group. This might be due to DRD2/ANKK1 TaqIA polymorphism [70]. Nuedexta, an FDA approved treatment for the pseudobulbar affect, was also utilized to treat MDD and BD. The purpose of adding dextromethorphan with quinidine in this combination is to inhibit the cytochrome P450 2D6 (CYP2D6) isoform, a dominant metabolic pathway of dextromethorphan, hence augmenting the bioavailability of dextromethorphan in CNS [112]. A proof-of-concept clinical trial demonstrated that after Nuedexta treatment, the response and remission rates in the patients with treatment resistant depression were 45% and 35%, respectively (NCT01882829). In a retrospective chart review, Nuedexta induced significant improvement in Clinical Global Impression (CGI) in depressed patients with treatment resistant bipolar disorder, implying its possible effectiveness in the BD treatment [71].

AVP-786, another dextromethorphan-based compound, is in conjunction with quinidine and deuterium to decrease the metabolism of dextromethorphan in the liver and hence increase its blood exposure. Following FDA Fast-Track designation for agitation in AD [113], four AD-related clinical studies of AVP-786 are underway (NCT02442765, NCT02442778, NCT02446132, and NCT03393520). In patients with MDD and schizophrenia, the efficacy, safety, and tolerability of AVP-786 were evaluated in the clinical studies (NCT02153502 and NCT03896945). AXS-05 (Axsome) is in combination with dextromethorphan and bupropion, which acts as an inhibitor of CYP2D6 to enhance the bioavailability of dextromethorphan [114]. In the AXS-05 treatment of agitation in patients with AD, the efficacy and safety of AXS-05 will be compared to placebo (NCT04797715). Three phase III clinical studies on the safety and efficacy of AXS-05 in patients with MDD were conducted without results posted to date (NCT02741791, NCT04019704, and NCT04039022).

(R,S)-Ketamine, an anesthetic and analgesic via intravenous administration, and its derivates (S)-ketamine (esketamine) and (R)-ketamine (arketamine) open a new era for glutamatergic rapid-acting antidepressant. At high doses (1-2 mg/kg), ketamine inhibits NMDAR as an uncompetitive antagonist to produce anesthesia, while at low doses, ketamine induces analgesia against both acute and chronic pain (0.25–0.5 mg/kg). Importantly, rapid-acting antidepressant effects of ketamine at moderate doses (0.5 mg/kg) have been proved in preclinical and clinical studies [3]. In most clinical studies of MDD, (R,S)-ketamine administration decreased depression severity with robust and rapid antidepressant effects [72], in accordance with studies of BD [73] and anxiolytic effects in anxiety disorders [74]. The (S+) enantiomer of ketamine was approved by FDA for adults with MDD with acute suicidal ideation or behavior. Esketamine improved depressive symptoms and delayed relapse in many studies [75], but did not demonstrate significant improvement as an adjunctive therapy with oral antidepressants in elderly patients with treatment-resistant depression [115]. In the study of treatment-resistant bipolar depression, the efficacy, safety, and pharmacokinetics of inhaled esketamine are still being evaluated (NCT03965871). Another enantiomer of ketamine, arketamine, is a less potent NMDAR uncompetitive antagonist, but displays greater and longer antidepressant effects than esketamine without psychotomimetic side effects [116]. In an open-label pilot study, intravenous arketamine generated fast-onset and sustained antidepressant effects in depressed patients [117], and the larger study is underway (NCT04108234).

Neramexane, a moderate-affinity NMDAR open-channel blocker, possesses similar kinetics and voltage-dependency to memantine. Although it was well tolerated at all administered doses in clinical studies, phase II/III clinical trials for moderate-to-severe AD yielded contradictory results [76]. Nitrous oxide, an uncompetitive NMDAR antagonist, is an inhaled anesthetic often used in obstetrics or dentistry [118]. One recently published research demonstrated that compared with 50% nitrous oxide, 25% nitrous oxide provides comparable antidepressant effects with a markedly lower rate of adverse effects [77]. Other studies are underway to evaluate the efficacy and safety of nitrous oxide in MDD (NCT03869736 and NCT03932825). Nitrous oxide acted as a pharmacologic treatment for lumbar puncture/other procedure-related anxiety (NCT02243826).

3.2.2 Indirect NMDAR blockers

Lamotrigine, inhibiting voltage-dependent Na^+, Ca^{2+}, and K^+ channels, acts as a presynaptic glutamate release inhibitor [119]. FDA approved lamotrigine for the maintenance treatment of BD. Lamotrigine failed to achieve clinical improvement in five clinical studies of MDD, while it induced higher response rate than placebo in BD studies [52]. In a comprehensive meta-analysis, lamotrigine performed better than placebo in improving unipolar and bipolar depressive symptoms [78]. Five of nine clinical trials of lamotrigine in schizophrenia revealed clinical improvement in a range of outcome measures [67].

Riluzole (BHV-0223), a glutamate release inhibitor, was approved by the US FDA for the treatment of amyotrophic lateral sclerosis. The mechanisms that reduce extracellular glutamate by riluzole includes reduced glutamate release through presynaptic inhibition of voltage-gated sodium channels (VGSCs), increased glutamate uptake by astroglial cells, and enhanced AMPA trafficking [120]. In a current clinical study of AD, riluzole decreased the reduction in cerebral glucose metabolism, a positive correlation with cognitive measures [79]. Additionally, riluzole only ameliorated depressive symptoms in one of four placebo-controlled MDD studies, and failed to reach clinical improvement in a BD study [52]. In one trial of anxiety disorders, eighty percent subjects responded positively to riluzole [80], and the following functional neuroimaging studies proved the alterations in hippocampal N-acetylaspartate (NAA) concentrations and volumes were in correlation with riluzole-induced improvement on anxiety scales [121]. Troriluzole (BHV-4157), a tripeptide prodrug conjugate of riluzole, has been developed to improve the bioavailability, safety, and dosing of riluzole. As a glutamate modulator, troriluzole decreases the level of synaptic glutamate via strengthening glutamate uptake, mainly through excitatory amino acid transporters (i.e., EAAT2) located on glial cells. Both in clinical studies of AD and anxiety, the clinical efficacy of troriluzole is under assessment (NCT03605667 and NCT03829241).

4. Conclusions

Not only does the discovery of ketamine to act as a novel rapid-acting antidepressant trigger a strong interest in developing novel NMDAR-modulating agents by a variety of proof-of-concept studies for CNS disorders, but also, after exploring the potential pathological mechanisms for the major CNS disorders as described above, the aberrant NMDAR activity shows to play a pivotal role in regulating clinical symptoms, hence facilitating the development of positive and negative NMDAR modulators against those pathological aberrances in NMDAR activity. Interestingly, but not surprisingly, monotherapy of single NMDAR modulators often failed in clinical studies, boosting the prosperity of combination treatment with multiple modulators, or even with the standard treatments, further implying the intricate mechanisms underlying the CNS pathology.

To date, numerous clinical studies of NMDAR modulators are still underway. With more successful clinical improvement by NMDAR modulators in clinical studies, the mysterious puzzles of CNS disorders could be dissolved gradually, further refining the utilization of NMDAR modulators as optimal treatment with less undesirable side effects for the sophisticated CNS disorders that involve vulnerability in NMDA homeostasis.

Acknowledgements

The authors thank Hung-Chun Liu and Cheng-Shen Lee for their assistance in preparation of the manuscript.

Conflict of interest

The corresponding author is the CEO of SyneuRx International Corp., which is developing CNS therapeutics.

Author details

Chih-Hung Lin[1], Po-Chang Shih[1] and Guochuan Emil Tsai[1,2]*

1 SyneuRx, New Taipei City, Taiwan

2 Department of Psychiatry and Biobehavioral Sciences, School of Medicine, UCLA, CA, USA

*Address all correspondence to: tsaimdphd@ucla.edu

References

[1] Tsai GE. Ultimate Translation: Developing Therapeutics Targeting on N-Methyl-d-Aspartate Receptor. 1st ed. Vol. 76, Advances in Pharmacology. Elsevier Inc.; 2016. 257-309 p.

[2] Hansen KB, Yi F, Perszyk RE, Menniti FS, Traynelis SF. NMDA receptors in the central nervous system. Vol. 1677, Methods in Molecular Biology. 2017. 1-80 p.

[3] Kohtala S. Ketamine—50 years in use: from anesthesia to rapid antidepressant effects and neurobiological mechanisms. Pharmacol Reports. 2021 Apr 1;73(2):323.

[4] Kantrowitz JT, Epstein ML, Lee M, Lehrfeld N, Nolan KA, Shope C, et al. Improvement in mismatch negativity generation during d-serine treatment in schizophrenia: Correlation with symptoms. Schizophr Res. 2018 Jan 1;191:70-79.

[5] Adell A. Brain NMDA receptors in schizophrenia and depression. Biomolecules. 2020;10(6):1-27.

[6] Li CT, Yang KC, Lin WC. Glutamatergic dysfunction and glutamatergic compounds for major psychiatric disorders: Evidence from clinical neuroimaging studies. Front Psychiatry. 2019;10(JAN):1-11.

[7] McKhann GM, Knopman DS, Chertkow H, Hyman BT, Jack CR, Kawas CH, et al. The diagnosis of dementia due to Alzheimer's disease: Recommendations from the National Institute on Aging-Alzheimer's Association workgroups on diagnostic guidelines for Alzheimer's disease. Alzheimer's Dement. 2011.

[8] Huang Y-J, Lin C-H, Lane H-Y, Tsai GE. NMDA Neurotransmission Dysfunction in Behavioral and Psychological Symptoms of Alzheimer's Disease. Curr Neuropharmacol. 2012 Oct 2;10(3):272.

[9] Lacor PN, Buniel MC, Furlow PW, Clemente AS, Velasco PT, Wood M, et al. Aβ oligomer-induced aberrations in synapse composition, shape, and density provide a molecular basis for loss of connectivity in Alzheimer's disease. J Neurosci. 2007.

[10] Li S, Jin M, Koeglsperger T, Shepardson NE, Shankar GM, Selkoe DJ. Soluble a β oligomers inhibit long-term potentiation through a mechanism involving excessive activation of extrasynaptic NR2B-containing NMDA receptors. J Neurosci. 2011;31(18):6627-6638.

[11] Xia P, Chen HSV, Zhang D, Lipton SA. Memantine preferentially blocks extrasynaptic over synaptic NMDA receptor currents in hippocampal autapses. J Neurosci. 2010.

[12] Li S, Mallory M, Alford M, Tanaka S, Masliah E. Glutamate transporter alterations in Alzheimer disease are possibly associated with abnormal APP expression. J Neuropathol Exp Neurol. 1997.

[13] Fernández-Tomé P, Brera B, Arévalo MA, De Ceballos ML. β-amyloid25-35 inhibits glutamate uptake in cultured neurons and astrocytes: Modulation of uptake as a survival mechanism. Neurobiol Dis. 2004.

[14] Jankovic J, Tan EK. Parkinson's disease: Etiopathogenesis and treatment. J Neurol Neurosurg Psychiatry. 2020.

[15] Dickson DW. Neuropathology of Parkinson disease. Park Relat Disord. 2018.

[16] Guo H, Camargo LM, Yeboah F, DIgan ME, Niu H, Pan Y, et al. A NMDA-receptor calcium influx assay sensitive to stimulation by glutamate and glycine/D-serine. Sci Rep. 2017.

[17] Mellone M, Stanic J, Hernandez LF, Iglesias E, Zianni E, Longhi A, et al. NMDA receptor gluN2A/gluN2B subunit ratio as synaptic trait of levodopa-induced dyskinesias: From experimental models to patients. Front Cell Neurosci. 2015.

[18] Schmitz Y, Castagna C, Mrejeru A, Lizardi-Ortiz JE, Klein Z, Lindsley CW, et al. Glycine transporter-1 inhibition promotes striatal axon sprouting via NMDA receptors in dopamine neurons. J Neurosci. 2013.

[19] Paulsen JS. Cognitive impairment in Huntington disease: Diagnosis and treatment. Curr Neurol Neurosci Rep. 2011.

[20] Davies S, Ramsden DB. Huntington's disease. Journal of Clinical Pathology - Molecular Pathology. 2001.

[21] Beal MF, Kowall NW, Ellison DW, Mazurek MF, Swartz KJ, Martin JB. Replication of the neurochemical characteristics of Huntington's disease by quinolinic acid. Nature. 1986.

[22] Tsapakis EM, Travis MJ. Glutamate and psychiatric disorders. Adv Psychiatr Treat. 2002.

[23] Frye MA, Tsai GE, Huggins T, Coyle JT, Post RM. Low Cerebrospinal Fluid Glutamate and Glycine in Refractory Affective Disorder. Biol Psychiatry. 2007;61(2):162-166.

[24] World Health Organization (WHO). Suicide worldwide in 2019: global health estimates. 2021. Licence: CC BY-NC-SA 3.0 IGO.

[25] Jesulola E, Micalos P, Baguley IJ. Understanding the pathophysiology of depression: From monoamines to the neurogenesis hypothesis model - are we there yet? Behavioural Brain Research. 2018.

[26] Nemeroff CB, Owens MJ. Treatment of mood disorders. Nat Neurosci. 2002;5(11s):1068-1070.

[27] Trullas R, Skolnick P. Functional antagonists at the NMDA receptor complex exhibit antidepressant actions. Eur J Pharmacol. 1990.

[28] Sanacora G, Treccani G, Popoli M. Towards a glutamate hypothesis of depression: An emerging frontier of neuropsychopharmacology for mood disorders. Neuropharmacology. 2012.

[29] Taylor MJ, Mannie ZN, Norbury R, Near J, Cowen PJ. Elevated cortical glutamate in young people at increased familial risk of depression. Int J Neuropsychopharmacol. 2011.

[30] Beneyto M, Meador-Woodruff JH. Lamina-specific abnormalities of NMDA receptor-associated postsynaptic protein transcripts in the prefrontal cortex in schizophrenia and bipolar disorder. Neuropsychopharmacology. 2008.

[31] Huang C-C, Wei I-H, Huang C-L, Chen K-T, Tsai M-H, Tsai P, et al. Inhibition of Glycine Transporter-I as a Novel Mechanism for the Treatment of Depression. Biol Psychiatry. 2013 Nov 15;74(10):734-741.

[32] Javitt DC. Glutamate as a therapeutic target in psychiatric disorders. Molecular Psychiatry. 2004.

[33] Fleischhacker WW. New drugs for the treatment of schizophrenic patients. Acta Psychiatr Scand. 1995.

[34] Kim JS, Kornhuber HH, Schmid-Burgk W, Holzmüller B. Low cerebrospinal fluid glutamate in schizophrenic patients and a new

hypothesis on schizophrenia. Neurosci Lett. 1980.

[35] Gilmour G, Dix S, Fellini L, Gastambide F, Plath N, Steckler T, et al. NMDA receptors, cognition and schizophrenia - Testing the validity of the NMDA receptor hypofunction hypothesis. Neuropharmacology. 2012.

[36] Lin CH, Lane HY, Tsai GE. Glutamate signaling in the pathophysiology and therapy of schizophrenia. Pharmacol Biochem Behav. 2012 Feb 1;100(4):665-677.

[37] Long KD, Mastropaolo J, Rosse RB, Manaye KF, Deutsch SI. Modulatory effects of d-serine and sarcosine on NMDA receptor-mediated neurotransmission are apparent after stress in the genetically inbred BALB/c mouse strain. Brain Res Bull. 2006.

[38] Hui C, Tsai GE. Inhibition of Glycine Transporter-1 Improves the Functional Outcome of Schizophrenia. Brain Prot Schizophr Mood Cogn Disord. 2010;9789048185535:577-610.

[39] Grande I, Berk M, Birmaher B, Vieta E. Bipolar disorder. The Lancet. 2016.

[40] Chitty KM, Lagopoulos J, Lee RSC, Hickie IB, Hermens DF. A systematic review and meta-analysis of proton magnetic resonance spectroscopy and mismatch negativity in bipolar disorder. European Neuropsycho pharmacology. 2013.

[41] De Sousa RT, Loch AA, Carvalho AF, Brunoni AR, Haddad MR, Henter ID, et al. Genetic Studies on the Tripartite Glutamate Synapse in the Pathophysiology and Therapeutics of Mood Disorders. Neuropsychopharmacology. 2017.

[42] Andreasen JT, Gynther M, Rygaard A, Bøgelund T, Nielsen SD, Clausen RP, et al. Does increasing the ratio of AMPA-to-NMDA receptor mediated neurotransmission engender antidepressant action? Studies in the mouse forced swim and tail suspension tests. Neurosci Lett. 2013.

[43] Martucci L, Wong AHC, De Luca V, Likhodi O, Wong GWH, King N, et al. N-methyl-d-aspartate receptor NR2B subunit gene GRIN2B in schizophrenia and bipolar disorder: Polymorphisms and mRNA levels. Schizophr Res. 2006.

[44] Bandelow B, Michaelis S, Wedekind D. Treatment of anxiety disorders. Dialogues Clin Neurosci. 2017.

[45] Muscatello MR, Spina E, Bandelow B, Baldwin DS. Clinically relevant drug interactions in anxiety disorders. Human Psycho pharmacology. 2012.

[46] Stahl MMS, Lindquist M, Pettersson M, Edwards IR, Sanderson JH, Taylor NFA, et al. Withdrawal reactions with selective serotonin re-uptake inhibitors as reported to the WHO system. Eur J Clin Pharmacol. 1997.

[47] Tovote P, Fadok JP, Lüthi A. Neuronal circuits for fear and anxiety. Nature Reviews Neuroscience. 2015.

[48] Wolosker H, Balu DT. D-Serine as the gatekeeper of NMDA receptor activity: implications for the pharmacologic management of anxiety disorders. Translational Psychiatry. 2020.

[49] Barkus C, McHugh SB, Sprengel R, Seeburg PH, Rawlins JNP, Bannerman DM. Hippocampal NMDA receptors and anxiety: At the interface between cognition and emotion. European Journal of Pharmacology. 2010.

[50] Amaral OB, Roesler R. Targeting the NMDA receptor for fear-related

disorders. Recent patents on CNS drug discovery. 2008.

[51] Kalia L V., Kalia SK, Salter MW. NMDA receptors in clinical neurology: excitatory times ahead. Lancet Neurol. 2008 Aug;7(8):742-755.

[52] Małgorzata P, Paweł K, Iwona ML, Brzostek T, Andrzej P. Glutamatergic dysregulation in mood disorders: opportunities for the discovery of novel drug targets. Expert Opin Ther Targets. 2020;24(12):1187-209.

[53] Leiderman E, Zylberman I, Zukin SR, Cooper TB, Javitt DC. Preliminary investigation of high-dose oral glycine on serum levels and negative symptoms in schizophrenia: an open-label trial. Biol Psychiatry. 1996 Feb 1;39(3):213-215.

[54] Tsai GE, Yang P, Chang Y-C, Chong M-Y. D-Alanine Added to Antipsychotics for the Treatment of Schizophrenia. Biol Psychiatry. 2006 Feb 1;59(3):230-234.

[55] Tsai GE, Falk WE, Gunther J, Coyle JT. Improved cognition in Alzheimer's disease with short-term D-cycloserine treatment. Am J Psychiatry. 1999 Mar;156(3):467-469.

[56] Forsyth JK, Bachman P, Mathalon DH, Roach BJ, Ye E, Asarnow RF. Effects of Augmenting N-Methyl-D-Aspartate Receptor Signaling on Working Memory and Experience-Dependent Plasticity in Schizophrenia: An Exploratory Study Using Acute d-cycloserine. Schizophr Bull. 2017 Sep 1;43(5):1123-1133.

[57] Tiihonen J, Tanskanen A, Hoti F, Vattulainen P, Taipale H, Mehtälä J, et al. Pharmacological treatments and risk of readmission to hospital for unipolar depression in Finland: a nationwide cohort study. The Lancet Psychiatry. 2017 Jul 1;4(7):547-553.

[58] Gammon D, Cheng C, Volkovinskaia A, Baker GB, Dursun SM. Clozapine: Why Is It So Uniquely Effective in the Treatment of a Range of Neuropsychiatric Disorders? Biomolecules. 2021.

[59] Delgado A, Velosa J, Zhang J, Dursun SM, Kapczinski F, de Azevedo Cardoso T. Clozapine in bipolar disorder: A systematic review and meta-analysis. J Psychiatr Res. 2020 Jun 1;125:21-27.

[60] Lane H-Y, Lin C-H, Huang Y-J, Liao C-H, Chang Y-C, Tsai GE. A randomized, double-blind, placebo-controlled comparison study of sarcosine (N-methylglycine) and d-serine add-on treatment for schizophrenia. Int J Neuropsychopharmacol. 2010 May 1;13(4):451-460.

[61] Lin C-H, Chen P-K, Chang Y-C, Chuo L-J, Chen Y-S, Tsai GE, et al. Benzoate, a D-Amino Acid Oxidase Inhibitor, for the Treatment of Early-Phase Alzheimer Disease: A Randomized, Double-Blind, Placebo-Controlled Trial. Biol Psychiatry. 2014 May 1;75(9):678-685.

[62] Lai C-H, Lane H-Y, Tsai GE. Clinical and Cerebral Volumetric Effects of Sodium Benzoate, a D-Amino Acid Oxidase Inhibitor, in a Drug-Naïve Patient with Major Depression. Biol Psychiatry. 2012.

[63] O'Suilleabhain P, Dewey RB. A Randomized Trial of Amantadine in Huntington Disease. Arch Neurol. 2003 Jul 1;60(7):996-998.

[64] Herrmann N, Cappell J, Eryavec GM, Lanctôt KL. Changes in Nursing Burden Following Memantine for Agitation and Aggression in Long-Term Care Residents with Moderate to Severe Alzheimer's Disease. CNS Drugs . 2012 Aug 29;25(5):425-33.

[65] Vanle B, Olcott W, Jimenez J, Bashmi L, Danovitch I, IsHak WW.

NMDA antagonists for treating the non-motor symptoms in Parkinson's disease. Transl Psychiatry. 2018 Dec 1;8(1):117.

[66] Zarate CA, Singh JB, Quiroz JA, De Jesus G, Denicoff KK, Luckenbaugh DA, et al. A Double-Blind, Placebo-Controlled Study of Memantine in the Treatment of Major Depression. Am J Psychiatry. 2006 Jan 1;163(1):153-155.

[67] Zhand N, Attwood DG, Harvey PD. Glutamate modulators for treatment of schizophrenia. Pers Med Psychiatry. 2019 Jul 1;15-16:1-12.

[68] Anand A, Gunn AD, Barkay G, Karne HS, Nurnberger JI, Mathew SJ, et al. Early antidepressant effect of memantine during augmentation of lamotrigine inadequate response in bipolar depression: a double-blind, randomized, placebo-controlled trial. Bipolar Disord. 2012 Feb 1;14(1):64-70.

[69] Feusner J, Kerwin L, Saxena S, Bystritsky A. Differential efficacy of memantine for obsessive-compulsive disorder vs. generalized anxiety disorder: an open-label trial. Psychopharmacol Bull. 2009;42(1):81-93.

[70] Lee SY, Chen SL, Chang YH, Chen SH, Chu CH, Huang SY, et al. The DRD2/ANKK1 gene is associated with response to add-on dextromethorphan treatment in bipolar disorder. J Affect Disord. 2012 May 1;138(3):295-300.

[71] Kelly TF, Lieberman DZ. The utility of the combination of dextromethorphan and quinidine in the treatment of bipolar II and bipolar NOS. J Affect Disord. 2014 Oct 1;167:333-335.

[72] Domany Y, Bleich-Cohen M, Tarrasch R, Meidan R, Litvak-Lazar O, Stoppleman N, et al. Repeated oral ketamine for out-patient treatment of resistant depression: randomised, double-blind, placebo-controlled, proof-of-concept study. Br J Psychiatry. 2019 Jan 1;214(1):20-26.

[73] Zarate CA, Brutsche NE, Ibrahim L, Franco-Chaves J, Diazgranados N, Cravchik A, et al. Replication of Ketamine's Antidepressant Efficacy in Bipolar Depression: A Randomized Controlled Add-On Trial. Biol Psychiatry. 2012 Jun 1;71(11):939-946.

[74] Glue P, Medlicott NJ, Harland S, Neehoff S, Anderson-Fahey B, Le Nedelec M, et al. Ketamine's dose-related effects on anxiety symptoms in patients with treatment refractory anxiety disorders. J Psychopharmacol. 2017 Apr 26;31(10):1302-1305.

[75] Popova V, Daly EJ, Trivedi M, Cooper K, Lane R, Lim P, et al. Efficacy and Safety of Flexibly Dosed Esketamine Nasal Spray Combined With a Newly Initiated Oral Antidepressant in Treatment-Resistant Depression: A Randomized Double-Blind Active-Controlled Study. Am J Psychiatry. 2019 May 21;176(6):428-438.

[76] Rammes G. Neramexane: a moderate-affinity NMDA receptor channel blocker: new prospects and indications. Expert Rev Clin Pharmacol. 2014;2(3):231-8.

[77] Nagele P, Palanca BJ, Gott B, Brown F, Barnes L, Nguyen T, et al. A phase 2 trial of inhaled nitrous oxide for treatment-resistant major depression. Sci Transl Med. 2021 Jun 9;13(597).

[78] Solmi M, Veronese N, Zaninotto L, van der Loos MLM, Gao K, Schaffer A, et al. Lamotrigine compared to placebo and other agents with antidepressant activity in patients with unipolar and bipolar depression: a comprehensive meta-analysis of efficacy and safety outcomes in short-term trials. CNS Spectr. 2016 Oct 1;21(5):403-418.

[79] Matthews DC, Mao X, Dowd K, Tsakanikas D, Jiang CS, Meuser C, et al.

Riluzole, a glutamate modulator, slows cerebral glucose metabolism decline in patients with Alzheimer's disease. Brain. 2021 Jun 18.

[80] Mathew SJ, Amiel JM, Coplan JD, Fitterling HA, Sackeim HA, Gorman JM. Open-Label Trial of Riluzole in Generalized Anxiety Disorder. Am J Psychiatry. 2005 Dec 1;162(12):2379-2381.

[81] Collingridge GL, Volianskis A, Bannister N, France G, Hanna L, Mercier M, et al. The NMDA receptor as a target for cognitive enhancement. Neuropharmacology. 2013 Jan;64:13.

[82] Peyrovian B, Rosenblat JD, Pan Z, Iacobucci M, Brietzke E, McIntyre RS. The glycine site of NMDA receptors: A target for cognitive enhancement in psychiatric disorders. Prog Neuro-Psychopharmacology Biol Psychiatry. 2019;92:387-404.

[83] Tsai G, Yang P, Chung L-C, Lange N, Coyle JT. D-serine added to antipsychotics for the treatment of schizophrenia. Biol Psychiatry. 1998 Dec 1;44(11):1081-1089.

[84] Tsai GE, Yang P, Chung LC, Tsai IC, Tsai CW, Coyle JT. D-serine added to clozapine for the treatment of schizophrenia. Am J Psychiatry. 1999 Nov;156(11):1822-1825.

[85] Schade S, Paulus W. D-Cycloserine in Neuropsychiatric Diseases: A Systematic Review. Int J Neuropsychopharmacol. 2016 Apr 1;19(4):1-7.

[86] Schwartz BL, Hashtroudi S, Herting RL, Schwartz P, Deutsch SI. d-Cycloserine enhances implicit memory in Alzheimer patients. Neurology. 1996 Feb 1;46(2):420-424.

[87] Tsai GE, Falk WE, Gunther J. A preliminary study of D-cycloserine treatment in Alzheimer's disease. J Neuropsychiatry Clin Neurosci. 1998;10(2):224-226.

[88] Heresco-Levy U, Gelfin G, Bloch B, Levin R, Edelman S, Javitt DC, et al. A randomized add-on trial of high-dose d-cycloserine for treatment-resistant depression. Int J Neuropsycho pharmacol. 2013 Apr 1;16(3):501-506.

[89] Goff DC, Tsai G, Manoach DS, Coyle JT. Dose-finding trial of D-cycloserine added to neuroleptics for negative symptoms in schizophrenia. Am J Psychiatry. 1995;152(8):1213-1215.

[90] Goff DC, Herz L, Posever T, Shih V, Tsai G, Henderson DC, et al. A six-month, placebo-controlled trial of d-cycloserine co-administered with conventional antipsychotics in schizophrenia patients. Psychopharmacol. 2004 Oct 21;179(1):144-150.

[91] Baker JF, Cates ME, Luthin DR. D-cycloserine in the treatment of posttraumatic stress disorder. Ment Heal Clin. 2017;7(2):88-94.

[92] Fasipe OJ. The emergence of new antidepressants for clinical use: Agomelatine paradox versus other novel agents. IBRO Reports. 2019 Jun 1;6:95-110.

[93] Alberati D, Moreau JL, Lengyel J, Hauser N, Mory R, Borroni E, et al. Glycine reuptake inhibitor RG1678: A pharmacologic characterization of an investigational agent for the treatment of schizophrenia. Neuropharmacology. 2012 Feb 1;62(2):1152-1161.

[94] Bugarski-Kirola D, Iwata N, Sameljak S, Reid C, Blaettler T, Millar L, et al. Efficacy and safety of adjunctive bitopertin versus placebo in patients with suboptimally controlled symptoms of schizophrenia treated with antipsychotics: results from three phase 3, randomised, double-blind, parallel-group, placebo-controlled, multicentre

studies in the SearchLyte clinical trial programme. The Lancet Psychiatry. 2016 Dec 1;3(12):1115-1128.

[95] Lane H-Y, Huang C-L, Wu P-L, Liu Y-C, Chang Y-C, Lin P-Y, et al. Glycine Transporter I Inhibitor, N-methylglycine (Sarcosine), Added to Clozapine for the Treatment of Schizophrenia. Biol Psychiatry. 2006 Sep 15;60(6):645-649.

[96] Lin C-Y, Liang S-Y, Chang Y-C, Ting S-Y, Kao C-L, Wu Y-H, et al. Adjunctive sarcosine plus benzoate improved cognitive function in chronic schizophrenia patients with constant clinical symptoms: A randomised, double-blind, placebo-controlled trial. World J Biol Psychiatry. 2015 Jul 4;18(5):357-368.

[97] V. Ferraris D, Tsukamoto T. Recent Advances in the Discovery of D-Amino Acid Oxidase Inhibitors and Their Therapeutic Utility in Schizophrenia. Curr Pharm Des. 2011 Mar 21;17(2):103-111.

[98] Matsuura A, Fujita Y, Iyo M, Hashimoto K. Effects of sodium benzoate on pre-pulse inhibition deficits and hyperlocomotion in mice after administration of phencyclidine. Acta Neuropsychiatr. 2015 Jan 20;27(3):159-167.

[99] Lane H-Y, Lin C-H, Green MF, Hellemann G, Huang C-C, Chen P-W, et al. Add-on Treatment of Benzoate for Schizophrenia: A Randomized, Double-blind, Placebo-Controlled Trial of d-Amino Acid Oxidase Inhibitor. JAMA Psychiatry. 2013 Dec 1;70(12): 1267-1275.

[100] Paoletti P, Bellone C, Zhou Q. NMDA receptor subunit diversity: Impact on receptor properties, synaptic plasticity and disease. Nat Rev Neurosci. 2013;14(6):383-400.

[101] Murrough JW, Abdallah CG, Mathew SJ. Targeting glutamate signalling in depression: Progress and prospects. Nat Rev Drug Discov. 2017;16(7):472-486.

[102] Kemp JA, Foster AC, Leeson PD, Priestley T, Tridgett R, Iversen LL, et al. 7-Chlorokynurenic acid is a selective antagonist at the glycine modulatory site of the N-methyl-D-aspartate receptor complex. Proc Natl Acad Sci U S A. 1988;85(17):6547.

[103] Zanos P, Piantadosi SC, Wu H-Q, Pribut HJ, Dell MJ, Can A, et al. The Prodrug 4-Chlorokynurenine Causes Ketamine-Like Antidepressant Effects, but Not Side Effects, by NMDA/GlycineB-Site Inhibition. J Pharmacol Exp Ther. 2015 Oct 1;355(1):76-85.

[104] Park LT, Kadriu B, Gould TD, Zanos P, Greenstein D, Evans JW, et al. A Randomized Trial of the N-Methyl-d-Aspartate Receptor Glycine Site Antagonist Prodrug 4-Chlorokynurenine in Treatment-Resistant Depression. Int J Neuropsychopharmacol. 2020 Jul 29;23(7):417-425.

[105] Doody RS, Gavrilova SI, Sano M, Thomas RG, Aisen PS, Bachurin SO, et al. Effect of dimebon on cognition, activities of daily living, behaviour, and global function in patients with mild-to-moderate Alzheimer's disease: a randomised, double-blind, placebo-controlled study. Lancet (London, England). 2008;372(9634):207-15.

[106] Kieburtz K, McDermott MP, Voss TS, Corey-Bloom J, Deuel LM, Dorsey ER, et al. A randomized, placebo-controlled trial of latrepirdine in Huntington disease. Arch Neurol. 2010 Feb;67(2):154-160.

[107] Fogaça M V., Fukumoto K, Franklin T, Liu RJ, Duman CH, Vitolo O V., et al. N-Methyl-D-aspartate receptor antagonist d-methadone produces rapid, mTORC1-dependent antidepressant effects. Neuropsychopharmacology. 2019.

[108] Ibrahim L, Diazgranados N, Jolkovsky L, Brutsche N, Luckenbaugh DA, Joseph Herring W, et al. A randomized, placebo-controlled, crossover pilot trial of the oral selective NR2B antagonist MK-0657 in patients with treatment-resistant major depressive disorder. J Clin Psychopharmacol. 2012 Aug;32(4):551-557.

[109] Ory-Magne F, Corvol J-C, Azulay J-P, Bonnet A-M, Brefel-Courbon C, Damier P, et al. Withdrawing amantadine in dyskinetic patients with Parkinson disease. Neurology. 2014 Jan 28;82(4):300-307.

[110] Rammes G, Danysz W, Parsons CG. Pharmacodynamics of Memantine: An Update. Curr Neuropharmacol. 2008 Mar 4;6(1):55-78.

[111] Ballard C, Thomas A, Gerry S, Yu L-M, Aarsland D, Merritt C, et al. A double-blind randomized placebo-controlled withdrawal trial comparing memantine and antipsychotics for the long-term treatment of function and neuropsychiatric symptoms in people with Alzheimer's disease (MAIN-AD). J Am Med Dir Assoc. 2015;16(4):316-322.

[112] Taylor CP, Traynelis SF, Siffert J, Pope LE, Matsumoto RR. Pharmacology of dextromethorphan: Relevance to dextromethorphan/ quinidine (Nuedexta®) clinical use. Pharmacol Ther. 2016 Aug 1;164:170-182.

[113] Garay RP, Grossberg GT. AVP-786 for the treatment of agitation in dementia of the Alzheimer's type. Expert Opin Investig Drugs. 2017 Jan 2;26(1):121-32.

[114] Hecking J, Davoudian PA, Wilkinson ST. Emerging Therapeutics Based on the Amino Acid Neurotransmitter System: An Update on the Pharmaceutical Pipeline for Mood Disorders. Chronic stress (Thousand Oaks). 2021 Jun 2;5.

[115] Ochs-Ross R, Daly EJ, Zhang Y, Lane R, Lim P, Foster K, et al. S114. Efficacy and Safety of Intranasal Esketamine Plus an Oral Antidepressant in Elderly Patients With Treatment-Resistant Depression. Biol Psychiatry. 2018 May 1;83(9):S391.

[116] Morris PJ, Moaddel R, Zanos P, Moore CE, Gould TD, Zarate CA, et al. Synthesis and N-Methyl-d-aspartate (NMDA) Receptor Activity of Ketamine Metabolites. Org Lett. 2017 Sep 1;19(17):4572-4575.

[117] Leal GC, Bandeira ID, Correia-Melo FS, Telles M, Mello RP, Vieira F, et al. Intravenous arketamine for treatment-resistant depression: open-label pilot study. Eur Arch Psychiatry Clin Neurosci. 2020 Feb 20;271(3):577-582.

[118] Jevtović-Todorović V, Todorovć SM, Mennerick S, Powell S, Dikranian K, Benshoff N, et al. Nitrous oxide (laughing gas) is an NMDA antagonist, neuroprotectant and neurotoxin. Nat Med. 1998 Apr;4(4):460-463.

[119] Grunze H, von Wegerer J, Greene RW, Walden J. Modulation of Calcium and Potassium Currents by Lamotrigine. Neuropsychobiology. 1998 Oct;38(3):131-138.

[120] Zarate CA, Manji HK. Riluzole in psychiatry: a systematic review of the literature. Expert Opin Drug Metab Toxicol. 2008 Sep;4(9):1223-1234.

[121] Abdallah CG, Coplan JD, Jackowski A, Sato JR, Mao X, Shungu DC, et al. A pilot study of hippocampal volume and N-acetylaspartate (NAA) as response biomarkers in riluzole-treated patients with GAD. Eur Neuropsychopharmacol. 2013 Apr 1;23(4):276-284.

Chapter 10

Emergence of Ketamine as a Rapid Acting Antidepressant: Mechanistic Insights and Future Directions

Atamjit Singh and Preet Mohinder Singh Bedi

Abstract

Ketamine is a phencyclidine derivative and N-methyl-D-aspartate receptor antagonist, widely popular as a dissociative anesthetic. Its use as an anesthetic in humans was progressively fallen out due to its associated adverse effects and the emergence of newer and safer anesthetics. In recent few decades, various reports related to its efficacy in the treatment of resistant depression with anti-suicidal potential draw significant attention from researchers around the globe. The rapid clinical effect of ketamine within hours as compared to traditional antidepressants that take several weeks makes it a hot topic in antidepressant research. Studies conducted in the recent past suggest its mechanism of action through glutamate modulation via receptors like NMDA, AMPA as well as downregulation of BDNF etc. This chapter will shed light on the various mechanisms of ketamine related to antidepressant activity. Along with that its pharmacokinetics, toxicology and ongoing clinical trials will also be discussed.

Keywords: ketamine, depression, antidepressant, NMDA, BDNF

1. Introduction

From last few decades with rapid development and modernization, significant improvements in the lifestyle of humans has been observed but with pros there are associated cons and so is major depressive disorder (MDD) which is affecting teenagers to adults and majorly observed in young working professionals. It is emerging as major contributor in global disease burden and reported as the second leading causes for disability [1]. According to the study conducted by mental health in Canada, MDD has lifetime prevalence of 11.3% [2]. Besides being a major challenge for healthcare system its pathophysiology is still not uncovered completely. One hypothesis based on monoamines suggest that it may resulted from functional deficiency of neurotransmitters named serotonin and/or noradrenaline which is widely utilized for categorization of antidepressant drugs [3]. But conflict is also standstill with the time frame of the effect and dose administration as clinical symptoms are observed after several weeks from the onset of therapy and only half are noted to have actual clinical response [4–7]. Apart from that one-third patients suffers from treatment resistant depression (TRD) that are nonresponsive to currently approved medications [8]. Non-responsiveness of currently available therapy especially for TRD arise the emergency need of more effective and safer antidepressant therapy.

Ketamine is a phencyclidine derivative and N-methyl-D-aspartate (NMDA) receptor antagonist, widely popular as a dissociative anesthetic. Ketamine was first reported for its efficacy in depression in year 2000, when sub-anesthetic intravenous dose of ketamine rapidly reduced the symptoms of MDD and effect continued up to 72 hours [9]. Taking lead from this, further clinical trials were conducted which showcase its efficacy in TRD patients with 60–70% response rate [10–14]. Onset of action was reported within 2–4 hours and last for 1 week with singe infusion while repeated infusions have effect up to 18–19 days. Clinical data also suggest the responsiveness of ketamine up to 44% on patients with comorbidities and ultra-resistant depression [15, 16]. In addition to this ketamine has been reported for its anti-suicidal and anti-anhedonic properties [14, 17, 18]. All this reports points toward the different mechanism of ketamine form traditional antidepressants.

2. Basic chemistry, pharmacology and pharmacokinetics of ketamine

Recently discovered antidepressant and anti-suicidal action of ketamine significantly attracted the researchers working in the field of psychiatry [9, 11, 19]. Ketamine is a phencyclidine derivative and a mixture of R(−) and S(+) enantiomers. Both R(−) and S(+) enantiomers has been explored widely and it was observed that S(+) enantiomer has higher potency than R(−) enantiomer (R-ketamine) for phencyclidine site on glutamate NMDA receptor along with stronger analgesic activity [20–24]. Inspired form these outputs, S(+) enantiomer also known as esketamine is now under investigations for antidepressant potential [25]. However

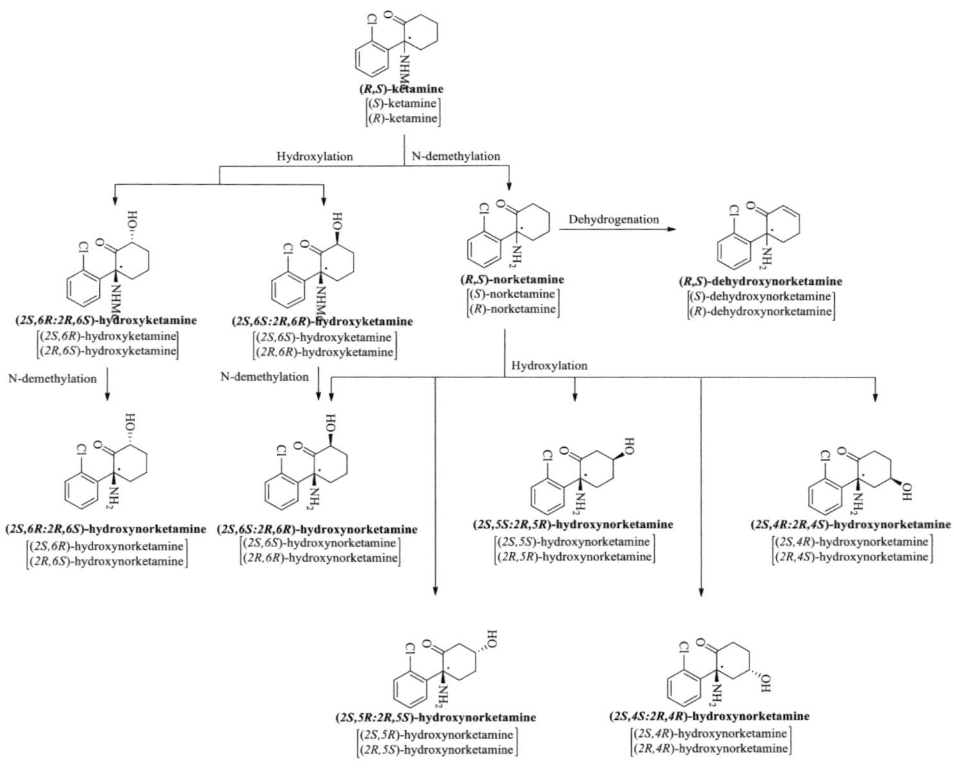

Figure 1.
General layout of metabolic pathway of ketamine showcasing stereoseletive metabolism through various cytochrome P450 enzymes.

conflict between these two is also exist with the side effects profile of both enantiomers related to dissociation, psychoses and cognition [26]. Reports suggest the rapid onset of antidepressant effects with R-ketamine but higher side effects than esketamine [27–34]. Ketamine undergo metabolism through CYP2B6- and CYP3A4-mediated N-demethylation resulting norketamine which further catabolized into hydroxynorketamines (HNKs) and dehyronorketamine (**Figure 1**). Investigations was also carried out on metabolites of ketamine. 2R,6R-HNK has been observed to have antidepressant like efficacy with nil side effects on rat models while several contradictory reports are also available [35–43]. Specifically, metabolite of esketamine i.e. S-norketamine showed antidepressant like properties with lesser side effects as with esketamine [44]. When talk about bioavailability, ketamine has varying bioavailability profile with different routes i.e. 100% with intravenous, 45% with intranasal, 30% with sublingual, 20% with oral, 93% with intramuscular while 30% with rectal route [24, 30, 44].

3. Overview of the status of clinical trials with ketamine and its enantiomers

Report on antidepressant efficacy of ketamine by Berman group in 2000 [9] initiated series of studies related to antidepressant activity of ketamine all around the globe. Multiple meta-analysis now established the candidature of ketamine against major depressive episodes in both bipolar as well as unipolar depression while efficacy was higher in unipolar as compared to bipolar depression [45–50]. In addition to this, numerous studies reported its effect last up to a week only for unipolar while it is up to 3–4 days in case of bipolar depression [46, 47, 49]. Randomized Controlled trials (RCT) exist in which effect of repeated infusions of ketamine for depression is studied but there is still lack of long term trial [51–53]. Studies on different routes of administration were also conducted that majorly include intranasal, sublingual and intramuscular [54–57]. In fact intranasal esketaminerecently got FDA clearance for TRD which was based on three acute-phase and two maintenance phase studies. These acute studies were conducted on severely depressed patients [58]. Maintenance trials were conducted up to 88 weeks where patient was administered esketamine weekly or every second week showcase reduced after relapse risk and also assured safety up to a year [59, 60]. A phase three trial consisted of 200 patients suggest the significant improvements in depression with ketamine adjuvant to an antidepressant [61]. There is another 5 year ongoing trial by Janssen for safety [62]. Keeping in view the antidepressant efficacy if R-ketamine, a phase I trial was started by Perception Pharmaceuticals but results are not processed yet [28].

4. Mechanistic insight into the antidepressant activity of ketamine

4.1 AMPA, BDNF and mTOR

Glutamate is one of the major excitatory neurotransmitters in central nervous system of human body that mainly acts on NMDA, ionotropic α-amino-3-hydroxy-5-methyl-4-isoxazolepropionic acid (AMPA) receptors (co-localized with NMDA) and metabotropic glutamate receptors. Glutamate activates AMPA receptors at synaptic cleft, which permit the entry of sodium ions into postsynaptic membrane. Entry of sodium ions results in depolarization of postsynaptic membrane that cause removal of NMDA receptor channel voltage-dependent magnesium ion block that activate NMDA receptor which allow the entry of sodium as well as calcium ions. Ketamine is a well-established non-competitive type NMDA receptor antagonist. Brain-derived neurotrophic factor (BDNF) and mTOR are two major proteins that are suspected to be involved in mechanistic window of ketamine. BDNF is a growth factor protein in central nervous system that promote neurogenesis and synaptogenesis along with support in survival of existing neurons. On the other hand, mTOR is suggested to have major role in neuronal development and circuit formation. mTOR further made two sub complexes known as mTOR complex 1 (mTORC1) and mTOR, from which mTORC1 is a target of ketamine [63, 64].

It has been observe that glutamatergic neurotransmission is deregulated in MDD and enhanced levels of glutamate levels in serum and plasma were observed in patient's dealing with MDD that why plasma glutamate levels are directly correlated with severity of depression [65–68]. Enhanced glutamate cause by loss of glial cells in MDD increases extra synaptic glutamate levels that suppressglutamatergic neurotransmission via activation of metabotropic glutamate receptor 2 (mGluR2) autoreceptors. A study suggest that change in depression symptoms by non-ketamine NMDA receptor antagonists like traxoprodil, lanicemine and rapastinel was much lower ass compared to ketamine [34, 69–71]. Ketamine good antagonistic activity for NMDA receptors present on γ-aminobutyric acid (GABA) that prevent activation of GABA interneurons resulting in downstream disinhibition of glutamatergic neurons that cause glutamate surge. Elevated levels of glutamate initiates activation of postsynaptic AMPA receptors that potentiate BDNF andmTORC1 signaling pathways. Ketamine demonstrated activate glutamate release and transmission in rat prefrontal cortex (RPC) [72]. Ketamine was also observed to enhance AMPA-evoked electrophysiological responses in the rat hippocampus and medial PFC pointing toward the involvement of ketamine in AMPA receptor transmission [73–77]. In a mouse model, ketamine was observed to increase the expression levels of two subunits of AMPA receptor known as GluA1 and GluA2 [34, 78].

Increased levels of BDNF and mTOR in rat hippocampus were observed within 30 minutes of treatment with ketamine [73, 79, 80]. Important to mention here that analgesic tramadol enhanced the effect of ketamine on force swim test along with upregulation of mTOR in the PFC and hippocampus of rat [81]. It is interesting to observe that increased BDNF and mTOR levels in hippocampal and RFC are controlled by AMPA because in a study treatment with AMPA receptor antagonist increased forced-swim test immobility time with reduced levels of BDNF and mTOR while with agonist immobility time reduced along with increased levels of both BDNF and mTOR [82]. Reports were also observed that suggest the nullification of antidepressant activity of ketamine with pre-treatment of rapamycin an mTORC1 inhibitor [83].

Numerous reports are present in the literature suggesting the possibility of ketamine's antidepressant activity via BDNF. No antidepressant activity was observed on treatment of ketamine in genetically modified mice lacking BDNF [73]. It is proposed that antagonism of NMDA through ketamine deactivates the eukaryotic elongation of factor 2 (eEF2) kinase that de-supress the translation of BDNF. Mice having Val66Met single-nucleotide polymorphism in BDNF gene showed impairment in BDNF release and mRNA trafficking. Administration of ketamine in these mice showed reduced antidepressant activity [84]. Reversal of anhedonicbehaviour with ketamine was observed in rats with chronic mild stress along with complete restoration of dendritic atrophy and dendritiv BDNF mRNA trafficking [85]. In social defeat stress model of mice, ketamine lessen reduction in BDNF, spine density of dendrites, synaptogenesis markers (GluA1 and PSD-95) in PFC, CA3 and dentate gyrus region of hippocampus at 8th day of treatment [86]. Elevated levels of BDNF were supposed to be associated with the lower severity

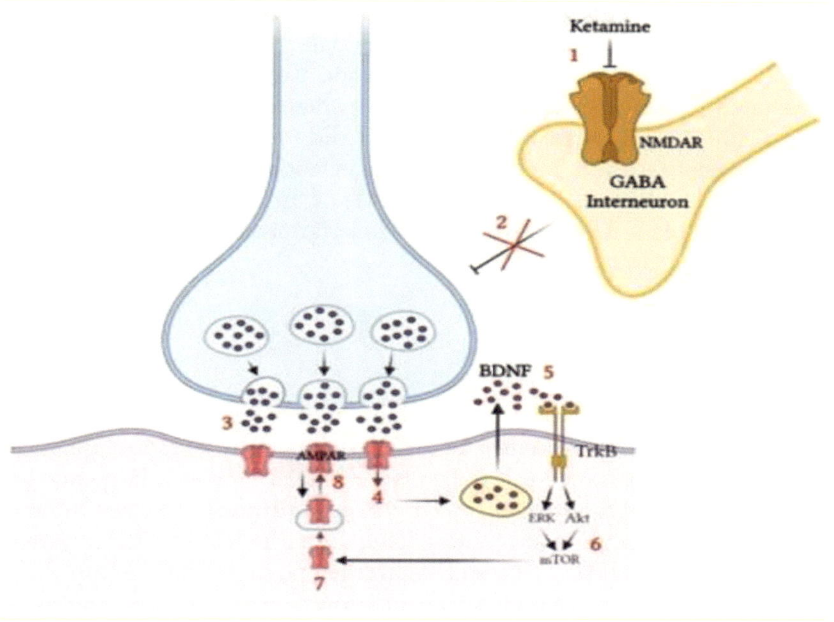

Figure 2.
Flow diagram of antidepressant activity of ketamine. (1) ketamine binds with N-methyl-d-aspartate receptors (NMDARs) and reduce excitability of γ-aminobutyric acid (GABA) ergic interneurons that results, (2) non-inhibition of glutamatergic neurons, (3) that further increase glutamate release which binds with α-amino-3-hydroxy-5-methyl-4-isoxazole-propionic acid (AMPA) receptors resulting inflow of sodium and calcium into cell, (4) cause activation of voltage gated calcium channels, (5) that further triggers the release of brain-derived neurotrophic factor (BDNF) into glutamate synapse. (6) BDNF from synapse binds with tropomyosin receptor kinase B (TrkB) resulting activation of MEK–ERK and PI3K-Akt signaling cascades that converge on to mTOR lead to (7) increased synaptic protein translation. (8) increased proteins in synapse lead to increased AMPAR-mediated synaptic transmission causing elevated synaptogenesis. All these events are hypothesized to restore disrupted connectivity between key brain regions and can be the possible reason of rapid and sustained antidepressant action of ketamine.

of depression like symptoms on rating scale [87, 88]. A study carried out on three depressed patients, suggest their response to ketamine and have increased levels of plasma mTOR expression and eEF2 phosphorylaton [89]. It is worth to note that in a trial conducted on 20 patients, pre-treatment with rapamycin tripled the response rate after 2 weeks from treatment thus may be due to targeting of rapamycin on neuroinflammation through its immunisupressant activity or may be due to promotion of haemostatsis of synaptic density (**Figure 2**) [90].

4.2 D-serine

D-serine is a potential co-agonist at NMDA receptor which is a possible biomarker in depression. Numerous studies highlighted the abnormality of D-serine levels in depression highlighting the antidepressant properties of D-serine [91–95]. Ketamine was found to inhibitor the transport of D-serine while ketamine metabolites were observed to decrease intracellular (PC-12 cells) concentrations of D-serine thus increasing plasma D-serine levels which is possible prediction related to its to antidepressant action [96–99].

4.3 Opioid system

Ketamine also have capability to bind with opioid receptors (mu, delta and kappa), monoaminergic receptors and transporters, and muscarinic and nicotinic cholinergic receptors [100]. Proposition is made that anti-suicidal as well as antidepressant actions of ketamine is related to the opioid system which is confirmed from the pre-treatment of naltrexone after that antidepressant effect was attenuated in patients [100, 101]. However many discrepancies are also exist along with [102, 103] because buprenorphine and methadone both are agonists to the opioid receptors and does not have any effect on antidepressant properties of ketamine [103]. These results rebels the role of opioid system in ketamine's antidepressant effects. Thus role of opioid in ketamine's antidepressant effects is yet unclear and controversial.

5. Future trends

With unique mechanism of action as compared to traditional antidepressants along with anti-suicidal properties, ketamine successfully attracted the researchers and physiologists toward itself in last two decades. However large mechanism of actions are still need to uncover thus it will be continue to be a hot topic and active area of research in psychiatry. There if a dire need to investigate the appropriate safety to efficacy ration of ketamine in depression therapy along with establishment of appropriate regimens for maintenance of therapy and discontinuation too. Reliable biomarkers are also needed to properly predict the response and adverse effects of ketamine. Numerous reports are also present in literature that caution the utilization of ketamine as an antidepressant in clinical practice [76, 104–108]. Keeping these thing apart, currently ketamine is emerging as a promising approach for treatment of patients suffering from TRD. Ketamine and its related neurochemical biomarkers can act as leads for development of future antidepressants.

6. Conclusion

Rapid antidepressant effect of ketamine depression therapy and important discovery in depression research. Its efficacy against TRD and anti-suicidal potential is a boon in depression research but at the same time its negative side effects and potential for being abuse is not to be neglected. However pathways like BDNF, mTOR, AMPA along D-serine and opioid receptors provided sufficient understanding but large portion of its mechanisms are still need to uncover. Even some studies create conflict to each other which is needed to be resolved. Overall analysis suggest that there is an important need to discover all aspects of ketamine in depression therapy to efficient use of this drug as an antidepressant in clinical practice. Moreover, ketamine can act as a lead for the development of new class of rapidly acting future antidepressant agents.

Acknowledgements

The authors are also thankful to Guru Nanak Dev University, Amritsar for providing various facilities to carry out the work.

Conflict of interest

The authors declare no conflict of interest.

Author details

Atamjit Singh[1] and Preet Mohinder Singh Bedi[1,2]*

1 Department of Pharmaceutical Sciences, Guru Nanak Dev University, Amritsar, Punjab, India

2 Drug and Pollution Testing Laboratory, Guru Nanak Dev University, Amritsar, Punjab, India

*Address all correspondence to: preet.pharma@gndu.ac.in

References

[1] Ferrari AJ, Charlson FJ, Norman RE, Patten SB, Freedman G, Murray CJ, Vos T, Whiteford HA. Burden of depressive disorders by country, sex, age, and year: Findings from the global burden of disease study 2010. PLoS medicine. 2013 Nov 5;10(11):e1001547.

[2] Patten SB, Williams JV, Lavorato DH, Wang JL, McDonald K, Bulloch AG. Descriptive epidemiology of major depressive disorder in Canada in 2012. The Canadian Journal of Psychiatry. 2015 Jan;60(1):23-30.

[3] Matveychuk D, Thomas RK, Swainson J, Khullar A, MacKay MA, Baker GB, Dursun SM. Ketamine as an antidepressant: Overview of its mechanisms of action and potential predictive biomarkers. Therapeutic Advances in Psychopharmacology. 2020 May;10:2045125320916657.

[4] Hirschfeld RM. History and evolution of the monoamine hypothesis of depression. Journal of clinical psychiatry. 2000 Mar 31;61(6):4-6.

[5] Liu B, Liu J, Wang M, Zhang Y, Li L. From serotonin to neuroplasticity: Evolvement of theories for major depressive disorder. Frontiers in cellular neuroscience. 2017 Sep 28;11:305.

[6] Undurraga J, Baldessarini RJ. Randomized, placebo-controlled trials of antidepressants for acute major depression: Thirty-year meta-analytic review. Neuropsychopharmacology. 2012 Mar;37(4):851-864.

[7] Fava M, Davidson KG. Definition and epidemiology of treatment-resistant depression. Psychiatric Clinics of North America. 1996 Jun 1;19(2):179-200.

[8] Nemeroff CB. Prevalence and management of treatment-resistant depression. Journal of Clinical Psychiatry. 2007 Jul 16;68(8):17.

[9] Berman RM, Cappiello A, Anand A, Oren DA, Heninger GR, Charney DS, Krystal JH. Antidepressant effects of ketamine in depressed patients. Biological psychiatry. 2000 Feb 15;47(4):351-354.

[10] Murrough JW, Iosifescu DV, Chang LC, Al Jurdi RK, Green CE, Perez AM, Iqbal S, Pillemer S, Foulkes A, Shah A, Charney DS. Antidepressant efficacy of ketamine in treatment-resistant major depression: A two-site randomized controlled trial. American Journal of Psychiatry. 2013 Oct;170(10):1134-1142.

[11] Zarate CA, Singh JB, Carlson PJ, Brutsche NE, Ameli R, Luckenbaugh DA, Charney DS, Manji HK. A randomized trial of an N-methyl-D-aspartate antagonist in treatment-resistant major depression. Archives of general psychiatry. 2006 Aug 1;63(8):856-864.

[12] Diazgranados N, Ibrahim L, Brutsche NE, Newberg A, Kronstein P, Khalife S, Kammerer WA, Quezado Z, Luckenbaugh DA, Salvadore G, Machado-Vieira R. a randomized add-on trial of an N-methyl-D-aspartate antagonist in treatment-resistant bipolar depression. Archives of general psychiatry. 2010 Aug 1;67(8):793-802.

[13] Coyle CM, Laws KR. The use of ketamine as an antidepressant: A systematic review and meta-analysis. Human Psychopharmacology: Clinical and Experimental. 2015 May;30(3): 152-163.

[14] Wilkinson ST, Ballard ED, Bloch MH, Mathew SJ, Murrough JW, Feder A, Sos P, Wang G, Zarate Jr CA, Sanacora G. The effect of a single dose of intravenous ketamine on suicidal ideation: A systematic review and individual participant data meta-analysis. American journal of psychiatry. 2018 Feb 1;175(2):150-158.

[15] Thomas RK, Baker G, Lind J, Dursun S. Rapid effectiveness of intravenous ketamine for ultraresistant depression in a clinical setting and evidence for baseline anhedonia and bipolarity as clinical predictors of effectiveness. Journal of psychopharmacology. 2018 Oct;32(10): 1110-1117.

[16] Thomas, R., Baker, G. and Dursun, S., 2017, November. Rapid Efficacy and Antisuicidal Actions of Intravenous Ketamine for Ultraresistant Depression in a Clinical Setting: A Retrospective, Database Study. In Neuropsychopharmacology (Vol. 43, Pp. S174-S174). Macmillan Building, 4 Crinan St, London N1 9xw, England: Nature Publishing Group.

[17] Grunebaum MF, Galfalvy HC, Choo TH, Keilp JG, Moitra VK, Parris MS, Marver JE, Burke AK, Milak MS, Sublette ME, Oquendo MA. Ketamine for rapid reduction of suicidal thoughts in major depression: A midazolam-controlled randomized clinical trial. American Journal of Psychiatry. 2018 Apr 1;175(4):327-335.

[18] Zanos P, Thompson SM, Duman RS, Zarate CA, Gould TD. Convergent mechanisms underlying rapid antidepressant action. CNS drugs. 2018 Mar;32(3):197-227.

[19] DiazGranados N, Ibrahim LA, Brutsche NE, Ameli R, Henter ID, Luckenbaugh DA, Machado-Vieira R, Zarate Jr CA. Rapid resolution of suicidal ideation after a single infusion of an N-methyl-D-aspartate antagonist in patients with treatment-resistant major depressive disorder. The Journal of clinical psychiatry. 2010 Jul 13;71(12):1605-1611.

[20] Muller J, Pentyala S, Dilger J, Pentyala S. Ketamine enantiomers in the rapid and sustained antidepressant effects. Therapeutic advances in psychopharmacology. 2016 Jun;6(3):185-192.

[21] Pfenninger EG, Durieux ME, Himmelseher S. Cognitive impairment after small-dose ketamine isomers in comparison to equianalgesic racemic ketamine in human volunteers. The Journal of the American Society of Anesthesiologists. 2002 Feb 1;96(2): 357-366.

[22] Andrade C. Ketamine for depression, 3: Does chirality matter?. The Journal of clinical psychiatry. 2017 Jun 28;78(6): e674-e676.

[23] Muller J, Pentyala S, Dilger J, Pentyala S. Ketamine enantiomers in the rapid and sustained antidepressant effects. Therapeutic advances in psychopharmacology. 2016 Jun;6(3): 185-192.

[24] Peltoniemi MA, Hagelberg NM, Olkkola KT, Saari TI. Ketamine: A review of clinical pharmacokinetics and pharmacodynamics in anesthesia and pain therapy. Clinical pharmacokinetics. 2016 Sep;55(9):1059-1077.

[25] Kim J, Farchione T, Potter A, Chen Q, Temple R. Esketamine for treatment-resistant depression-first FDA-approved antidepressant in a new class. N Engl J Med. 2019 Jul 4;381(1):1-4.

[26] Hashimoto K. Rapid-acting antidepressant ketamine, its metabolites and other candidates: A historical overview and future perspective. Psychiatry and clinical neurosciences. 2019 Oct;73(10):613-627.

[27] Lane RM, Baker GB. Chirality and drugs used in psychiatry: Nice to know or need to know?. Cellular and molecular neurobiology. 1999 Jun;19(3):355-372.

[28] Hashimoto K, Yang C. Is (S)-norketamine an alternative antidepressant for esketamine?. European archives of psychiatry and clinical neuroscience. 2019 Oct;269(7):867-868.

[29] Zhang JC, Li SX, Hashimoto K. R (−)-ketamine shows greater potency

and longer lasting antidepressant effects than S (+)-ketamine. Pharmacology Biochemistry and Behavior. 2014 Jan 1;116:137-141.

[30] Yang C, Shirayama Y, Zhang JC, Ren Q, Yao W, Ma M, Dong C, Hashimoto K. R-ketamine: A rapid-onset and sustained antidepressant without psychotomimetic side effects. Translational psychiatry. 2015 Sep;5(9):e632.

[31] Yang C, Han M, Zhang JC, Ren Q, Hashimoto K. Loss of parvalbumin-immunoreactivity in mouse brain regions after repeated intermittent administration of esketamine, but not R-ketamine. Psychiatry research. 2016 May 30;239:281-283.

[32] Fukumoto K, Toki H, Iijima M, Hashihayata T, Yamaguchi JI, Hashimoto K, Chaki S. Antidepressant potential of (R)-ketamine in rodent models: Comparison with (S)-ketamine. Journal of Pharmacology and Experimental Therapeutics. 2017 Apr 1;361(1):9-16.

[33] Hashimoto K, Kakiuchi T, Ohba H, Nishiyama S, Tsukada H. Reduction of dopamine D 2/3 receptor binding in the striatum after a single administration of esketamine, but not R-ketamine: A PET study in conscious monkeys. European archives of psychiatry and clinical neuroscience. 2017 Mar 1;267(2):173-176.

[34] Yang C, Yang J, Luo A, Hashimoto K. Molecular and cellular mechanisms underlying the antidepressant effects of ketamine enantiomers and its metabolites. Translational psychiatry. 2019 Nov 7;9(1):1-1.

[35] Zanos P, Moaddel R, Morris PJ, Georgiou P, Fischell J, Elmer GI, Alkondon M, Yuan P, Pribut HJ, Singh NS, Dossou KS. NMDAR inhibition-independent antidepressant actions of ketamine metabolites. Nature. 2016 May;533(7604):481-486.

[36] Chaki S. Is metabolism of (R)-ketamine essential for the antidepressant effects?. International Journal of Neuropsychopharmacology. 2018 Feb;21(2):154-156.

[37] Li L, Vlisides PE. Ketamine: 50 years of modulating the mind. Frontiers in human neuroscience. 2016 Nov 29;10:612.

[38] Mion G, Villevieille T. Ketamine pharmacology: An update (pharmacodynamics and molecular aspects, recent findings). CNS neuroscience & therapeutics. 2013 Jun;19(6):370-380.

[39] Zanos P, Highland JN, Liu X, Troppoli TA, Georgiou P, Lovett J, Morris PJ, Stewart BW, Thomas CJ, Thompson SM, Moaddel R. (R)-ketamine exerts antidepressant actions partly via conversion to (2R, 6R)-hydroxynor-ketamine, while causing adverse effects at sub-anaesthetic doses. British journal of pharmacology. 2019 Jul;176(14): 2573-2592.

[40] Fukumoto K, Fogaça MV, Liu RJ, Duman C, Kato T, Li XY, Duman RS. Activity-dependent brain-derived neurotrophic factor signaling is required for the antidepressant actions of (2R, 6R)-hydroxynorketamine. Proceedings of the National Academy of Sciences. 2019 Jan 2;116(1):297-302.

[41] Chou D, Peng HY, Lin TB, Lai CY, Hsieh MC, Wen YC, Lee AS, Wang HH, Yang PS, Chen GD, Ho YC. (2R, 6R)-hydroxynorketamine rescues chronic stress-induced depression-like behavior through its actions in the midbrain periaqueductal gray. Neuropharmacology. 2018 Sep 1;139:1-2.

[42] Xiong Z, Fujita Y, Zhang K, Pu Y, Chang L, Ma M, Chen J, Hashimoto K. Beneficial effects of (R)-ketamine, but not its metabolite (2R, 6R)-hydroxynor-ketamine, in the depression-like phenotype, inflammatory bone markers, and bone mineral density in a

chronic social defeat stress model. Behavioural brain research. 2019 Aug 5;368:111904.

[43] Yamaguchi JI, Toki H, Qu Y, Yang C, Koike H, Hashimoto K, Mizuno-Yasuhira A, Chaki S. (2 R, 6 R)-Hydroxynorketamine is not essential for the antidepressant actions of (R)-ketamine in mice. Neuropsychopharmacology. 2018 Aug;43(9): 1900-1907.

[44] Yang Y, Cui Y, Sang K, Dong Y, Ni Z, Ma S, Hu H. ketamine blocks bursting in the lateral habenula to rapidly relieve depression. Nature. 2018 Feb;554(7692): 317-322.

[45] Zhang K, Hashimoto K. An update on ketamine and its two enantiomers as rapid-acting antidepressants. Expert review of neurotherapeutics. 2019 Jan 2;19(1):83-92.

[46] Kishimoto T, Chawla JM, Hagi K, Zarate CA, Kane JM, Bauer M, Correll CU. Single-dose infusion ketamine and non-ketamine N-methyl-d-aspartate receptor antagonists for unipolar and bipolar depression: A meta-analysis of efficacy, safety and time trajectories. Psychological medicine. 2016 May;46(7):1459-1472.

[47] Lee EE, Della Selva MP, Liu A, Himelhoch S. Ketamine as a novel treatment for major depressive disorder and bipolar depression: A systematic review and quantitative meta-analysis. General hospital psychiatry. 2015 Mar 1;37(2):178-184.

[48] McGirr A, Berlim MT, Bond DJ, Fleck MP, Yatham LN, Lam RW. A systematic review and meta-analysis of randomized, double-blind, placebo-controlled trials of ketamine in the rapid treatment of major depressive episodes. Psychological medicine. 2015 Mar; 45(4):693-704.

[49] Romeo B, Choucha W, Fossati P, Rotge JY. Meta-analysis of short-and mid-term efficacy of ketamine in unipolar and bipolar depression. Psychiatry research. 2015 Dec 15; 230(2):682-688.

[50] Fond G, Loundou A, Rabu C, Macgregor A, Lançon C, Brittner M, Micoulaud-Franchi JA, Richieri R, Courtet P, Abbar M, Roger M. Ketamine administration in depressive disorders: A systematic review and meta-analysis. Psychopharmacology. 2014 Sep;231(18): 3663-3676.

[51] Phillips JL, Norris S, Talbot J, Hatchard T, Ortiz A, Birmingham M, Owoeye O, Batten LA, Blier P. Single and repeated ketamine infusions for reduction of suicidal ideation in treatment-resistant depression. Neuropsychopharmacology. 2020 Mar;45(4):606-612.

[52] Albott CS, Lim KO, Forbes MK, Erbes C, Tye SJ, Grabowski JG, Thuras P, Batres-y-Carr TM, Wels J, Shiroma PR. Efficacy, safety, and durability of repeated ketamine infusions for comorbid posttraumatic stress disorder and treatment-resistant depression. The Journal of clinical psychiatry. 2018 May 1;79(3):17m11634.

[53] Zheng W, Zhou YL, Liu WJ, Wang CY, Zhan YN, Li HQ, Chen LJ, Li MD, Ning YP. Rapid and longer-term antidepressant effects of repeated-dose intravenous ketamine for patients with unipolar and bipolar depression. Journal of psychiatric research. 2018 Nov 1;106:61-68.

[54] Lapidus KA, Levitch CF, Perez AM, Brallier JW, Parides MK, Soleimani L, Feder A, Iosifescu DV, Charney DS, Murrough JW. A randomized controlled trial of intranasal ketamine in major depressive disorder. Biological psychiatry. 2014 Dec 15;76(12):970-976.

[55] Gálvez V, Li A, Huggins C, Glue P, Martin D, Somogyi AA, Alonzo A, Rodgers A, Mitchell PB, Loo CK. Repeated intranasal ketamine for

treatment-resistant depression—The way to go? Results from a pilot randomised controlled trial. Journal of Psychopharmacology. 2018 Apr;32(4):397-407.

[56] Andrade C. Intranasal drug delivery in neuropsychiatry: Focus on intranasal ketamine for refractory depression. The Journal of clinical psychiatry. 2015 May 27;76(5):e628-e631.

[57] Loo CK, Gálvez V, O'keefe E, Mitchell PB, Hadzi-Pavlovic D, Leyden J, Harper S, Somogyi AA, Lai R, Weickert CS, Glue P. Placebo-controlled pilot trial testing dose titration and intravenous, intramuscular and subcutaneous routes for ketamine in depression. ActaPsychiatrica-Scandinavica. 2016 Jul;134(1):48-56.

[58] FDA. FDA report on esketamine for treatment resistant depression, https://www.fda.gov/media/121379/download (2021).

[59] Daly EJ, Trivedi MH, Janik A, Li H, Zhang Y, Li X, Lane R, Lim P, Duca AR, Hough D, Thase ME. Efficacy of esketamine nasal spray plus oral antidepressant treatment for relapse prevention in patients with treatment-resistant depression: A randomized clinical trial. JAMA psychiatry. 2019 Sep 1;76(9):893-903.

[60] Wajs E, Aluisio L, Morrison R, Daly E, Lane R, Lim P, Holder R, Sanacora G, Young AH, Kasper S, Sulaiman AH. Long-Term Safety of Esketamine Nasal Spray plus Oral Antidepressant in Patients with Treatment-Resistant Depression: Phase 3, Open-Label, Safety and Efficacy Study (SUSTAIN-2). InPosterpresentado en the Annual Meeting of the American Society of Clinical Psychopharmacology, Miami, US 2018 May 29.

[61] Popova V, Daly EJ, Trivedi M, Cooper K, Lane R, Lim P, Mazzucco C, Hough D, Thase ME, Shelton RC, Molero P. Efficacy and safety of flexibly dosed esketamine nasal spray combined with a newly initiated oral antidepressant in treatment-resistant depression: A randomized double-blind active-controlled study. American Journal of Psychiatry. 2019 Jun 1;176(6):428-438.

[62] Swainson J, Thomas RK, Archer S, Chrenek C, MacKay MA, Baker G, Dursun S, Klassen LJ, Chokka P, Demas ML. Esketamine for treatment resistant depression. Expert review of neurotherapeutics. 2019 Oct 3;19(10):899-911.

[63] Talbot J, Phillips JL, Blier P. Ketamine for chronic depression: Two cautionary tales. Journal of psychiatry & neuroscience: JPN. 2019 Nov;44(6):384.

[64] Saxton RA, Sabatini DM. mTOR signaling in growth, metabolism, and disease. Cell. 2017 Mar 9;168(6):960-976.

[65] Altamura C, Maes M, Dai J, Meltzer HY. Plasma concentrations of excitatory amino acids, serine, glycine, taurine and histidine in major depression. European Neuropsychopharmacology. 1995 Jan 1;5:71-75.

[66] Küçükibrahimoğlu E, Saygın MZ, Çalışkan M, Kaplan OK, Ünsal C, Gören MZ. The change in plasma GABA, glutamine and glutamate levels in fluoxetine-or S-citalopram-treated female patients with major depression. European journal of clinical pharmacology. 2009 Jun;65(6):571-577.

[67] Mitani H, Shirayama Y, Yamada T, Maeda K, Ashby Jr CR, Kawahara R. Correlation between plasma levels of glutamate, alanine and serine with severity of depression. Progress in Neuro-Psychopharmacology and Biological Psychiatry. 2006 Aug 30;30(6):1155-1158.

[68] Krystal JH, Sanacora G, Duman RS. Rapid-acting glutamatergic antidepressants: The path to ketamine and beyond. Biological psychiatry. 2013 Jun 15;73(12):1133-1141.

[69] Abdallah CG, Sanacora G, Duman RS, Krystal JH. Ketamine and rapid-acting antidepressants: A window into a new neurobiology for mood disorder therapeutics. Annual review of medicine. 2015 Jan 14;66:509-523.

[70] Aleksandrova LR, Phillips AG, Wang YT. Antidepressant effects of ketamine and the roles of AMPA glutamate receptors and other mechanisms beyond NMDA receptor antagonism. Journal of psychiatry & neuroscience: JPN. 2017 Jul;42(4):222.

[71] Strasburger SE, Bhimani PM, Kaabe JH, Krysiak JT, Nanchanatt DL, Nguyen TN, Pough KA, Prince TA, Ramsey NS, Savsani KH, Scandlen L. What is the mechanism of Ketamine's rapid-onset antidepressant effect? A concise overview of the surprisingly large number of possibilities. Journal of clinical pharmacy and therapeutics. 2017 Apr;42(2):147-154.

[72] Moghaddam B, Adams B, Verma A, Daly D. Activation of glutamatergic neurotransmission by ketamine: A novel step in the pathway from NMDA receptor blockade to dopaminergic and cognitive disruptions associated with the prefrontal cortex. Journal of Neuroscience. 1997 Apr 15;17(8):2921-2927.

[73] Autry AE, Adachi M, Nosyreva E, Na ES, Los MF, Cheng PF, Kavalali ET, Monteggia LM. NMDA receptor blockade at rest triggers rapid behavioural antidepressant responses. Nature. 2011 Jul;475(7354):91-95.

[74] Koike H, Iijima M, Chaki S. Involvement of AMPA receptor in both the rapid and sustained antidepressant-like effects of ketamine in animal models of depression. Behavioural brain research. 2011 Oct 10;224(1):107-111.

[75] Maeng S, Zarate Jr CA, Du J, Schloesser RJ, McCammon J, Chen G, Manji HK. Cellular mechanisms underlying the antidepressant effects of ketamine: Role of α-amino-3-hydroxy-5-methylisoxazole-4-propionic acid receptors. Biological psychiatry. 2008 Feb 15;63(4):349-352.

[76] El Iskandrani KS, Oosterhof CA, El Mansari M, Blier P. Impact of subanesthetic doses of ketamine on AMPA-mediated responses in rats: An in vivo electrophysiological study on monoaminergic and glutamatergic neurons. Journal of Psychopharmacology. 2015 Jul;29(7):792-801.

[77] Björkholm C, Jardemark K, Schilström B, Svensson TH. Ketamine-like effects of a combination of olanzapine and fluoxetine on AMPA and NMDA receptor-mediated transmission in the medial prefrontal cortex of the rat. European Neuropsychopharmacology. 2015 Oct 1;25(10):1842-1847.

[78] Nosyreva E, Szabla K, Autry AE, Ryazanov AG, Monteggia LM, Kavalali ET. Acute suppression of spontaneous neurotransmission drives synaptic potentiation. Journal of Neuroscience. 2013 Apr 17;33(16): 6990-7002.

[79] Li N, Lee B, Liu RJ, Banasr M, Dwyer JM, Iwata M, Li XY, Aghajanian G, Duman RS. mTOR-dependent synapse formation underlies the rapid antidepressant effects of NMDA antagonists. Science. 2010 Aug 20;329(5994):959-964.

[80] Yang C, Hu YM, Zhou ZQ, Zhang GF, Yang JJ. Acute administration of ketamine in rats increases hippocampal BDNF and mTOR levels during forced swimming test. Upsala journal of medical sciences. 2013 Mar 1;118(1):3-8.

[81] Yang C, Li WY, Yu HY, Gao ZQ, Liu XL, Zhou ZQ, Yang JJ. Tramadol pretreatment enhances ketamine-induced antidepressant effects and increases mammalian target of rapamycin in rat hippocampus and prefrontal cortex. Journal of

Biomedicine and Biotechnology. 2012 Oct;2012.

[82] Zhou W, Wang N, Yang C, Li XM, Zhou ZQ, Yang JJ. Ketamine-induced antidepressant effects are associated with AMPA receptors-mediated upregulation of mTOR and BDNF in rat hippocampus and prefrontal cortex. European Psychiatry. 2014 Sep;29(7):419-423.

[83] Li N, Liu RJ, Dwyer JM, Banasr M, Lee B, Son H, Li XY, Aghajanian G, Duman RS. Glutamate N-methyl-D-aspartate receptor antagonists rapidly reverse behavioral and synaptic deficits caused by chronic stress exposure. Biological psychiatry. 2011 Apr 15;69(8): 754-761.

[84] Liu RJ, Lee FS, Li XY, Bambico F, Duman RS, Aghajanian GK. Brain-derived neurotrophic factor Val66Met allele impairs basal and ketamine-stimulated synaptogenesis in prefrontal cortex. Biological psychiatry. 2012 Jun 1;71(11):996-1005.

[85] Tornese P, Sala N, Bonini D, Bonifacino T, La Via L, Milanese M, Treccani G, Seguini M, Ieraci A, Mingardi J, Nyengaard JR. Chronic mild stress induces anhedonic behavior and changes in glutamate release, BDNF trafficking and dendrite morphology only in stress vulnerable rats. The rapid restorative action of ketamine. Neurobiology of stress. 2019 Feb 1;10:100160.

[86] Dong C, Zhang JC, Yao W, Ren Q, Ma M, Yang C, Chaki S, Hashimoto K. Rapid and sustained antidepressant action of the mGlu2/3 receptor antagonist MGS0039 in the social defeat stress model: Comparison with ketamine. International Journal of Neuropsychopharmacology. 2017 Mar 1;20(3):228-236.

[87] Laje G, Lally N, Mathews D, Brutsche N, Chemerinski A, Akula N, Kelmendi B, Simen A, McMahon FJ, Sanacora G, Zarate Jr C. Brain-derived neurotrophic factor Val66Met polymorphism and antidepressant efficacy of ketamine in depressed patients. Biological psychiatry. 2012 Dec 1;72(11):e27.

[88] Chen MH, Lin WC, Wu HJ, Cheng CM, Li CT, Hong CJ, Tu PC, Bai YM, Tsai SJ, Su TP. Antisuicidal effect, BDNF Val66Met polymorphism, and low-dose ketamine infusion: Reanalysis of adjunctive ketamine study of Taiwanese patients with treatment-resistant depression (AKSTP-TRD). Journal of affective disorders. 2019 May 15;251:162-169.

[89] Yang C, Zhou ZQ, Gao ZQ, Shi JY, Yang JJ. Acute increases in plasma mammalian target of rapamycin, glycogen synthase kinase-3β, and eukaryotic elongation factor 2 phosphorylation after ketamine treatment in three depressed patients. Biological psychiatry. 2013 Jun 15;73(12):e35-e36.

[90] Abdallah CG, Averill LA, Gueorguieva R, Goktas S, Purohit P, Ranganathan M, D'Souza DC, Formica R, Southwick SM, Duman RS, Sanacora G. Rapamycin, an immunosuppressant and mTORC1 inhibitor, triples the antidepressant response rate of ketamine at 2 weeks following treatment: A double-blind, placebo-controlled, cross-over, randomized clinical trial. Biorxiv. 2018 Jan 1:500959.

[91] Ishiwata S, Hattori K, Sasayama D, Teraishi T, Miyakawa T, Yokota Y, Matsumura R, Nishikawa T, Kunugi H. Cerebrospinal fluid D-serine concentrations in major depressive disorder negatively correlate with depression severity. Journal of affective disorders. 2018 Jan 15;226:155-162.

[92] Hashimoto K, Yoshida T, Ishikawa M, Fujita Y, Niitsu T, Nakazato M, Watanabe H, Sasaki T, Shiina A, Hashimoto T, Kanahara N.

Increased serum levels of serine enantiomers in patients with depression. Actaneuropsychiatrica. 2016 Jun;28(3): 173-178.

[93] Malkesman O, Austin DR, Tragon T, Wang G, Rompala G, Hamidi AB, Cui Z, Young WS, Nakazawa K, Zarate Jr CA, Manji HK. Acute D-serine treatment produces antidepressant-like effects in rodents. International Journal of Neuropsychopharmacology. 2012 Sep 1;15(8):1135-1148.

[94] Wei IH, Chen KT, Tsai MH, Wu CH, Lane HY, Huang CC. Acute amino acid D-serine administration, similar to ketamine, produces antidepressant-like effects through identical mechanisms. Journal of agricultural and food chemistry. 2017 Dec 13;65(49) :10792-10803.

[95] Otte DM, Barcena de Arellano ML, Bilkei-Gorzo A, Albayram Ö, Imbeault S, Jeung H, Alferink J, Zimmer A. Effects of chronic D-serine elevation on animal models of depression and anxiety-related behavior. PloS one. 2013 Jun 21;8(6):e67131.

[96] Singh NS, Bernier M, Camandola S, Khadeer MA, Moaddel R, Mattson MP, Wainer IW. Enantioselective inhibition of d-serine transport by (S)-ketamine. British journal of pharmacology. 2015 Sep;172(18):4546-4559.

[97] Singh NS, Rutkowska E, Plazinska A, Khadeer M, Moaddel R, Jozwiak K, Bernier M, Wainer IW. Ketamine metabolites enantioselectively decrease intracellular D-serine concentrations in PC-12 cells. PloS one. 2016 Apr 20;11(4):e0149499.

[98] Moaddel R, Luckenbaugh DA, Xie Y, Villaseñor A, Brutsche NE, Machado-Vieira R, Ramamoorthy A, Lorenzo MP, Garcia A, Bernier M, Torjman MC. D-serine plasma concentration is a potential biomarker of (R, S)-ketamine antidepressant response in subjects with treatment-resistant depression. Psychopharmacology. 2015 Jan;232(2):399-409.

[99] Hashimoto K. Blood D-serine levels as a predictive biomarker for the rapid antidepressant effects of the NMDA receptor antagonist ketamine. Psychopharmacology. 2014 Oct;231(20): 4081-4082.

[100] Williams NR, Heifets BD, Bentzley BS, Blasey C, Sudheimer KD, Hawkins J, Lyons DM, Schatzberg AF. Attenuation of antidepressant and antisuicidal effects of ketamine by opioid receptor antagonism. Molecular psychiatry. 2019 Dec;24(12):1779-1786.

[101] Williams NR, Heifets BD, Blasey C, Sudheimer K, Pannu J, Pankow H, Hawkins J, Birnbaum J, Lyons DM, Rodriguez CI, Schatzberg AF. Attenuation of antidepressant effects of ketamine by opioid receptor antagonism. American Journal of Psychiatry. 2018 Dec 1;175(12):1205-1215.

[102] Yoon G, Petrakis IL, Krystal JH. Association of combined naltrexone and ketamine with depressive symptoms in a case series of patients with depression and alcohol use disorder. JAMA psychiatry. 2019 Mar 1;76(3):337-338.

[103] Marton T, Barnes DE, Wallace A, Woolley JD. Concurrent use of buprenorphine, methadone, or naltrexone does not inhibit ketamine's antidepressant activity. Biological psychiatry. 2019 Jun 15;85(12):e75-e76.

[104] Molero P, Ramos-Quiroga JA, Martin-Santos R, Calvo-Sánchez E, Gutiérrez-Rojas L, Meana JJ. Antidepressant efficacy and tolerability of ketamine and esketamine: A critical review. CNS drugs. 2018 May;32(5): 411-420.

[105] Ho RC, Zhang MW. Ketamine as a rapid antidepressant: The debate and implications. BJPsych Advances. 2016 Jul;22(4):222-233.

[106] Short B, Fong J, Galvez V, Shelker W, Loo CK. Side-effects associated with ketamine use in depression: A systematic review. The Lancet Psychiatry. 2018 Jan 1;5(1):65-78.

[107] Schatzberg AF. A word to the wise about intranasal esketamine. American Journal of Psychiatry. 2019 Jun 1;176(6): 422-424.

[108] Sanacora G, Frye MA, McDonald W, Mathew SJ, Turner MS, Schatzberg AF, Summergrad P, Nemeroff CB, American Psychiatric Association. A consensus statement on the use of ketamine in the treatment of mood disorders. JAMA psychiatry. 2017 Apr 1;74(4):399-405.

Chapter 11

Perspective Chapter: Ketamine, Depression, and Gender Bias

Tahani K. Alshammari, Sarah Alseraye, Nouf M. Alrasheed, Anfal F. Bin Dayel, Asma S. Alonazi, Jawza F. Al Sabhan and Musaad A. Alshammari

Abstract

Our knowledge regarding pathological and treatment resistance mechanisms involved in depression is far from understood. Sexual dimorphism in this topic is well acknowledged. However, the need to highlight sex-based discrepancies is unmet. Ketamine, the dissociative anesthetic, has emerged as a rapid antidepressant. This chapter reviewed sexual dimorphism in pharmacological and genetic models of depression, emphasizing ketamine-related antidepressant effects. Aiming by this report, we would extend our knowledge, highlight gender as one of the vital factors in examining depression in preclinical studies, and elucidate complex antidepressant effects associated with ketamine administration. Our central goal is to encourage neuroscientists to consider gender in their studies of mood disorders.

Keywords: ketamine, depression, sexual dimorphism, ketamine isomers

1. Introduction

The physiological and pharmacological applications of Ketamine's evolved historically. In the mid-1950s, it was initially introduced as an anesthetic agent, and it was short-acting with better post-operational effects compared to phencyclidine. Phencyclidine by itself is linked to multiple undesirable effects, including severe and prolonged post-surgery hallucinations, agitation, and delirium that made it undesirable for human use [1, 2]. Functionally, ketamine is a safer derivative of phencyclidine [3]. Both are psychoactive arylcyclohexamines agents, a unified feature of these compounds is their molecular antagonism of the N-methyl-D-aspartate (NMDA) receptor [4]. Ketamine lacks the complete unconsciousness state and is characterized by catatonia, catalepsy, and amnesia [3]. However, ketamine still retains some adverse events, such as abuse potentials and dissociative effects, and neurotoxicity when administered through the spinal cord.

In the seventies, the Food and Drug Administration (FDA) approved ketamine, and it became commercially available as a rapid and short-acting anesthetic agent [3]. Among other anesthetics, ketamine is characterized by a more significant safety, which makes it advantageous compared to other anesthetics. On the level of circuitry, as an agent, it does not elevate the blood pressure. Additionally, physiologically, it is not linked to respiratory depression in both intravenous doses of 1–2 mg/kg or intramuscular doses of 4–11 mg/kg [3, 5]. At subanesthetic doses, ketamine

IntechOpen

exhibited an analgesic effect and can be clinically used in numerous conditions associated with pain in a mechanism similar to opioids but with less respiratory depressive effects [3]. Overall, high-priced patient-monitoring tools and equipment are not necessary for clinical applications of ketamine. Thus, it is a good anesthetic of choice, especially in the middle- and low-income countries. Due to the fact ketamine, clinical applications were indispensable. It has been listed on the World Health Organization (WHO) Essential Medicines List since 1985 [6]. Also, ketamine was reported sedation in individuals with severe behavioral disturbances in clinical settings. In some cases, agitated patients may require police interference to handle them, and in comparison, to the standard sedative induction protocol, ketamine was found to be effective in parenteral relatively low doses (about 5 mg/kg) [7].

The chronic use of ketamine is linked to abuse liabilities and issues with the urinary tract system [8]. The illicit use of ketamine is well-acknowledged. However, ketamine overdose is not a common event. According to the recommendations of the WHO Expert Committee on Drug Dependence in 2016, ketamine should not be listed in the international drug control conventions [6].

In general, multiple uncovered potential novel uses of ketamine were identified including the neuroprotective effect of ketamine and its use in the management of epilepsy, chronic pain, migraine, inflammation, and tumors. Interestingly, in the past few years (the 2000s), ketamine has progressively received increased attention, and there has been significant research into the potential use of ketamine as an expeditiously acting treatment for MDD, treatment-resistant depression (TRD), and suicidality [6, 9]. Intranasal (S)-ketamine has recently been approved for depression by the FDA [10]. However, it is currently too expensive for the widespread use and is unlikely to be cost-effective for the management of TRD in the United States unless its price falls by more than 40% [11].

The chemical basis of ketamine is a similar composition of a racemic mixture, in a ratio of 1:1. This mixture is composed of arketamine (R-ketamine) and esketamine (S-ketamine) [12]. Functionally, these enantiomers are different. In the mid-eighties, white and his colleagues [13] conducted the first comparative study to examine the clinical differences between ketamine isomers using the electroencephalographic monitoring of brain activity in healthy volunteers. They observed that the arketamine exhibited less hypnotic and analgesic effects compared to the esketamine. The arketamine was associated with a faster recovery rate, regarded as the reduced central nervous system depressant effects [13]. Subsequent studies reported more functional and pharmacological differences. For example, the esketamine has greater potency toward the NMDA receptors (as an antagonist), and thus it is pharmacologically more active than the R-ketamine. Additionally, the arketamine exhibits higher potency toward the μ-opioid receptor (an agonist) [14].

In clinical settings, the esketamine was found to be as twice as potent in anesthetic effect compared to the racemic mixture and as threefold potent compared to arketamine [3, 14]. Furthermore, esketamine is described as the less psychotomimetic and the greater analgesic enantiomer. In comparison to arketamine the esketamine is linked to reduced clinically significant side effects such as drowsiness, fatigue, and altered cognitive function [14]. In another clinical study, they examined the recovery effects of both isomers. One hour following the intravenous administration of ketamine isomers, individuals who received the esketamine exhibited better concentration and memory retention [15]. Accordingly, in analgesic and anesthetic applications, esketamine is more favored [14].

Besides, they exhibit neuroprotective differences. In primary cultured rat hippocampal neurons, the esketamine exerts neuroprotective effects. It prevents the release of arachidonic acid and modulates axonal outgrowth measured by the expression of microtubule-associated protein at different time points [16].

	Esketamine	Arketamine	References
Potency	This isomer is considered as functionally more potent than the racemic mixture (2× more than the racemic mixture, and 3× more than R-ketamine)	This isomer is a less active one.	[3, 14]
NMDAR antagonizing affinity	Greater affinity	Lower affinity	[20]
μ-Opioid receptor agonism Affinity	Greater affinity	Lower affinity	[20, 21]
Side effects (psychotomimetic, drowsiness, lethargy, and cognitive impairment, and abuse liabilities)	More side effects	less side effects	[12]

Table 1.
The main differences between ketamine isomers.

Interestingly, even if the potency is comparable among the isomers, the molecular mechanism may differ. In guinea pig histamine-mediated preconstricted strips, both isomers were found to mediate spasmolytic effects. Even though their potency was similar, the mechanism was quite different. The esketamine exerts more effects through adrenaline signaling, whereas arketamine spasmolytic modulation was through calcium signaling [17].

Preclinical evidence using various depression animal models suggests the potential antidepressant advantages of arketamine over esketamine. Despite the lower affinity of arketamine, NMDA receptors exhibited superior potency and more prolonged antidepressant effects than esketamine. For that reason, other molecular targets may play an essential role in mediating ketamine antidepressant effects [10, 18]. Importantly, arketamine also has fewer side effects than either (R, S)-ketamine or esketamine as it may not induce psychotomimetic side effects or exhibit abuse potential in rodents and monkeys [11, 14, 19].

A previous report examined the enantiomers' molecular targets selectivity and potency. Their impact on multiple neurotransmitter systems revealed that both isomers have similar effects. They increased the release of serotonin, dopamine, and noradrenaline neurotransmitters. The magnitude of their effects was quite different [18]. Arketamine showed a significant impact on the release of serotonin than esketamine. At the same time, esketamine increases dopamine release more than arketamine [19]. **Table 1** summarizes the main differences between ketamine isomers.

2. Ketamine, the antidepressant

Major depressive disorder (MDD) places a considerable burden on the community [22]. Among mood disorders, MDD is a common one, and it is considered one of the debilitating psychiatric disorders. Commonly prescribed antidepressants are of limited efficacy and take weeks to months to yield full therapeutic effects [21]. Most existing treatments have been found by serendipity. However, there are several limitations. First, the response to antidepressants is relatively heterogeneous; in fact, a considerable number of patients do not respond well to the treatment, the TRD [23]. An additional challenge is to distinguish TRD from inadequately treated depression [24]. Furthermore, differences are exhibited in patients' pharmacokinetic and pharmacodynamics characteristics, which could be a key reason for the discrepancy in sex-related efficacy [25]. Moreover, most drugs are intolerable [26, 27], frequent, and enduring [28]. For these reasons, there is a need to identify and develop effective and ideal antidepressant agents.

Recently, Ketamine gained a lot of attention in its fast-onset and effectiveness when applied to depressed patients. Overall, the ketamine efficacy was successfully recorded in severely depressed patients using different validated rating scales [14]. In early 2000, Berman and his colleagues recorded the fast, moderately persistent, and robust pharmacological effects in depressed patients [29]. The double-blinded trial showed that depressed patients were significantly improved 3 days following the ketamine administration, which opened a new avenue in the management of MDD. Over the last 20 years, studies have indicated the antidepressant properties of ketamine. As an antidepressant agent, it functions in quite different mechanisms and onset than conventional antidepressant agents. Of particular interest, it brings an antidepressant effect in patients with refractory depression [30].

The central nervous system pharmacological targets of ketamine are diverse and ubiquitous. One of the main pharmacological targets for ketamine is the excitatory NMDA receptors. It is believed that ketamine mediates the anesthetic and analgesic effects through the direct noncompetitive NMDA receptors antagonist. It stimulates glutamate release in preclinical [31], and clinical studies [32]. The in vivo magnetic resonance spectroscopy clinical studies indicated that the metabolism of the 13-C-glutamate is elevated in cortical brain regions [33, 34].

Additionally, ketamine act—in lower affinity—molecularly at the inhibitory receptor the γ-aminobutyric acid (GABA) [35]. In fact, a previous report suggested the deficit of both GABAergic and glutamatergic is a unified pathological feature of MDD [36].

The AMPA receptor is another target for ketamine. Functional activation of AMPA receptors is essential for recruiting multiple pathways in modulating ketamine-induced antidepressant effects [37]. Preclinical evidence has found that the activation of AMPA receptor is critical for mediating rapid and sustained ketamine-induced antidepressant effects [38]. Ketamine was reported to elevate the hippocampal expression of AMPA receptor subunits, the glutamate receptor (GluA)1 and 2 subunits [39]. A previous study indicated that the AMPA-mediated Ketamine-induced antidepressant effects involve the glycogen synthase kinase-3 [40]. Electrophysiological studies indicate that AMPA signaling is essential for mediating the ketamine-induced antidepressant effects [38, 41]. A meta-analysis study based on in vivo and ex vivo studies indicated that ketamine elevates the level of dopamine in different brain regions relevant to the pathology of depression, including the frontal cortex, striatum, and nucleus accumbens [42].

Another molecular target for ketamine is opioid signaling. Ketamine was reported to be a weak agonist to opioid receptors isoforms, including the mu, delta, and kappa. Studies indicated that the involvement of the opioid receptor is essential for ketamine-induced antidepressant effects [14, 43].

Additionally, in a double-blind clinical study using suicidality-specific rating scales, naltrexone—an opioid receptor antagonist—was found to weaken the anti-suicidality effects of ketamine. Indicating that opioid receptor activation plays a major role in the anti-suicidality effects of ketamine [43].

The dopaminergic, cholinergic, serotonergic, and opioid, receptors are implicated in ketamine-induced antidepressant effects [44]. Furthermore, ketamine acts on the hyperpolarization-activated cyclic nucleotide-gated (HCN) channels. Moreover, ketamine provides anti-inflammatory activities. It decreases the production of pro-inflammatory cytokines including the nuclear factor κB, the tumor necrosis factor-α, the interleukin 6 (IL-6), and the inducible nitric oxide synthase [3].

Another molecular target for ketamine is the glucocorticoids pathway. The administration of ketamine was found to stimulate the release of glucocorticoid downstream component, the Serum glucocorticoid kinase 1 (SGK1). Indicating that the pharmacological function of ketamine may recruit the glucocorticoid receptor pathway [45]. **Table 2** describes the primary molecular targets for ketamine-mediated antidepressants effects.

The pathway	Description of the action	The mechanism of actions	References
NMDAR	The disinhibition hypothesis	At subanesthetic doses, ketamine inhibits NMDARs on GABAergic interneurons	[29, 46]
		Leading to alteration in the disinhibition and the overall feedback and feed-forward mechanisms.	[47]
		Another consequence, changing the postsynaptic AMPARs activations.	[32, 37]
	Direct inhibition of extra-synaptic NMDARs	Ketamine directly prevents the extra-synaptic GluN2B. Leading to precluding the glutamate-induced activation of glutamatergic receptors. Overall, this would alter protein synthesis	[37]
	Blocking spontaneous NMDAR activation)	On principal cells—at rest—ketamine directly inhibits NMDARs	[32]
		Preventing the tonic activation leading to activation of other pathways such as eEF2 and BDNF signaling	[46]
AMPA receptor	The activation of AMPA receptor	ketamine-induced antidepressant effects are linked to the functional activation of AMPA receptors	[37]
		Preclinical evidence has found that AMPA receptor activation is critical for mediating rapid and sustained ketamine-induced antidepressant effects	[38]
BDNF	The activation of BDNF	Ketamine-induced behavioral antidepressant effects are mediated through BDNF release in hippocampal primary neuronal cultures	[48]
		Ketamine-induced cellular effects through BDNF release in rats.	[49]
		In a clinical setting, the level of plasma BDNF in treatment-resistant depressed patients correlates with the infused level of ketamine.	[50]
eEF2	The inhibition of eEF2	The ketamine glutamatergic-mediated mechanisms reduce eEF2 kinase activation, leading to alterations in synaptic plasticity	[32]
Monoamines	Increases monoamines levels	Ketamine prevents serotonin reuptake	[29]
		Ketamine prevents dopamine reuptake	[51]
		Ketamine prevents norepinephrine reuptake	
Opioid system	Opioid agonism	Weak agonistic effects are mediated toward multiple isoforms of opioid receptors, including the mu, delta, and kappa	[14]
		Multiple studies indicated that activation of the opioid receptor is essential for ketamine-induced antidepressant effects	[51]

NMDAR, N-methyl-D'aspartate receptor; AMPAR, α-amino-3-hydroxy-5-methyl-4-isoxazolepropionic acid receptors; mTORC1, mechanistic target of rapamycin complex 1; eEF2, eukaryotic elongation factor 2; BDNF, brain-derived neurotrophic factor.

Table 2.
The main molecular targets for ketamine-mediated antidepressants effects.

3. Ketamine sexually dimorphic antidepressant effects

The prevalence of depression is almost twice as high among women as men [46–48]. The clinical symptoms are also more prolonged and severe in women, with a high rate of recurrence compared to men [49]. Additionally, exposure to psychosocial stress is a significant risk factor for stress-related disorders, including depression. Most importantly, the physiological responses to stress are sexually dimorphic [50–52].

One possible explanation for sexually dimorphic stress responses is the locus coeruleus, a brain stem nucleus responsible for most of the noradrenergic system [53]. Triggering the locus coeruleus is a critical component of stress responses. A previous report demonstrated that neuronal populations within the locus coeruleus are substantially sensitive to the corticotropin-releasing factor in female rats compared to males [54]. We previously reported considerable evidence indicating that sexual dimorphism is a confounding factor facing a complete understanding of pathological mechanisms involved in depression and in finding an effective treatment [55].

Multiple studies have reported that ketamine-induced antidepressant effects are exerted in a sexually dimorphic manner. For instance, in a transgenic animal model, the intraperitoneal injection of ketamine exhibited sexually dimorphic molecular changes. It was found to elevate the mRNA level of Bdnf in females [56]. In another example, ketamine exhibited neurobehavioral and neurochemical alterations in a sex-dependent manner. A single sub-anesthetic ketamine dose was found to alter the 5-hydroxyindoleacetic acid to the 5-hydroxytryptamine ratio in the prefrontal cortex of female rats in 24 h post ketamine injection. While performing the forced-swim test in a behavioral setting, female rats exhibited more sensitivity to lower doses of ketamine than male rats [57]. Indicating the profound effects of hormones over the ketamine-mediated antidepressant effects. In line with this, another report found that ketamine-induced antidepressant effects were not observed in ovariectomized rats. Additionally, these effects were functionally observable following the administration of both estrogen and progesterone [58].

Interestingly, the sub-anesthetic ketamine dose was found to exhibit pharmacological dissociative effects in a sexually dimorphic manner. Whereas female rats were more sensitive and developed more significant ataxia in comparison to male rats. Besides, the magnitude of head weaving in female rats during their diestrus phase was more significant compared to females in their other stages of the estrous cycle [59]. Also, pharmacokinetics profiling of ketamine in rats indicated that both ketamine and ketamine-metabolites were presented in higher plasma concentrations in female rats than in males, suggesting the rate of hepatic clearance and metabolism might be affected by female hormones [60].

The effect of ketamine on neuroplasticity markers was examined at the proteomic level in the different brain regions following multiple ketamine bolus doses. Different bolus doses were found to induce the protein expression of c-Fos in the amygdala of female rats, not the male rats. Also, in the prefrontal cortex, this expression was modulated by the estrous cycle [61]. The administration of ketamine in female mice exposed to chronic unpredictable mild stress was reported to be mediated via the extracellular-signal-regulated kinase and glucose transporter 3 (ERK/GLUT3) signaling pathway [62].

The glucose transporter 3 (GLUT3) was found to be essential for modulating neuronal circuitry and metabolic functions [63]. This isoform of glucose transporters is predominantly expressed in neuronal populations [64]. Additionally, glut3 heterozygous mice exhibited seizures, cognitive impairments, and altered sociability behaviors in a sex-dependent manner [65].

On the other hand, ERK signaling is a crucial modulator of physiological roles affected by gender. For instance, a previous report indicated that the ERK pathway regulates the hypothalamic-pituitary-gonadal axis, and the functional maturation of the female reproduction system in pituitary-targeted ERK knockout mice is altered [66]. In line with this, in a model of psychiatric disorders, the neonatal ventral hippocampal lesion, a validated animal model of schizophrenia, the ERK signaling was reported to function in a sex-dependent manner. In the report, the content, and the phosphorylation level of different components of the ERK signaling was found to be sexually dimorphic [67].

The whole gender-related variable psychological, neurobehavioral, and molecular effects in clinical and preclinical studies are not a characteristic of ketamine alone. Other antidepressants function in a sexual-dimorphism manner. For example, males reported better outcomes than depressed females in response to tricyclic antidepressants, classical antidepressant agents. On the other hand, females exhibited better responses to selective serotonin reuptake inhibitors [68]. Indicating the significant role of gender and the hormonal system in the pathology of depression.

4. Organizational and activational hormonal effects

Whether a depression model is environmental [55], pharmacological, or genetic, organizational, and activational hormonal effects cannot be overlooked. The organizational and activational hypothesis was introduced in the late 1950s [69]. This hypothesis suggests that sex hormones regulate the central nervous system's organization, development, and function. Organizational effects refer to the effect of steroid hormones on the brain during early developmental stages. At the same time, activational effects are lifelong hormonal effects [70].

A review conducted by Arnold [71] proposed a framework for the organizational and activational hypothesis. In his report, this hypothesis's fundamentals include prenatal masculinization, where the prenatal exposure of female guinea pigs to testosterone alters their behavior later on. These females behaved like a male guinea pig. These changes were permanent, which could be mediated by the hormonal effect on neuronal development (the organizational effect), and that indicates the central nervous system's vulnerability during this critical period of development. Overall, this framework supports the notion that steroid hormones' cellular, molecular, and behavioral effects vary [71]. Extensive reports reviewed this hypothesis [71–73]. However, steroidal hormones' activational versus organizational effects have not yet been clearly characterized [74].

5. Conclusions

Further investigation into sexual dimorphism in the neurobiology of depression is quite essential. This knowledge could potentially improve the diagnosis and treatment of depression and provide a basis for sex-based interventions. These interventions could take into account the pharmacodynamic and pharmacokinetic differences between men and women. It can further consider molecular targets for each gender.

This can be achieved if sex-oriented research on the mechanism of depression in both sexes is conducted at clinical and pre-clinical levels. Despite their limitations, animal models provide a wealth of knowledge on depression neurobiology. This chapter aimed to review existing pre-clinical research on sex differences in the neurobiology of depression and, therefore, to highlight the unmet need to investigate depression with respect to gender as a variable and, most importantly, encourage researchers to establish disease-based studies.

Conflict of interest

The authors declare that there is no conflict of interest.

Author details

Tahani K. Alshammari[1*], Sarah Alseraye[1], Nouf M. Alrasheed[1], Anfal F. Bin Dayel[1], Asma S. Alonazi[1], Jawza F. Al Sabhan[2] and Musaad A. Alshammari[1]

1 Department of Pharmacology and Toxicology, College of Pharmacy, King Saud University, Riyadh, Saudi Arabia

2 Department of Clinical Pharmacy, King Saud University, Riyadh, Saudi Arabia

*Address all correspondence to: talshammary@ksu.edu.sa

References

[1] Hashimoto K. Rapid-acting antidepressant ketamine, its metabolites and other candidates: A historical overview and future perspective. Psychiatry and Clinical Neurosciences. 2019;**73**(10):613-627

[2] Alshammari TK. The ketamine antidepressant story: New insights. Molecules. 2020;**25**(23):5777

[3] Zanos P et al. Ketamine and ketamine metabolite pharmacology: Insights into therapeutic mechanisms. Pharmacological Reviews. 2018;**70**(3):621-660

[4] Salter MD and Gunja N. Chapter14—Arylcyclohexamines, in Novel Psychoactive Substances. 2nd ed. Dargan P and Wood D Editors. Boston: Academic Press; 2022. pp. 381-414

[5] Rosenbaum SB, Gupta V and Palacios JL. Ketamine. StatPearls Publishing LLC.Treasure Island, FL, United States of America. 2021

[6] WHO. Expert Committee on Drug Dependence. Fact File on Ketamine. Geneva, Switzerland: WHO; 2016

[7] Isbister GK et al, Ketamine as rescue treatment for difficult-to-sedate severe acute behavioral disturbance in the emergency department. Annals of Emergency Medicine. 2016;67(5): 581-587

[8] Srirangam S, Mercer J. Ketamine Bladder Syndrome: An Important Differential Diagnosis When Assessing a Patient With Persistent Lower Urinary Tract Symptoms. Vol. 2012. Tavistock Square, London: BMJ Case Reports; 2012. p. bcr2012006447

[9] Pribish A, Wood N, Kalava A. A review of nonanesthetic uses of ketamine. Anesthesiology Research and Practice. 2020;**2020**:5798285

[10] Wei Y, Chang L, Hashimoto K. A historical review of antidepressant effects of ketamine and its enantiomers. Pharmacology Biochemistry and Behavior. 2020;**190**:172870

[11] Ross EL, Soeteman DI. Cost-effectiveness of esketamine nasal spray for patients with treatment-resistant depression in the United States. Psychiatric Services. 2020;**71**(10): 988-997

[12] Yang CS, Zhang Y, Ren JC, Yao Q, Ma W, Cong MC, et al. R-ketamine: A rapid-onset and sustained antidepressant without psychotomimetic side effects. Translational Psychiatry. 2015;**5**(9): e632-e632

[13] White PF et al. Comparative pharmacology of the ketamine isomers. Studies in volunteers. British Journal of Anaesthesia. 1985;**57**(2):197-203

[14] Corriger A, Pickering G. Ketamine and depression: A narrative review. Drug Design, Development and Therapy. 2019;**13**:3051-3067

[15] Pfenninger EG, Durieux ME, Himmelseher S. Cognitive impairment after small-dose ketamine isomers in comparison to equianalgesic racemic ketamine in human volunteers. Anesthesiology. 2002;**96**(2):357-366

[16] Himmelseher S, Pfenninger E, Georgieff M. The effects of ketamine-isomers on neuronal injury and regeneration in rat hippocampal neurons. Anesthesia & Analgesia. 1996;**83**(3):505-512

[17] Hirota K et al. Relaxant effect of ketamine and its isomers on histamine-induced contraction of tracheal smooth muscle. British Journal of Anaesthesia. 1996;**76**(2):266-270

[18] Andrade C. Ketamine for depression, 3: Does chirality matter? The Journal of Clinical Psychiatry. 2017;**78**(6):e674-e677

[19] Ago Y et al. (R)-ketamine induces a greater increase in prefrontal 5-HT release than (S)-ketamine and ketamine metabolites via an AMPA receptor-independent mechanism. The International Journal of Neuropsychopharmacology. 2019;**22**(10):665-674

[20] Jelen LA, Young AH, Stone JM. Ketamine: A tale of two enantiomers. Journal of Psychopharmacology. 2020;**35**(2):109-123

[21] Abdallah CG et al. Ketamine's mechanism of action: A path to rapid-acting antidepressants. Depression and Anxiety. 2016;**33**(8):689-697

[22] Williams AV, Trainor BC. The impact of sex as a biological variable in the search for novel antidepressants. Frontiers in Neuroendocrinology. 2018;**50**:107-117

[23] Culpepper L. Why do you need to move beyond first-line therapy for major depression? The Journal of Clinical Psychiatry. 2010; **71**(Suppl. 1):4-9

[24] Nemeroff CB. Augmentation strategies in patients with refractory depression. Depression and Anxiety. 1996;**4**(4):169-181

[25] Sramek JJ, Murphy MF, Cutler NR. Sex differences in the psychopharmacological treatment of depression. Dialogues in Clinical Neuroscience. 2016;**18**(4):447-457

[26] Penn E, Tracy DK. The drugs don't work? Antidepressants and the current and future pharmacological management of depression. Therapeutic Advances in Psychopharmacology. 2012;**2**(5):179-188

[27] Pallanti S, Koran LM. Citalopram and sexual side effects of selective serotonin reuptake inhibitors. The American Journal of Psychiatry. 1999;**156**(5):796

[28] Papakostas GI. Limitations of contemporary antidepressants: Tolerability. The Journal of Clinical Psychiatry. 2007;**68**(Suppl. 10):11-17

[29] Kraus C et al. The influence of ketamine on drug discovery in depression. Drug Discovery Today. 2019;**24**(10):2033-2043

[30] Andrade C. Ketamine for depression, 1: Clinical summary of issues related to efficacy, adverse effects, and mechanism of action. The Journal of Clinical Psychiatry. 2017;**78**(4):e415-e419

[31] Lorrain DS et al. Effects of ketamine and N-methyl-D-aspartate on glutamate and dopamine release in the rat prefrontal cortex: Modulation by a group II selective metabotropic glutamate receptor agonist LY379268. Neuroscience. 2003;**117**(3):697-706

[32] Krystal JH et al. Ketamine: A paradigm shift for depression research and treatment. Neuron. 2019;**101**(5): 774-778

[33] Chowdhury GMI et al. 1H-[13C]-nuclear magnetic resonance spectroscopy measures of ketamine's effect on amino acid neurotransmitter metabolism. Biological Psychiatry. 2012;**71**(11):1022-1025

[34] Abdallah CG et al. The effects of ketamine on prefrontal glutamate neurotransmission in healthy and depressed subjects. Neuropsychopharmacology. 2018;**43**(10):2154-2160

[35] Wang DS, Penna A, Orser BA. Ketamine increases the function of γ-aminobutyric acid type a receptors in

hippocampal and cortical neurons. Anesthesiology. 2017;**126**(4):666-677

[36] Ren Z et al. Bidirectional homeostatic regulation of a depression-related brain state by gamma-aminobutyric acidergic deficits and ketamine treatment. Biological Psychiatry. 2016;**80**(6):457-468

[37] Zanos P, Gould TD. Mechanisms of ketamine action as an antidepressant. Molecular Psychiatry. 2018;**23**(4): 801-811

[38] Koike H, Iijima M, Chaki S. Involvement of AMPA receptor in both the rapid and sustained antidepressant-like effects of ketamine in animal models of depression. Behavioural Brain Research. 2011;**224**(1):107-111

[39] Matveychuk D et al. Ketamine as an antidepressant: Overview of its mechanisms of action and potential predictive biomarkers. Therapeutic Advances in Psychopharmacology. 2020;**10**:2045125320916657

[40] Beurel E et al. Ketamine-induced inhibition of glycogen synthase kinase-3 contributes to the augmentation of α-amino-3-hydroxy-5-methylisoxazole-4-propionic acid (AMPA) receptor signaling. Bipolar Disorders. 2016;**18**(6):473-480

[41] Nosyreva E et al. Acute suppression of spontaneous neurotransmission drives synaptic potentiation. The Journal of Neuroscience. 2013;**33**(16):6990

[42] Kokkinou M, Ashok AH, Howes OD. The effects of ketamine on dopaminergic function: Meta-analysis and review of the implications for neuropsychiatric disorders. Molecular Psychiatry. 2018;**23**(1):59-69

[43] Williams NR et al. Attenuation of antidepressant and antisuicidal effects of ketamine by opioid receptor antagonism. Molecular Psychiatry. 2019;**24**(12):1779-1786

[44] McMillan R, Muthukumaraswamy SD. The neurophysiology of ketamine: An integrative review. Reviews in the Neurosciences. 2020;**31**(5):457-503

[45] Wegman-Points L et al. Corticosterone as a potential confounding factor in delineating mechanisms underlying ketamine's rapid antidepressant actions. Frontiers in Pharmacology. 2020;**11**(1927):250

[46] Ma L et al. Sex differences in antidepressant effect of sertraline in transgenic mouse models. Frontiers in Cellular Neuroscience. 2019;**13**:24

[47] Weissman MM, Klerman GL. Sex differences and the epidemiology of depression. Archives of General Psychiatry. 1977;**34**(1):98-111

[48] Kessler RC et al. Sex and depression in the National Comorbidity Survey I: Lifetime prevalence, chronicity and recurrence. Journal of Affectice Disorders. 1993;**29**:85-96

[49] Kornstein SG et al. Gender differences in chronic major and double depression. Journal of Affective Disorders. 2000;**60**:1-11

[50] Goel N, Bale TL. Examining the intersection of sex and stress in modelling neuropsychiatric disorders. Journal of Neuroendocrinology. 2009;**21**(4):415-420

[51] Laman-Maharg A, Trainor BC. Stress, sex, and motivated behaviors. Journal of Neuroscience Research. 2017;**95**(1-2):83-92

[52] Verma R, Balhara YP, Gupta CS. Gender differences in stress response: Role of developmental and biological determinants. Industrial Psychiatry Journal. 2011;**20**(1):4-10

[53] Poe GR et al. Locus coeruleus: A new look at the blue spot. Nature Reviews Neuroscience. 2020;**21**(11): 644-659

[54] Curtis AL, Bethea T, Valentino RJ. Sexually dimorphic responses of the brain norepinephrine system to stress and corticotropin-releasing factor. Neuropsychopharmacology. 2006;**31**(3):544-554

[55] Alshammari TK. Sexual dimorphism in pre-clinical studies of depression. Progress in Neuro-Psychopharmacology & Biological Psychiatry. 2020;**105**:110120

[56] Herzog DP et al. Sexually dimorphic behavioral profile in a transgenic model enabling targeted recombination in active neurons in response to ketamine and (2R,6R)-hydroxynorketamine administration. International Journal of Molecular Sciences. 2020;**21**(6):e46729

[57] Franceschelli A et al. Sex differences in the rapid and the sustained antidepressant-like effects of ketamine in stress-naïve and "depressed" mice exposed to chronic mild stress. Neuroscience. 2015;**290**:49-60

[58] Carrier N, Kabbaj M. Sex differences in the antidepressant-like effects of ketamine. Neuropharmacology. 2013;**70**:27-34

[59] Radford KD et al. Sex-related differences in intravenous ketamine effects on dissociative stereotypy and antinociception in male and female rats. Pharmacology Biochemistry and Behavior. 2020;**199**:173042

[60] Saland SK, Kabbaj M. Sex differences in the pharmacokinetics of low-dose ketamine in plasma and brain of male and female rats. Journal of Pharmacology and Experimental Therapeutics. 2018;**367**(3):393

[61] Zhang M et al. Effects of subanesthetic intravenous ketamine infusion on neuroplasticity-related proteins in male and female Sprague-Dawley rats. IBRO Neuroscience Reports. 2021;**11**:42-51

[62] Ouyang X et al. Ketamine ameliorates depressive-like behaviors in mice through increasing glucose uptake regulated by the ERK/GLUT3 signaling pathway. Scientific Reports. 2021;**11**(1):18181

[63] Kuo MH et al. Glucose transporter 3 is essential for the survival of breast cancer cells in the brain. Cell. 2019;**8**(12):e45367

[64] Mantych GJ et al. Cellular localization and characterization of glut 3 glucose transporter isoform in human brain. Endocrinology. 1992;**131**(3): 1270-1278

[65] Dai Y et al. Sex-specific life course changes in the neuro-metabolic phenotype of Glut3 null heterozygous mice: Ketogenic diet ameliorates electroencephalographic seizures and improves sociability. Endocrinology. 2017;**158**(4):936-949

[66] Bliss SP et al. ERK signaling in the pituitary is required for female but not male fertility. Molecular Endocrinology (Baltimore, Md.). 2009;**23**(7):1092-1101

[67] Bychkov E, Ahmed MR, Gurevich EV. Sex differences in the activity of signalling pathways and expression of G-protein-coupled receptor kinases in the neonatal ventral hippocampal lesion model of schizophrenia. The International Journal of Neuropsychopharmacology. 2011;**14**(1):1-15

[68] LeGates TA, Kvarta MD, Thompson SM. Sex differences in antidepressant efficacy. Neuropsychopharmacology. 2019;**44**(1):140-154

[69] Phoenix CH et al. Organizing action of prenatally administered testosterone

propionate on the tissues mediating mating behavior in the female Guinea pig. Endocrinology. 1959;**65**:369-382

[70] Arnold AP, Breedlove SM. Organizational and activational effects of sex steroids on brain and behavior: A reanalysis. Hormones and Behavior. 1985;**19**(4):469-498

[71] Arnold AP. The organizational-activational hypothesis as the foundation for a unified theory of sexual differentiation of all mammalian tissues. Hormones and Behavior. 2009;**55**(5):570-578

[72] Schulz KM, Molenda-Figueira HA, Sisk CL. Back to the future: The organizational–activational hypothesis adapted to puberty and adolescence. Hormones and Behavior. 2009;**55**(5): 597-604

[73] McCarthy MM, Wright CL, Schwarz JM. New tricks by an old dogma: Mechanisms of the organizational/Activational hypothesis of steroid-mediated sexual differentiation of brain and behavior. Hormones and Behavior. 2009;**55**(5):655-665

[74] Lenz B et al. Sex hormone activity in alcohol addiction: Integrating organizational and activational effects. Progress in Neurobiology. 2012;**96**(1):136-163

Chapter 12

Ketamine Anesthesia in Electroconvulsive Therapy

Maiko Satomoto

Abstract

Electroconvulsive therapy (ECT) is highly effective both Major Depressive Disorder (MDD) and Bipolar Disorder (BD). Ketamine, an antagonist of the N-Methyl-D-aspartate receptor, has been described to have antidepressant properties. There is a hypothesis that ECT performed with anesthesia using ketamine is more effective than conventional ECT. Also, although ECT is the gold standard for BD and MDD, there are questions about which is more effective, ketamine treatment or ECT, and whether ketamine is more effective when used in combination with ECT. In this chapter, we review the current literature on the effectiveness of ECT and ketamine. Furthermore, we discuss whether ketamine can be an alternative treatment to ECT for patients with TRD.

Keywords: ketamine, electroconvulsive therapy, depression, side effect, cognitive impairment

1. Introduction

Major Depressive Disorder (MDD) and Bipolar Disorder (BD) are very popular psychiatric disorders that affect 10–15% of people in their lifetime. If symptoms do not improve during episodes of depression with at least two types of antidepressants, this condition is referred to as Treatment-Resistant Depression (TRD), which is observed in 12–20% of patients with depression [1]. The gold standard treatment for TRD is Electroconvulsive Therapy (ECT) [2]. ECT is a safe and effective treatment for TRD. Data shows that the efficacy rate is 79%, and the remission rate is 75% when ECT is used for patients with MDD [3]. Various oral treatments have been introduced since the 1990s. Tricyclic and tetracyclic antidepressants had emerged by the 1990s, and second-generation antidepressants such as selective serotonin reuptake inhibitors (SSRI) and serotonin-noradrenaline reuptake inhibitors (SNRI) were introduced at the end of the 1990s. Although the cause of depression is not clear, the monoamine hypothesis attributes depression to a decrease in neurotransmitters such as serotonin and noradrenaline, which are monoamines, and the action mechanism of the antidepressants is often explained based on the monoamine hypothesis. SSRI and SNRI have fewer side effects, such as dry mouth and dysuria, compared with tricyclic antidepressants, and internationally, they are recognized as the standard treatment. However, the availability of many antidepressants does not necessarily mean that the drug therapy for depression is adequate. STAR*D [4], a large-scale clinical trial investigating the efficacy of switching to the next stage of treatment in patients with depression showing inadequate response to antidepressant medication, found that about half of the total population responded to the initial SSRI treatment, with one-third achieving remission; the response and remission rates decreased with each switch to a different treatment.

Remission has been pointed out to be related to social functioning and prognosis, which is emphasized [5] as a therapeutic goal of depression treatment. According to the results of STAR*D [4], the cumulative remission rate is approximately 67% when medication is switched thrice. This finding suggests that a certain number of patients do not show an adequate response even after treatment with multiple antidepressants, and the limited efficacy of standard treatments is a clinical problem.

2. What is ECT?

Electroconvulsive therapy (ECT) is a treatment method in which generalized seizure activity is induced in the brain through electrical stimulation, producing neurobiological effects to improve clinical symptoms. The history of ECT can be traced back to 1938 when Cerletti U and Bini L of Italy developed a method to induce seizures by passing an electric current through the brain from the scalp on the head, which was the beginning of ECT. Since then, ECT has spread rapidly. Earlier in ECT, an electric current was passed without pretreatment, such as intravenous anesthesia, causing generalized tonic-clonic seizures, feeling of extreme fear experienced by patients, and side effects such as bone fractures or dislocations due to seizures were the problems posed by the treatment. For this reason, ECT was developed, in the 1950s, to pass an electric current without causing seizures of skeletal muscles by keeping patients on mechanical ventilation and administering a combination of anesthetics and muscle relaxants under the supervision of an anesthesiologist.

3. Indications for ECT

ECT is said to have no absolute contraindications. Relative contraindications include (1) intracranial lesions, (2) increased intracranial pressure, (3) recent myocardial infarction, (4) recent cerebral infarction, (5) unstable aneurysm or vascular malformation, (6) pheochromocytoma, and (7) patients with poor physical condition (physical status of 4 or 5 as per the American Society of Anesthesiologists, i.e., with severe threatening systemic disease or moribund). Although medical history interview (allergies, asthma, and history of surgery), blood biochemical tests, electrocardiogram, chest and abdominal X-rays, head CT, and electroencephalogram are performed and recorded before ECT, an echocardiogram, head MRI, and MRA should also be conducted. The cognitive function should also be evaluated in advance, as postictal delirium and transient cognitive impairment may occur, which are described later. ECT is indicated for psychiatric disorders such as depression, schizophrenia, and mania, and has also been shown to be effective in treating Parkinson's disease, malignant syndromes, and chronic pain. The effectiveness of ECT differs depending on the subtype of schizophrenia. At the same time, the treatment is effective for catatonic and acute onset paranoia cases, and there is little effect in hebephrenic and chronic cases. The primary use of ECT should be considered in the following situations: (1) severe symptoms, such as the high risk of suicide attempt or extreme agitation; (2) general deterioration of the patient's condition due to psychiatric symptoms, such as refusing food or catatonic condition; (3) high risk of other forms of treatment, such as in the case of elderly patients or pregnant women; (4) history of ECT treatment with a favorable response; and

(5) preference of the patient. The secondary use of ECT may be considered when the patient is resistant to drug therapy or the patient's tolerability to drug therapy is poor. The indication for ECT is determined based on a combination of diagnosis, symptom type, severity, treatment history, consideration of the expected risks and benefits of ECT with other treatments, and patient's preference.

4. Side effects of ECT

The most common side effects of ECT are postictal delirium and transient cognitive impairment. However, the stimulation dose can be adjusted according to the seizure threshold of each patient by using pulse wave therapy devices, which has significantly reduced seizures compared with conventional treatments. Although the parasympathetic nervous system is dominant immediately after an electric current is passed during ECT, the sympathetic nervous system subsequently becomes dominant. Therefore, bradycardia and sinus arrest may temporarily occur early on. Thereafter, tachycardia and elevated blood pressure are observed, and ventricular arrhythmias may also occur. Although tachycardia and elevated blood pressure are transient, patients with a history of hypertension or ischemic heart disease should be intravenously administered antihypertensive drugs. Even with using muscle relaxants in ECT, the masseter muscle contracts when an electric current passes and can damage the teeth and oral cavity. Although dentures are removed to prevent this, and a bite block is used, dental treatment may be required before ECT if the teeth shake significantly. Other side effects include headache, myalgia, nausea, and prolonged convulsions. Manic episodes may also occur in bipolar depression.

5. Procedure of ECT

ECT is performed in the operating theater under respiratory and circulatory management by an anesthesiologist. In addition to stimulation electrodes and Electroencephalogram (EEG) electrodes (two channels on the left and right) attached to the forehead, Electrocardiogram (ECG) electrodes and Electromyography (EMG) electrodes (on the dorsum of one foot) are attached, the vital signs of the patient are checked, and intravenous anesthesia is administered. When the patient falls asleep, the blood flow to the lower leg with the EMG electrodes is restricted by applying a pressure equal to or more than the systolic blood pressure using the manchette of a sphygmomanometer and a muscle relaxant is administered intravenously. After muscle relaxation is confirmed, a bite block is inserted in the patient's mouth. After passing an electric current, tonic-clonic seizures are observed only in the lower leg with restricted blood flow. The bag-valve-mask ventilation is used when the patient falls asleep until it is confirmed that the patient has resumed spontaneous breathing. The vital signs are rechecked after the patient is fully awake and taken out from the operating theater. Even after returning to the ward, a monitor is attached to the patient for around 1 hour to check the vital signs. This procedure is performed 2–3 times a week, for a total of 8–12 times.

6. Drugs commonly used in ECT

Short-acting intravenous anesthetics are used. Propofol and thiopental are commonly used. The higher the dose of the anesthetic drug, the less likely that seizures will occur; hence, the minimum dose of the intravenous anesthetic drug that puts the patient to sleep is administered. The muscle relaxant used is succinylcholine, which is a depolarizing muscle relaxant. Although non-depolarizing muscle relaxants may also be used to reduce myalgia and increased intragastric pressure, their long duration of action may lead to problems such as the need for a muscle relaxant antagonist [6] after ECT and residual muscle relaxation. Anesthesiologists are also aware that hyperventilation can lead to seizures.

7. Information on ketamine

Although ketamine is an old N-methyl-D-aspartate (NMDA) receptor antagonist, in recent years, the use of subanesthetic doses of ketamine as a therapeutic agent has been reported to have antidepressant effects. Some reports indicate remission rates exceeding 80% with the use of low doses of ketamine [7–10]. There have also been reports that the response to seizures was good when used as an adjunct to ECT, so we did a comprehensive study of the reports. Ketamine may be used independently or as an adjunct, in addition to propofol or thiopental.

We have cited reference Jankauskas et al., [11], which includes a summary up to 2017. Most studies show that when ketamine is used independently or in combination with non-barbiturates such as propofol at doses of 0.8 mg/kg or more during ECT, there is a faster improvement in symptoms and a significant improvement in depressive symptoms compared with the control group where ketamine is not used [12–16]. Seizures during ECT are longer in the intravenous anesthesia group with ketamine or ketamine alone than the intravenous anesthesia group without ketamine [14, 17, 18]. Ketamine was observed to significantly improve cognitive function in the original cases of cognitive decline [14]. Some results show a faster recovery in the ketamine group even if there is no change in the outcome [14, 19].

On the other hand, even if ketamine prolongs the duration of seizures, according to some reports, ketamine is not better than other anesthetics in reducing depressive symptoms or improving cognition [16, 20–23]. The effect of ketamine on the duration of seizures during ECT has been evaluated differently in each study, and the ECT protocols vary from institution to institution making efficacy assessment difficult [11]. The additional problem is that the assessment items (seizure duration, early stage of rapport, or cognitive improvement) do not match.

Since propofol suppresses the disadvantages of ketamine such as agitation, cardiotoxicity, nausea, and psychotomimetic effects, the combination of propofol and ketamine is good as propofol suppresses the disadvantages of ketamine without compromising its efficacy [13, 17]. Ketamine also reduces hypotension, a side effect of propofol, another reason for considering the combination as good [17]. Many reports indicate that the benefits of ketamine are not effective when used in combination with barbiturates due to the anti-seizure action of barbiturates and did not show a reduction effect for depression [12, 16, 20, 24].

Safety concerns with ECT include high rates of hypertension, prolonged QTc interval, transient arrhythmias, confusion or fear, and hallucinations that may occur upon awakening from the anesthetic [12, 13, 17, 20, 25–27]. The incidence of hallucinations has a positive correlation with the increase in ketamine dose, especially in the dose range of 0.8–2.0 mg/kg [13, 17, 20, 25–27]. Caution should be exercised when using ketamine in patients with cardiovascular diseases, as the drug increases blood pressure. Caution should also be exercised when using ketamine in patients with a history of psychomimetic episodes, as there is a possibility of psychotogenesis.

Concomitant use of propofol may be considered to mitigate some of these adverse effects [13]. However, the complexity and cost of the medication will increase. Most of the adverse effects such as agitation, cardiotoxicity, nausea, and psychotomimetic effects are temporary [12, 16]. Therefore, an analysis of individual risks and benefits needs to be considered.

8. Role of ketamine in ECT in recent years

Although studies of varying scales and assessment have continued, some studies have found the addition of ketamine to ECT to be effective [28, 29], and some have found the addition as not effective [30]. We will introduce one such study. A multi-site randomized, placebo-controlled, double-blind trial, "Ketamine-ECT study" was planned at the University of Newcastle in the United Kingdom to investigate whether the adjunctive use of ketamine can attenuate the cognitive impairment caused by ECT [31]. ECT continues to be the gold standard for severe and treatment-resistant depression. However, a significant limitation contributing to the declining use of ECT is its association with cognitive impairment, especially in anterograde and retrograde memory and functional impairment.

On the other hand, preliminary data suggest that ketamine, used either as the sole anesthetic drug or in addition to other anesthetics, may reduce or prevent cognitive impairment after ECT. A hypothesis has been postulated that ketamine protects from excess excitatory neurotransmitter stimulation during ECT through glutamate receptor antagonism. The primary aim of the "ketamine-ECT study" was to investigate whether the adjunctive use of ketamine can attenuate the cognitive impairment caused by ECT. The secondary aim was to examine if ketamine increases the speed of clinical improvement with ECT. The summary of the study is that moderately to severely depressed patients who had been prescribed ECT were randomly grouped on a 1:1 basis to receive either adjunctive ketamine or saline in addition to standard anesthesia for ECT. A 0.5 mg/kg dose of ketamine was administered as a bolus instead of continuous administration. The primary neuropsychological outcome is anterograde verbal memory (Hopkins Verbal Learning Test-Revised delayed recall task) after four ECT treatments. Secondary cognitive outcomes include verbal fluency, autobiographical memory, visuospatial memory, and digitization span. Efficacy was assessed using evaluation by observer and report of subjects on the depressive symptoms by patients.

This randomized trial validated the hypothesis that low doses of ketamine administered with a course of ECT treatment would improve outcomes in depression. We did not find significant evidence for cognitive and efficacy outcomes by administering a dose of 0.5 mg/kg ketamine as an adjunct in patients treated with ECT for depression.

However, the number of subjects was less than the number of patients recruited, which implies that the small to medium benefits and medium to extensive harms of ketamine cannot be ruled out. Therefore, it is not always possible to conclude based on only these results. It is also debated that evaluation in this field is complicated, especially the evaluation of cognitive function after ECT. For example, although patients recover most of the cognitive decline after ECT within a few days to a few weeks after the completion of treatment, it is challenging to accurately measure the recovery of retrograde autobiographical memory, which is the primary concern for patients. Although this paper has been discussed extensively, the study did not indicate that ketamine improved the outcome of depression. However, since treatment-resistant depression still exists and some papers have shown that ketamine is effective, we believe it is worth continuing research by evaluating various subgroups or using an optimal psychological index to determine the efficacy.

9. Future of ketamine in ECT

As introduced in Section 8, there are more than 130 papers on the adjunctive use of ketamine with ECT; however, only a few are definitive. Although well-conceived studies with sufficient resources are needed, they are not conducted, and the availability of funding is also not likely. Many papers have recognized the efficacy of ketamine with small-scale studies. ECT is an effective treatment method in clinical practice since patients showing resistance to treatment with only oral medication are high at 33%. Memory impairment caused by ECT is a significant problem faced by patients. The condition of patients with depression before ECT treatment varies widely; hence, it is necessary to divide them into subgroups. If there is a possibility that ECT can improve cognitive impairment, we consider that further studies are needed to evaluate the effects of ketamine by dividing patients into more specific subgroups.

10. Ketamine as an alternative to ECT

As described in Section 8, the decline in cognitive function after the ECT procedure causes significant distress to patients [32]. Unfortunately, additional ECT is sometimes required due to the frequent recurrence of TRD. The recurrence rate of TRD within 6 months of ECT is reported to be between 39% (with continued medication) and 84% (without continued medication) [33]. If patients become aware of their cognitive impairment even once, ECT treatment becomes unbearably painful for them [33]. There is a pressing need to develop a treatment with the same effectiveness as ECT but with fewer side effects and recurrences. Ketamine, an NMDA receptor antagonist, has repeatedly shown an immediate and strong antidepressant effect in patients with MDD [34, 35]. Ketamine demonstrates a positive effect even in patients with severe TRD [36]. Whether ketamine can be an alternative treatment to ECT for patients with TRD is discussed in this section. There are six papers at present [37]. While randomized control trials [38–40] are discussed in three papers, the other three cover open-label trials [41–43]. The results suggest that ketamine therapy develops antidepressant effects more quickly than ECT, but perhaps the effect is not sustained compared with ECT. Unlike ECT, cognitive impairment was found to be less with ketamine therapy. The sample size of the studies was limited, followed different treatment protocols, and long-term follow-up was lacking in most trials. The occurrence of assignment bias is high as the trials were not randomized, and performing ECT and ketamine therapy in double-blind trials is difficult. The results of the current studies do not provide convincing evidence to indicate that ketamine therapy is an equally effective alternative to ECT for patients with TRD. If ketamine is used in high doses for chronic cases because of its advantages over ECT during treatment at the initial stage, it may cause memory impairment [44]. Long-term maintenance therapy with ketamine may make patients prone to ketamine-related addiction. This risk should be considered when comparing ketamine therapy to ECT. The reported acute side effects of ketamine therapy are dizziness, headache, blurred vision, body numbness, depersonalization, vertigo, double vision, and nausea. The reasons for discontinuing ketamine were dissociative symptoms, hypertension, and unpleasant experience. The impact of acute and chronic adverse events attributable to ketamine therapy needs to be compared with the common side effects of ECT treatment, such as cognitive impairment, myalgia, arthralgia, headache, and risks associated with general anesthesia. Studies with larger sample sizes and longer follow-up duration are needed.

11. Conclusions

ECT is still the gold standard for severe and treatment-resistant depression patients, but cognitive dysfunction after ECT is the problem. Although the antidepressant effect of ketamine has been attracting attention in recent years, it cannot be said that ketamine is an effective treatment alternative to ECT at this stage. Many studies have shown that adding small amounts of ketamine during ECT is effective with small-scale studies. Although well-conceived studies with sufficient resources are needed, they are not conducted.

Acknowledgements

This work was supported by Grants-in-Aid for Scientific Research (KAKENHI) Grants No. 19 K18308.

Conflict of interest

The author declares no conflict of interest.

Author details

Maiko Satomoto
Department of Anesthesiology, Toho University Omori Medical Center, Tokyo, Japan

*Address all correspondence to: maiko.satomoto@med.toho-u.ac.jp

References

[1] Mrazek DA, Hornberger JC, Altar CA, Degtiar I. A review of the clinical, economic, and societal burden of treatment-resistant depression: 1996-2013. Psychiatric Services. 2014;**65**:977-987. DOI: 10.1176/appi.ps.201300059

[2] UK ECT Review Group. Efficacy and safety of electroconvulsive therapy in depressive disorders: A systematic review and meta-analysis. Lancet. 2003;**361**:799-808. DOI: 10.1016/S0140-6736(03)12705-5

[3] Tang YL, Jiang W, Ren YP, Ma X, Cotes RO, McDonald WM. Electroconvulsive therapy in China: Clinical practice and research on efficacy. The Journal of ECT. 2012;**28**:206-212. DOI: 10.1097/YCT.0b013e31825957b1

[4] Rush AJ, Trivedi MH, Wisniewski SR, Nierenberg AA, Stewart JW, Warden D, et al. Acute and longer-term outcomes in depressed outpatients requiring one or several treatment steps: A STAR*D report. American Journal of Psychiatry. 2006;**163**:1905-1917. DOI: 10.1176/ajp.2006.163.11.1905

[5] Rush AJ, Kraemer HC, Sackeim HA, Fava M, Trivedi MH, Frank E, et al. Report by the ACNP Task Force on response and remission in major depressive disorder. Neuropsychopharmacology. 2006;**31**:1841-1853. DOI: 10.1038/sj.npp.1301131

[6] Kadoi Y, Nishida A, Saito S. Recovery time after sugammadex reversal of rocuronium-induced muscle relaxation for electroconvulsive therapy is independent of cardiac output in both young and elderly patients. The Journal of ECT. 2013;**29**:33-36. DOI: 10.1097/YCT.0b013e31826cf348

[7] aan het Rot M, Collins KA, Murrough JW, Perez AM, Reich DL, Charney DS, et al. Safety and efficacy of repeated-dose intravenous ketamine for treatment-resistant depression. Biological Psychiatry. 2010;**67**:139-145. DOI: 10.1016/j.biopsych.2009.08.038

[8] Rasmussen KG, Lineberry TW, Galardy CW, Kung S, Lapid MI, Palmer BA, et al. Serial infusions of low-dose ketamine for major depression. Journal of Psychopharmacology. 2013;**27**:444-450. DOI: 10.1177/0269881113478283

[9] Shiroma PR, Johns B, Kuskowski M, Wels J, Thuras P, Albott CS, et al. Augmentation of response and remission to serial intravenous subanesthetic ketamine in treatment resistant depression. Journal of Affective Disorders. 2014;**155**:123-129. DOI: 10.1016/j.jad.2013.10.036

[10] Naughton M, Clarke G, O'Leary OF, Cryan JF, Dinan TG. A review of ketamine in affective disorders: Current evidence of clinical efficacy, limitations of use and pre-clinical evidence on proposed mechanisms of action. Journal of Affective Disorders. 2014;**156**:24-35. DOI: 10.1016/j.jad.2013.11.014

[11] Jankauskas V, Necyk C, Chue J, Chue P. A review of ketamine's role in ECT and non-ECT settings. Neuropsychiatric Disease and Treatment. 2018;**14**:1437-1450. DOI: 10.2147/NDT.S157233

[12] Jarventausta K, Chrapek W, Kampman O, Tuohimaa K, Björkqvist M, Häkkinen H, et al. Effects of S-ketamine as an anesthetic adjuvant to propofol on treatment response to electroconvulsive therapy in treatment-resistant depression: A randomized pilot study. The Journal of ECT. 2013;**29**:158-161. DOI: 10.1097/YCT.0b013e318283b7e9

[13] Wang X, Chen Y, Zhou X, Liu F, Zhang T, Zhang C. Effects of propofol

and ketamine as combined anesthesia for electroconvulsive therapy in patients with depressive disorder. The Journal of ECT. 2012;**28**:128-132

[14] Yoosefi A, Sepehri AS, Kargar M, Akhondzadeh S, Sadeghi M, Rafei A, et al. Comparing effects of ketamine and thiopental administration during electroconvulsive therapy in patients with major depressive disorder: A randomized, double-blind study. The Journal of ECT. 2014;**30**:15-21. DOI: 10.1097/YCT.0b013e31824d1d02

[15] Rybakowski JK, Bodnar A, Krzywotulski M, Chlopocka-Wozniak M, Michalak M, Rosada-Kurasinska J, et al. Ketamine anesthesia, efficacy of electroconvulsive therapy, and cognitive functions in treatment-resistant depression. The Journal of ECT. 2016;**32**(3):164-168. DOI: 10.1097/YCT.0000000000000317

[16] Zhong X, He H, Zhang C, Wang Z, Jiang M, Li Q, et al. Mood and neuropsychological effects of different doses of ketamine in electroconvulsive therapy for treatment-resistant depression. Journal of Affective Disorders. 2016;**201**:124-130. DOI: 10.1016/j.jad.2016.05.011

[17] Yalcin S, Aydogan H, Selek S, Kucuk A, Yuce HH, Karababa F, et al. Ketofol in electroconvulsive therapy anesthesia: Two stones for one bird. Journal of Anesthesia. 2012;**26**:562-567. DOI: 10.1007/s00540-012-1378-6

[18] Erdil F, Begec Z, Kayhan GE, Yologlu S, Ersoy MO, Durmus M. Effects of sevoflurane or ketamine on the QTc interval during electroconvulsive therapy. Journal of Anesthesia. 2015;**29**:180-185. DOI: 10.1007/s00540-014-1899-2

[19] Salehi B, Mohammadbeigi A, Kamali AR, Taheri-Nejad MR, Moshiri I. Impact comparison of ketamine and sodium thiopental on anesthesia during electroconvulsive therapy in major depression patients with drug-resistant; a double-blind randomized clinical trial. Annals of Cardiac Anaesthesia. 2015;**18**:486-490. DOI: 10.4103/0971-9784.166444

[20] Kuscu OO, Karacaer F, Biricik E, Gulec E, Tamam L, Gunes Y. Effect of ketamine, thiopental and ketamine-thiopental combination during electroconvulsive therapy for depression. Turkish Journal of Anaesthesiology and Reanimation. 2015;**43**:313-317. DOI: 10.5152/TJAR.2015.92668

[21] Fernie G, Currie J, Perrin JS, Stewart CA, Anderson V, Bennett DM, et al. Ketamine as the anaesthetic for electroconvulsive therapy: The KANECT randomised controlled trial. The British Journal of Psychiatry. 2017;**210**:422-428. DOI: 10.1192/bjp.bp.116.189134

[22] Rasmussen KG, Kung S, Lapid MI, Oesterle TS, Geske JR, Nuttall GA, et al. A randomized comparison of ketamine versus methohexital anesthesia in electroconvulsive therapy. Psychiatry Research. 2014;**215**:362-365. DOI: 10.1016/j.psychres.2013.12.027

[23] Loo CK, Katalinic N, Garfield JB, Sainsbury K, Hadzi-Pavlovic D, Mac-Pherson R. Neuropsychological and mood effects of ketamine in electroconvulsive therapy: A randomised controlled trial. Journal of Affective Disorders. 2012;**142**:233-240. DOI: 10.1016/j.jad.2012.04.032

[24] Abdallah CG, Fasula M, Kelmendi B, Sanacora G, Ostroff R. Rapid antidepressant effect of ketamine in the electroconvulsive therapy setting. The Journal of ECT. 2012;**28**:157-161. DOI: 10.1097/YCT.0b013e31824f8296

[25] Erdil F, Ozgul U, Colak C, Cumurcu B, Durmus M. Effect of the

addition of ketamine to sevoflurane anesthesia on seizure duration in electroconvulsive therapy. The Journal of ECT. 2015;**31**:182-185. DOI: 10.1097/YCT.0000000000000225

[26] Lenze EJ, Farber NB, Kharasch E, Schweiger J, Yingling M, Olney J, et al. Ninety-six hour ketamine infusion with co-administered clonidine for treatment-resistant depression: A pilot randomised controlled trial. The World Journal of Biological Psychiatry. 2016;**17**:230-238. DOI: 10.3109/15622975.2016.1142607

[27] Ibrahim L, Diazgranados N, Franco-Chaves J, Schweiger J, Yingling M, Olney J, et al. Course of improvement in depressive symptoms to a single intravenous infusion of ketamine vs add-on riluzole: Results from a 4-week, double-blind, placebo-controlled study. Neuropsychopharmacology. 2012;**37**:1526-1533. DOI: 10.1038/npp.2011.338

[28] Altinay M, Karne H, Anand A. Administration of sub-anesthetic dose of ketamine and electroconvulsive treatment on alternate week days in patients with treatment resistant depression: A double blind placebo controlled trial. Psychopharmacology Bulletin. 2019;**49**:8-16

[29] Zhang M, Rosenheck R, Lin X, Li Q, Zhou Y, Xiao Y, et al. A randomized clinical trial of adjunctive ketamine anesthesia in electro-convulsive therapy for depression. Journal of Affective Disorders. 2018;**227**:372-378. DOI: 10.1016/j.jad.2017.11.034

[30] Gamble JJ, Bi H, Bowen R, Weisgerber G, Sanjanwala R, Prasad R, et al. Ketamine-based anesthesia improves electroconvulsive therapy outcomes: A randomized-controlled study. Canadian Journal of Anesthesia. 2018;**65**:636-646. DOI: 10.1007/s12630-018-1088-0

[31] Anderson IM, Blamire A, Branton T, Clark R, Downey D, Dunn G, et al. Ketamine augmentation of electroconvulsive therapy to improve neuropsychological and clinical outcomes in depression (ketamine-ECT): A multicentre, double-blind, randomised, parallel-group, superiority trial. The Lancet Psychiatry. 2017;**4**:365-377. DOI: 10.1016/S2215-0366(17)30077-9

[32] Verwijk E, Obbels J, Spaans HP, Sienaert P. Doctor, will I get my memory back? Electroconvulsive therapy and cognitive side-effects in daily practice. Tijdschrift Voor Psychiatrie. 2017;**59**:632-637

[33] Sackeim HA, Haskett RF, Mulsant BH, Thase ME, Mann JJ, Pettinati HM, et al. Continuation pharmacotherapy in the prevention of relapse following electroconvulsive therapy: A randomized controlled trial. JAMA. 2001;**285**:1299-1307. DOI: 10.1001/jama.285.10.1299

[34] Han Y, Chen J, Zou D, Zheng P, Li Q, Wang H, et al. Efficacy of ketamine in the rapid treatment of major depressive disorder: A meta-analysis of randomized, double-blind, placebo-controlled studies. Neuropsychiatric Disease and Treatment. 2016;**12**:2859-2867. DOI: 10.2147/NDT.S117146

[35] Kishimoto T, Chawla JM, Hagi K, Zarate CA, Kane JM, Bauer M, et al. Single-dose infusion ketamine and non-ketamine N-methyl-d-aspartate receptor antagonists for unipolar and bipolar depression: A meta-analysis of efficacy, safety and time trajectories. Psychological Medicine. 2016;**46**:1459-1472. DOI: 10.1017/S0033291716000064

[36] Ruberto VL, Jha MK, Murrough JW. Pharmacological treatments for patients with treatment-resistant depression. Pharmaceuticals (Basel). 2020;**13**:116. DOI: 10.3390/ph13060116

[37] Veraart JKE, Smith-Apeldoorn SY, Spaans HP, Kamphuis J, Schoevers RA. Is ketamine an appropriate alternative to ECT for patients with treatment resistant depression? A systematic review. Journal of Affective Disorders. 2021;**281**:82-89. DOI: 10.1016/j.jad.2020.11.123

[38] Ghasemi M, Kazemi MH, Yoosefi A, Ghasemi A, Paragomi P, Amini H, et al. Rapid antidepressant effects of repeated doses of ketamine compared with electroconvulsive therapy in hospitalized patients with major depressive disorder. Psychiatry Research. 2014;**215**:355-361. DOI: 10.1016/j.psychres.2013.12.008

[39] Kheirabadi G, Vafaie M, Kheirabadi D, Mirlouhi Z, Hajiannasab R. Comparative effect of intravenous ketamine and electroconvulsive therapy in major depression: A randomized controlled trial. Advanced Biomedical Research. 2019;**8**:25. DOI: 10.4103/abr.abr_166_18

[40] Sharma RK, Kulkarni G, Kumar CN, Arumugham SS, Sudhir V, Mehta UM, et al. Antidepressant effects of ketamine and ECT: A pilot comparison. Journal of Affective Disorders. 2020;**276**:260-266. DOI: 10.1016/j.jad.2020.07.066

[41] Allen AP, Naughton M, Dowling J, Walsh A, Ismail F, Shorten G, et al. Serum BDNF as a peripheral biomarker of treatment-resistant depression and the rapid antidepressant response: A comparison of ketamine and ECT. Journal of Affective Disorders. 2015;**186**:306-311. DOI: 10.1016/j.jad.2015.06.033

[42] Basso L, Bönke L, Aust S, Gärtner M, Heuser-Collier I, Otte C, et al. Antidepressant and neurocognitive effects of serial ketamine administration versus ECT in depressed patients. Journal of Psychiatric Research. 2020;**123**:1-8. DOI: 10.1016/j.jpsychires.2020.01.002

[43] Loureiro JRA, Leaver A, Vasavada M, Sahib AK, Kubicki A, Joshi S, et al. Modulation of amygdala reactivity following rapidly acting interventions for major depression. Human Brain Mapping. 2020;**41**(7):1699-1710. DOI: 10.1002/hbm.24895

[44] Morgan CJ, Dodds CM, Furby H, Pepper F, Fam J, Freeman TP, et al. Long-term heavy ketamine use is associated with spatial memory impairment and altered hippocampal activation. Frontiers in Psychiatry. 2014;**5**:149. DOI: 10.3389/fpsyt.2014.00149

Section 5

Special Situations

Chapter 13

Ketamine for Anesthetic Premedication in Children: Pearls, Pitfalls and Review of Clinical Utility

Shahla Haleem

Abstract

Ketamine, since its difficult introduction into clinical practice nearly half a millennium ago, has now become widely utilized as an anesthetic agent, especially in adults. Its efficacy in procedural anesthesia and pain management, along with its safety, has been proven in several clinical studies. This book chapter reviews the clinical utility of ketamine when used in young individuals. Premedication is an essential component of anesthetic protocol for parents and children to overcome emotional or psychological distress. Preoperative anxiety, being associated with greater pain during postoperative recovery in children, calls for the effective use of premedicants. This chapter describes how the cognizance of perioperative pain and the use of ketamine in children has become especially popular over the past few decades. It also discusses how intramuscular ketamine as a premedicant in subanaesthetic doses has a special role in the management of highly uncooperative children. As a potent analgesic, ketamine has a complex mechanism of action, producing a state of sedation, immobility, analgesia, amnesia, and dissociation from the environment. Some institutions are using ketamine in infants over 7 months and toddlers as part of premedication protocols for preoperative sedation, prevention of response to separation and intravenous access, and postoperative pain control in infants. This chapter also discusses the pearls and pitfalls in using ketamine in these challenging populations.

Keywords: ketamine, procedural sedation, analgesia, dissociative anesthesia, preanesthetic drug, premedication

1. Introduction

Ketamine, since its difficult introduction into clinical practice nearly half a millennium ago, has now become widely utilized as an anesthetic agent, especially in adults. Its efficacy in procedural anesthesia and pain management, along with its safety, has been proven in several clinical studies. This book chapter reviews the clinical utility of ketamine when used in young individuals as a premedicant.

Surgical interventions are not merely physically stressful but are an emotionally distressful process for both children and their parents. In a scheduled surgical operation, the preoperative period is a traumatic and challenging experience for younger patients; which is often taken casually. This usually leads to preoperative anxiety, postoperative distress, prolonged child illness, and hospitalization. Excessive preoperative anxiety has been reported to result in more pain, negative postoperative outcomes as fear of anesthesia, and long-term behavioral problems [1].

Approximately 70% of the children exhibit significant stress and anxiety before surgery [2]. Preanesthetic medications are highly required in pediatric surgical patients for the management of preoperative anxiety, to help in iv cannulation, mask acceptance, and prevent long-term psychological/behavioral disturbances.

Approximately 84–100% of anesthesiologists now use the premedicants [3]. As part of the anesthetic technique, these premedicant drugs are given before the administration of an anesthetic agent, to make anesthesia safer and more agreeable to the patient. To alleviate anxiety and fear of surgery and anesthesia a premedicant is usually required before anesthesia.

2. Criteria for selection of premedication

Various factors have to be considered while selecting the premedication. The premedicant must be able:

1. To provide sedation and hypnosis have an amnesiac effect

2. To allay anxiety and apprehension

3. Have an anticholinergic effect

4. Have anti-emetic effect

5. Have an additive or synergistic effect on induction, for instance, ensuring a smoother and more rapid induction of anesthesia

6. To inhibit the parasympathetic nervous system

7. Reducing the dosage of anesthetic agents

8. Counteract certain adverse effects of the anesthetic drug

9. To relieve pain

2.1 Choice of premedicant

It is found that if preoperative apprehension of the child is not relieved, leads to psychic trauma, struggling, prolonged stormy induction, sometimes hypoxemia, or even anoxia owing to inadequate induction and relaxation finally airway obstruction, thereby anesthetic risk is increased or multiply. It is an unforgettable situation for children and even adults and permanent psychological trauma. The choice of premedicant is usually individualized, chosen for a particular patient and technique of anesthesia. They should relieve anxiety and central nervous system (CNS) depressants are necessary for psychic sedation.

3. Commonly used premedicant and their comparison with ketamine

They are fentanyl, midazolam, promethazine pheniramine maleate and dexmedetomidine have their own merits and demerits. Narcotics and benzodiazepines may produce respiratory depression and require close monitoring. Barbiturate, a hypnotic, is also used as a premedicant when basal narcotic doses are required. Such doses produce unconsciousness with respiratory and circulatory depression. Antisecretory agents, the anticholinergics are commonly used with premedicant drugs in children, considered mandatory in new-born and infants due to the following reasons: they suppress secretions or dry up secretion, prevent bradycardia, prevent laryngospasm (may produce due to excessive secretion), produce bronchodilatation and have an antiemetic effect. The most common method of administration of anticholinergic drugs in the past was the intramuscular route now they are used intravenously [4].

3.1 Comparison with phenothiazines

In comparison to ketamine the phenothiazine derivatives as chlorpromazine (the prototype), prochlorperazine, trimeprazine, and promethazine (phenergan), enhance the effects of other central nervous system depressants. They are neuroleptics and dopamine antagonists having antihistaminic, antiadrenergic, anticholinergic, and antiemetic activity.

Contrary to ketamine phenothiazines are sympatholytic and ganglioplegic, can cause hypotension due to alpha-1-adrenergic blockade and peripheral vasodilation; contraindicated in shock, hypotensive, or anemic patients. Phenothiazines possess antiarrhythmic properties, and promethazine of this group has the least side effects and is often recommended. In the past, trimeprazine and promethazine were the most commonly used premedicant in children. Furthermore, they lack any generalized hypnotic effect and do not produce analgesia, instead are ant analgesia. A large dose can depress ventilation, when combined with opioids and hypnotics, due to additive effects, thus respiratory depression may occur.

Contrarily, ketamine is sympathomimetic, a potent analgesic, and has anti-inflammatory, antidepressant, and antiemetic effects through its action centrally on the chemoreceptor trigger zone as well on the vomiting center of the CNS.

Metabolism of phenothiazine is by biotransformation in the liver with glucuronic acid. If overdosed, metabolites are excreted in the urine for several days, as no specific antagonist is available. Phenothiazines can be given, orally, subcutaneously, intramuscularly, or intravenously.

3.2 Comparison with benzodiazepines

The sedative-hypnotic drugs are usually essential premedicants in children, as a struggling child is often challenging to provide anesthesia to. A drowsy or sleepy child makes the process easier. The benzodiazepines are the most common premedicant in this group used in infants and children apart from adult patients because of their good anxiolytic properties coupled with fewer side effects. It was used approximately in 83% population to get smooth induction of anesthesia along with sedation and amnesia. In the past, temazepam or diazepam have been used in children when using ether-based or chloroform-based anesthetic protocols. Temazepam is most frequently used due to its short half-life as compared to diazepam [4]. Midazolam is a benzodiazepine believed to be a good choice for premedication due to its anxiolytic, sedative, anticonvulsant, antiemetic, rapid onset, and relatively short duration of action [5], but several studies have shown that satisfactory results are seen only in 60–80% of cases [6].

However, these drugs are less frequently used by some anesthetists probably due to concern of delayed recovery from anesthesia and respiratory depression following intravenous injection, which requires close monitoring.

The antagonist agent to benzodiazepines is flumazenil which is not frequently used in most parts of the world due to the high cost involved. Flumazenil injection is indicated for a complete or partial reversal of the sedative effects of benzodiazepines in conscious sedation and general anesthesia in both adult and pediatric populations.

3.3 Comparison with alpha 2 adrenergic agonists

In uncooperative children, clonidine or dexmedetomidine can also be used as a premedicant due to its anxiolytic property. They can reduce the need for rescue analgesics, reduce emergence agitation, postoperative nausea and vomiting, and postoperative shivering [7]. Dexmedetomidine being highly selective having sympatholytic properties provides sedation, analgesia, and anxiolysis without causing respiratory depression. It can be used as an adjunct for premedication, especially for those patients who are susceptible to preoperative stress [8].

Thus, children treated with dexmedetomidine are more adequately sedated at the time of arrival in the PACU and a less volatile anesthetic is required to achieve hemodynamic endpoints. This allows rapid recovery from anesthesia with greater overall cardiovascular stability and fewer episodes of tachycardia in the perioperative period [8].

4. Use of ketamine as a premedicant

Ketamine as a premedicant in children is not a very popular practice. It is a non-barbiturate anesthetic, meeting most of the criteria of ideal premedicant produces balanced sedation with intact airway reflexes, immobility, analgesia, amnesia, and dissociation from the environment. The incidence of agitation, anxiety at parental separation, and reaction to insertion of the intravenous catheter were very low while adverse side effects were seen rarely. There is less respiratory depression and no myocardial depression. The cardiovascular changes including changes in blood pressure (BP) or heart rate (HR) are significant when used alone. However, its effects on intracranial pressure and intraocular pressure have been concerning overtime.

5. Routes of administration of ketamine

The use of ketamine as a premedicant in children has not been a very popular practice historically. However, its oral preparations have been reported to be used by some authors in the past [5, 9–11].

Ketamine is rapidly absorbed after intravenous, intramuscular, or intranasal administrations. It was found that when it is given through the intranasal or intravenous routes, pharmacokinetic parameters were similar [12]. In general, drug absorption is mainly determined by its physicochemical properties. Ketamine's formulation as the ketamine is highly lipid-soluble which is five times higher than thiopentone. It has an extensive distribution in the body and has low binding to plasma proteins, being approximately 10–30% [13, 14].

Bioavailability of ketamine depends largely on the route of administration as 20% oral; 93–90% intravenous or intramuscular; 25% rectal; 50% intranasal [15, 16].

After the intravenous route of administration, action is achieved within 1 min as it reaches the receptors very quickly with a transfer half-life of less than 1 min. On i.m. administration, the plasma peak concentration attained within 5 min. It is found that on intramuscular injection, the absorption occurs very fast in children as compared to adults. Children's muscles are not well developed as compared to adults and the regional flow is different.

Ketamine has a lipid-soluble structure, which diffuses more rapidly than non-lipid soluble drugs across cell membranes. On oral administration, it diffuses across a cell membrane from a region of high concentration such as gastrointestinal fluids to low concentration as blood. Apart from the flow following diffusion gradient and lipid solubility, it also depends on size, degree of ionization, and absorptive surface area. After oral administration, most of the ketamine is destroyed in the acidic media of the gastrointestinal tract, degraded by its secretions and enzymes. Despite the large surface area of the stomach, not much of the drug is absorbed from the stomach due to the thick mucus layer. Furthermore, owing to its parasympatholytic effect it has a short transit time hence gets less time for absorption. Thus, a large part of the drug gets destroyed on oral administration as compared to intramuscular or intravenous [3].

The intrarectal ketamine bioavailability is 25% while intranasal has 50%. It is found that nor ketamine plasma concentration achieved higher as compared to ketamine on identical dose [3].

5.1 Common clinical practice regarding the route of administration

Despite faster absorption by intravenous and intramuscular routes, it was most commonly used by the oral route in the past. Oral transmucosal ketamine (OTK) in the form of a lollipop was also used in the past.

In our hospital, we use ketamine as premedication either intravenous or intramuscular route.

Figure 1 summarizes the decision-making behind choosing between the two routes of ketamine.

The effectiveness of ketamine as premedication may be assessed based on Epstein et al. [17] scoring system, i.e. the Five Points-Sedation Score.

1. Asleep,

2. Not readily arousable,

3. Asleep, but arousable,

4. Calm but awake,

5. Restless, agitated

With ketamine, we should be getting a score of either 1 or 2 indicating the adequacy of sedation.

Regarding the score for acceptance of separation from parents (scoring = 1. easy, 2. slightly resistant, 3. markedly resistant) we get the score of 1 usually, representing competence of ketamine as premedication.

For mask acceptance (1. easy, 2. slightly resistant, 3. markedly resistant) again, the score with ketamine is usually 1, signifying the capability of ketamine as premedication.

	Ketamine IV	Ketamine IM
Dose	1-2 mg/kg slow IV push.	4-5 mg/kg IM
Onset	1-5 min	4-5 min
Duration	Approx. 20min	Approx. 25 min
Benefits	**1.** Provides Analgesia, Sedation and Amnesia **2.** Predictable onset and offset. **3.** Does not decrease respiratory drive.	Same as IV
Side-effects	Emesis Laryngospasm Emergence reaction	Similar IV but higher rate of emesis
Recovery	Approx. 60 min	Approx. 90-120 min

Figure 1.
Comparison of intravenous and intramuscular dosing of ketamine. Figure adapted from Emergency Medicine Cases website. Available from: https://emergencymedicinecases.com/pediatric-procedural-sedation/, Creative Commons License.

6. Standard protocol for ketamine as premedicant

Prerequisite for ketamine premedication includes the readily available all resuscitation equipment, emergency drugs anesthesia machine, or Ambu resuscitator for positive pressure ventilation and continuous oxygen source.

Preanesthetic evaluation to be done before ketamine administration. Children under 3 months of age are an absolute contraindication and age between 3 and 6 months is a relative contraindication to ketamine-based anesthesia. Pulmonary as current upper respiratory infection or neurologic disease as psychosis were not considered fit for ketamine premedication. Children with cardiovascular diseases where increased heart rate and cardiac workload is present as hypertension, ischaemic heart disease, cardiac failure are also cases where ketamine is contraindicated. Thyroid disease, and acute globe injury or glaucoma are considered as a contraindication to ketamine anesthesia.

The procedure should be explained to the parents including sedation and even about rare unpleasant emergence phenomena. Informed consent must be obtained before the use of ketamine premedication. Baseline vitals to be checked including

BP, HR, RR, and O_2 saturation. If the administration is planned apart from an oral route, then topical anesthetic cream should be applied approximately 45–60 min before the start of the intravenous line.

Anticholinergics as glycopyrrolate or atropine are necessary with ketamine premedication to prevent the excessive salivation associated with ketamine use, which may lead to blockage of the endotracheal tube due to drooling of saliva. However, in oral or intramuscular ketamine premedication, anticholinergic is usually given after sedation, following the start of the intravenous line. Intravenous ketamine premedication is started with anticholinergic as glycopyrrolate/atropine depending upon pediatric age, infants, or grown-up child. Benzodiazepines such as midazolam are usually given simultaneously in a low dose with ketamine via i.v. or i.m. route to prevent its psychomimetic effects like agitation, hypertension, hyperthermia, and seizures [18].

Anesthetic adjunctive agent as ondansetron may be considered before the start of ketamine sedation, in children over 8 years of age [19].

Standard monitoring includes pulse oximetry, non-invasive blood pressure, heart rate and respiratory rates (RR) along with close observation of the airway and chest movements are required. The intravenous line usually sets in after achieving sedation and analgesia.

The oral ketamine dose is 4–6 mg/kg, usually, 5 mg/kg is adequate. Intravenous dose is 1–2 mg/kg, usually, 1.5 mg/kg, given slowly (over 1–2 min) as rapid administration may lead to respiratory depression, clinical onset is 1–2 min. The intramuscular dose is 2–4 mg/kg, clinical onset 3–4 min, effective sedation is achieved within 5 min. Intranasal is 3–5 mg/kg onset 10–15 min and buccal/transmucosal is 5–6 mg/kg onset is also 10–15 min. Per-rectal ketamine usually 5–10 mg/kg is given. 10 mg/kg may lead to delayed emergence from anesthesia [20].

In our institution, we prefer the intramuscular route for ketamine premedication in an uncooperative or frightened child or when it is difficult to put IV line or where no intravenous access has been secured before the transfer of the child to the preoperative preparation room. If there is already an IV line then it is a reasonable approach to administer ketamine intravenously. However, rapid injection through the intravenous route has also been associated with respiratory depression [21].

7. Side effects of ketamine premedication

Ketamine does have side effects. Most commonly these are seen as vocalization, random purposeless movements, muscle twitching, and hypersalivation, and transient tachycardia and/or hypertension.

Hypersalivation needs essential anticholinergic in premedication and may require oral suctioning. Excessive salivation and bronchial secretions may sometimes lead to occasional laryngospasm (incidence of 0.3%) which needed immediate positive pressure ventilation, or rapid sequence intubation (RSI) [22]. Respiratory depression (0.4%) or even transient apnoea may occur, assisted mask ventilation may be needed. Vomiting is common in older children usually over 8 years of age. In short surgical procedures where oral ketamine is used as premedicant unpleasant emergence, phenomena may be seen beyond mid-adolescence, which resolve after some time in a calm and quiet environment with minimal or no stimulation.

Generally, the side effects are related to doses, larger doses take less onset time but longer time for metabolism and excretion, finally more chances of residual effects as hallucination, emergence, and vomiting. Orally administered ketamine of 6 mg/kg have an onset of action to produce sedation 10 min as compared to 3 mg/kg takes 20 min [23, 24].

8. Use of co-medication with ketamine

The combination of ketamine with other drugs has also been used in several studies, with the co-medication helping to overcome the side effects and increases bioavailability by affecting the drug disposition and its pharmacokinetics [12].

8.1 Combination of ketamine with midazolam

It is reported that when a combination of ketamine and midazolam administered orally produces 90% successful anxiolysis as compared to <75% when either drug is given alone. This oral mixture produces a better quality of sedation and amnesia and requires less IV propofol as compared to intramuscular meperidine, promethazine, and chlorpromazine for pediatric cardiac catheterization [25].

8.2 Combination of ketamine with dexmedetomidine

The combination of dexmedetomidine with ketamine reduces its cardiovascular effects and slower the elimination, as dexmedetomidine is a strong inhibitor of the N-demethylation of ketamine to norketamine.

9. Conclusions

As a potent analgesic, ketamine has a complex mechanism of action, producing a state of sedation, immobility, analgesia, amnesia, and dissociation from the environment. Ketamine as a premedicant especially in subanaesthetic doses and in combination with midazolam produces prompt sedation. Some institutions are using ketamine in infants over 7 months and toddlers as part of premedication protocols for preoperative sedation, prevention of response to separation and intravenous access, and postoperative pain control in infants. This helps in smooth separation from parents and the child accepts the face mask easily, is immobile, is dissociated from the environment. There is little incidence of emergence phenomenon on recovery. The patient is somewhat sedated without any respiratory depression or suppression of protective reflexes or any other untoward side effects with good postoperative analgesia. Intramuscular ketamine as a premedicant in subanaesthetic doses has a special role in the management of uncooperative children.

Conflict of interest

The authors declare no conflict of interest.

Author details

Shahla Haleem
Faculty of Medicine, Department of Anaesthesiology and Critical Care,
J.N. Medical College, AMU, Aligarh, India

*Address all correspondence to: shahlahaleem@yahoo.co.in

References

[1] Deshmukh PV, Kulkarni SS, Parchandekar MK, Sikchi SP. Comparison of preanesthetic sedation in pediatric patients with oral and intranasal midazolam. Journal of Anaesthesiology Clinical Pharmacology. 2016;**32**(3):353-358

[2] Kain ZN, Mayes LC, O'Connor TZ, Cicchetti DV. Preoperative anxiety in children. Predictors and outcomes. Archives of Pediatrics and Adolescent Medicine. 1996;**150**:1238-1245

[3] Mion G, Villevieille T. Ketamine pharmacology: An update (pharmacodynamics and molecular aspects, recent findings). CNS Neuroscience & Therapeutics. 2013;**19**:370-380

[4] Mirakhur RK. Preanaesthetic medication: A survey of current usage. Journal of the Royal Society of Medicine. 1991;**84**:481

[5] Funk W, Jakob W, Riedl T, et al. Oral preanaesthetic medication for children: Double-blind randomized study of a combination of midazolam and ketamine vs midazolam or ketamine alone. British Journal of Anaesthesia. 2000;**84**:335-340

[6] Kogan A, Katz J, Efrat R, Eidelman LA. Premedication with midazolam in young children: A comparison of four routes of administration. Pediatric Anaesthesia. 2002;**12**:685-689

[7] Nishina K, Mikawa K. Clonidine in paediatric anaesthesia. Current Opinion in Anaesthesiology. 2002;**15**:309-316

[8] Bhana N, Goa KL, McClellan KJ. Dexmedetomidine. Drugs. 2000;**59**(2): 263-268

[9] Gutstein HB, Johnson KL, Heard HB, Gregory GA. Oral ketamine preanesthetic medication in children. Anesthesiology. 1992;**76**:28-33

[10] Gingrich BK. Difficulties encountered in a comparative study of orally administered midazolam and ketamine. Anesthesiology. 1994;**80**:1414-1415

[11] Ashwani K, Anuradha AS, Rakesh G, Mridu PN. Comparative evaluation of ketamine, midazolam and combination of both as oral premedicants in children. Journal of Anaesthesiology Clinical Pharmacology. 2009;**25**:449-453

[12] Vlerick L, Devreese M, Peremans K, Dockx R, Croubels S, Duchateau L, et al. Pharmacokinetics, absolute bioavailability and tolerability of ketamine after intranasal administration to dexmedetomidine sedated dogs. PLoS One. 2020;**15**(1):e0227762. DOI: 10.1371/journal.pone.0227762

[13] Drug Absorption—Clinical Pharmacology—MSD Manuals. Available from: https://www.msdmanuals.com

[14] Clements JA, Nimmo WS, Grant IS. Bioavailability, pharmacokinetics, and analgesic activity of ketamine in humans. Journal of Pharmaceutical Sciences. 1982;**71**(5):539-542. DOI: 10.1002/jps.2600710516

[15] Fanta S, Kinnunen M, Backman JT, Kalso E. Population pharmacokinetics of *S*-ketamine and norketamine in healthy volunteers after intravenous and oral dosing. European Journal of Clinical Pharmacology. 2015;**71**:441-447

[16] Malinovsky JM, Servin F, Cozian A, Lepage JY, Pinaud M. Ketamine and norketamine plasma concentrations after i.v., nasal and rectal administration in children. British Journal of Anaesthesia. 1996;**77**:203-207

[17] Epstein RH, Mendel HG, Witkowski TA, Waters R, Guarniari KM, Marr AT, et al. The safety and efficacy of oral transmucosal fentanyl citrate for preoperative sedation in young children. Anesthesia and Analgesia. 1996;**83**: 1200-1205

[18] Rabie ME. Combination of oral ketamine and midazolam versus midazolam alone as a premedication in children undergoing tonsillectomy. Alexandria Journal of Anaesthesia and Intensive Care. 2005;**8**(3):58-64

[19] Langston WT, Wathen JE, Roback MG, Bajaj L. Effect of ondansetron on the incidence of vomiting associated with ketamine sedation in children: A double-blind, randomized, placebo-controlled trial. Annals of Emergency Medicine. 2008;**52**(1):30-34

[20] Tanaka M, Sato M, Saito A, Nishikawa T. Reevaluation of rectal ketamine premedication in children: Comparison with rectal midazolam. Anesthesiology. 2000;**93**(5):1217-1224. DOI: 10.1097/00000542-200011000-00014

[21] Deasy C, Babl EF. Intravenous vs intramuscular ketamine for pediatric procedural sedation by emergency medicine specialists: A review. Pediatric Anesthesia. 2010;**20**:787-796

[22] Green SM, Johnson NE. Ketamine sedation for pediatric procedures: Part 2, review and implications. Annals of Emergency Medicine. 1990;**19**:1033-1046

[23] Filatov SM, Baer GA, Rorarius MG, Oikkonen M. Efficacy and safety of premedication with oral ketamine for day-case adenoidectomy compared with rectal diazepam/diclofenac and EMLA. Acta Anaesthesiologica Scandinavica. 2000;**44**:118-124

[24] Sekerci CM, Donmez A, Ates Y, Okten F. Oral ketamine premedication in children (placebo controlled double blind study). European Journal of Anaesthesiology. 1996;**13**:606-611

[25] Auden SM, Sobczyk WL, Solinger RE, Goldsmith LJ. Oral ketamine/midazolam is superior to intramuscular meperidine, promethazine, and chlorpromazine for pediatric cardiac catheterization. Anesthesia and Analgesia. 2000;**90**: 299-305

Chapter 14

Uses of Ketamine in the Paediatric Population

Bhagyalakshmi Ramesh

Abstract

General anesthesia in pediatric patients can vary from light sedation to complete anesthesia with unconsciousness, amnesia and muscle relaxation. A wide variety of procedures are done under general anesthesia in children ranging from surgeries done for correction of congenital defects, cardiac surgeries, scoliosis surgery, hernia surgery etc. to procedures done outside the operating room (OR) for diagnostic and therapeutic purposes. Non-Operating room Anesthesia (NORA) may include painless procedures like CT scan, MRI, radiotherapy for cancer treatment etc. or painful procedures like biopsy, lumbar puncture, securing IV access, insertion of central line etc. done in ICU which requires a cooperative child. Ketamine has an important role in the pediatric population, both as an induction agent and as a sedative-analgesic drug especially in countries where newer drugs are not readily available. Ketamine helps to alleviate separation anxiety. Even procedures done under regional techniques in some older children require use of sedation. Ketamine can be administered through various routes-IV, IM, intranasal etc. It can be used along with other groups of drugs like Benzodiazepines, Barbiturates, Alpha 2 agonists, Propofol etc. Thus Ketamine is a versatile drug with various indications for use in the pediatric population which will be discussed in the current chapter.

Keywords: conscious sedation, ketamine, intranasal, propofol, paediatric

1. Introduction

Ketamine was first synthesised in 1962 and put into clinical practice in 1970. It has a chiral structure and consists of two optical isomers S (+) and R (−) forms. Ketamine is commonly used for anaesthesia in the paediatric population. A recent survey identified standard induction agents used in children varied from Etomidate in 26.9% (7/26), propofol in 19.2% (5/26), a combination of benzodiazepines and ketamine in 19.2% (5/26), and barbiturates in 11.5% (3/26) [1]. The use of anaesthesia in paediatric age group outside the OR includes dental offices, endoscopy suites, cardiac catheterization laboratory, radiology facilities, radiation oncology departments, paediatric intensive care units (PICUs), and emergency departments. Patients aged less than 3 years routinely require anaesthesia prior to any procedure. By 7 years of age however most children can tolerate non-painful exams and treatments without anaesthesia support [2, 3]. In the OR Ketamine may be used for sedating the child prior to inducing GA in order to decrease anxiety due to parental separation. However the psychological side effects of Ketamine as well as availability of other agents made Ketamine less popular as an induction agent. Induction technique preferred in children is usually inhalational route especially with the availability of Sevoflurane.

2. Ketamine for conscious sedation

The American Society of Anaesthesiology (ASA) defines four levels of sedation (**Table 1**): minimal (anxiolysis), moderate (conscious), deep (purposeful response to vigorous stimulation), and general anaesthesia (unresponsive). A variety of pharmacologic agents are available to sedate and anaesthetise patients. Conscious sedation can be defined as, "A controlled state of depressed consciousness that allows the protective reflexes to be maintained, retaining the patient's ability to maintain a patent airway independently and continuously and allows appropriate response by the patient to physical stimulation or verbal command." A patient can progress from one level to another during sedation given in various doses. Hence continuous monitoring and vigilance is of utmost importance. The drugs used must be titrated to achieve the desired effect, prevent overdose and sudden loss of consciousness. Prior to even short procedures requiring sedation, the child must be evaluated thoroughly –check for any comorbidities like seizure history, previous surgeries, allergic reactions, birth history, developmental milestones attained etc. Airway should be examined to anticipate any difficult airway-enlarged tonsils, congenital defects etc. The blood investigations necessary should be ordered as per need just like prior to a child for major surgical procedure. Adequate fasting guidelines should be explained and ensured. An understanding of the pharmacodynamics and pharmacokinetic effects of sedating drugs which are going to be used is essential. Appropriate sized airway equipment, venous access, appropriate intraoperative monitoring equipment, properly equipped staff in recovery area and proper discharge criteria should also be checked. Sedation drugs can be administered through various routes—oral, nasal, intramuscular, intravenous (IV), subcutaneous, and inhalational routes.

For conscious sedation drugs are used in sub anaesthetic doses and titrated to obtain adequate effect. Various drugs have been used for conscious sedation in paediatric age group which includes Ketamine. The doses of drugs used for Conscious sedation is given in **Table 2**.

	Mild	**Moderate**	**Deep sedation**	**General anaesthesia**
Response to verbal stimulus	Normal	Only responds purposefully	Response seen only on repeated painful stimulation	No response even to painful stimulus
Airway	Not affected	Usually able to maintain airway without intervention	May not be able to maintain airway reflexes	Airway adjuncts like supraglottic airway device or endotracheal intubation required
Spontaneous Ventilation	Maintains spontaneous respiration	Adequate	May be inadequate	Frequently inadequate
Cardiovascular Function	No cardiovascular depression	Usually normal	Usually normal	Cardiovascular depression may occur

Table 1.
ASA levels of sedation.

Drug	Route of administration
Midazolam	IV/Intranasal
Ketamine	IV/IM/rectal/oral/intranasal
Dexmedetomidine	IV
Propofol	IV
Ketofol	IV
Opioids (Fentanyl/Remifentanyl)	IV

Table 2.
Drugs used for conscious sedation.

3. Clinical effects of ketamine

Ketamine is a phencyclidine derivative which acts as an N-methyl-D-aspartate (NMDA) receptor antagonist at the dorsal horn of the spinal cord [2, 4]. It induces dissociative amnesia and analgesia [5]. Ketamine has the advantage of various routes of administration available for use. Administration routes include intravenous (1–2 mg/kg), intramuscular (2–10 mg/kg), oral (3–6 mg/kg), intranasal (2–4 mg/kg), and rectal (5–10 mg/kg) (Refer **Table 3**) [6]. Ketamine has many advantages over other drugs especially due to its relative cardiovascular steadiness and restricted effect on the respiratory mechanics. Recovery occurs within 30–120 min, and this allows the patient to be discharged on the same day as the procedure. It has a dose dependent cardiovascular stimulant effect. In children with congenital heart disease, it causes only minor increases in heart rate and mean pulmonary artery pressure during cardiac catheterization procedures [1]. It has various effects on the other systems in the body some of which are listed in **Table 4**.

Route	Dose
IV	1–2 mg/kg
IM	2–10 mg/kg
Oral	3–6 mg/kg
Intranasal	2–4 mg/kg
Sedation	0.2–0.75 mg/kg IV or 2–4 mg/kg IM

Table 3.
Dosages of ketamine.

Organ system	Effect
Cardiovascular	Increases heart rate, blood pressure, cardiac output
Respiratory	Increases the oral secretions, bronchodilator, maintains the airway reflexes
Neurologic	Dissociative anaesthesia Increase in intracranial pressure, excitatory effects on thalamus and limbic systems, increase in intraocular pressure, increase in cerebral metabolism, increase in cerebral oxygen consumption Emergence delirium

Table 4.
Effects of ketamine on various systems.

Adverse reactions associated with ketamine include dreams, hallucinations, delirium, agitation, vomiting, increased salivation, and laryngospasm [7]. It causes increase in intraocular and intracranial pressures after its administration. Hence it is not used in patients with glaucoma, open globe injuries, or elevated intracranial pressure [5]. Clinically, ketamine is frequently used to facilitate short, painful procedures in the emergency department [4, 8]. Sedation can be achieved with minimal respiratory depression. However when higher doses are used, one can easily induce general anaesthesia [5].

Ketamine causes hyper salivation and thus needs to be administered with an antisialagogue like Atropine or glycopyrrolate. To prevent hallucinations and delirium it is often combined with short acting benzodiazepines like midazolam.

4. Ketofol

The combination of ketamine and propofol, known as ketofol is also a popular drug used for procedural sedation. The two drugs when combined act synergistically and thus helps to decrease the dose of each drug independently. The side effects of ketamine which includes vomiting, laryngospasm, and emergence delirium, can be decreased by adding propofol. In the same way using ketamine along with propofol decreases the risk of propofol-induced respiratory depression and hypotension. The combination also provides for analgesia [9]. There is no standard combination mentioned but usually Ketamine and Propofol are mixed in a 1:1 ratio (mg) [10]. According to a prospective randomised controlled study involving paediatric patients undergoing cardiac catheterization, using a propofol: ketamine combination in the ratio of 10:2 (mg) preserved mean arterial pressure without affecting recovery time [11]. Studies which have compared ketofol with propofol have shown that ketofol produces consistent depth of sedation. Patient satisfaction scores were also found to be similar. Propofol causes pain on injection but the combination of propofol with Ketamine reduces pain on injection. The risk of airway and respiratory complications were similar in both groups [12–15]. Ketofol decreases the requirements of both opioids and propofol. Ketofol is thus an acceptable choice for short procedures in the emergency department or critical care setting [10]. The efficacy, safety, pharmacokinetics, and pharmacodynamics require further evaluation with additional prospective trials in the paediatric population.

With currently available IV anaesthetic agents such as Propofol, barbiturates, opioids etc. which are used frequently in combination with Ketamine for procedures done outside the OR, the complication rates has declined from 23% [16] seen in the 1980s to 1–2%. This is somewhat similar to the complication rates in the ORs [17–19]. A current study by Owusu-Agyemang et al. [3] showed that use of propofol either alone or in combination with Dexmedetomidine and Fentanyl lowered complication rates to 0.05%.Some newer drugs like Fospropofol have been approved by FDA for sedation purposes. Some drugs like Remimazolam and other Etomidate derivatives are still in clinical trial stages. Some centres have seen the resurgence of inhalational anaesthetic nitrous oxide.

5. Ketamine use in cancer pain management

Cancer pain management, especially in terminal stages, can be challenging. Cancer pain is mediated through various pathways, including visceral, nociceptive, neuropathic and central. Currently used agents have limited role in addressing each component and have significant adverse events. The safety profile of Ketamine has been evaluated in a number of trials. The WHO ladder for pain management includes acetaminophen, non-steroidal anti-inflammatory drugs, weak opioids like tramadol and the strong opioids like morphine for cancer pain management. In addition to this, topical local anaesthetics like lignocaine can also be used. However US FDA approval for many of these medications is lacking for use in the paediatric age group.

Safety and efficacy as an anaesthetic and analgesic has been well documented; however, ketamine has not yet been approved as an analgesic agent by the US FDA. This may prevent its free use by many for cancer pain management [20–23]. When Ketamine is used in doses <1 mg/kg it has minimal depressant effects on cardiovascular and respiratory systems as it produces only minimal sedation (Refer **Table 1**) [20, 24]. However it produces analgesia and modulate central sensitization, hyperalgesia, and opioid tolerance. Hence the National Comprehensive Cancer Network guidelines has recommended considering oral or intravenous (IV) ketamine for pain not responding to other analgesics [20, 25]. Ketamine has been used through various routes of administration-IV, IM, oral, sublingual Intranasal rectal and even epidural in patients with malignancy. The bioavailability of intranasal Ketamine was found to be 45–50% [26, 27].

A review of five studies of ketamine for cancer pain in children showed that patients treated with oral and IV ketamine had only few adverse events reported. However, these studies were all retrospective. Participants' cancer diagnoses include acute myelogenous leukaemia, myelodysplastic syndrome, osteosarcoma, metastatic giant malignant mesenchymal tumour, glioblastoma multiforme, neuroblastoma, Ewing sarcoma, spindle cell sarcoma, synovial cell sarcoma, and Wilm's tumour [28]. There are several very small case series or individual case reports of children being treated with ketamine for pain with promising results. For example, at Melbourne, a protocol for IV ketamine administration is being used to treat children who have been unresponsive to two doses of morphine. Additional dose of ketamine (0.1 mg/kg) given as a bolus has helped to achieve effective pain control. These doses have not been associated with hallucinations or dysphoria. However, this report does not enumerate percentages of patients with adequate pain control after treatment with ketamine [29]. A prospective phase I trial of oral ketamine in the dose of 0.25–1 mg/kg given in divided doses in children with chronic noncancer pain has been undertaken [30].

Children with severe cancer pain have been treated with ketamine in doses of 3 mg/kg/day given orally [31] and 0.1–1 mg/kg/h given intravenously. In a retrospective review, 8 of the 11 (73%) children and adolescents had decreased need for opioids and improved pain control [32]. The results of these reports suggest that pain control may be achieved with the use of ketamine in children with cancer pain. These doses were well tolerated by the children between 3 and 17 years of age with cancer pain without nausea, sedation, hallucination, respiratory distress, or psychotomimetic effects.

6. Side effects of ketamine

The common side effects of ketamine include nausea, vomiting, occurrence of bizarre dreams, hallucinations, emergence agitation, seizures. It causes tachycardia and hypertension and thus is contraindicated in patients with cardio vascular illnesses. It also increases in intra ocular pressure and is thus contraindicated in open eye injuries.

Some studies have shown lorazepam given along with Ketamine to decrease the psychotomimetic side effects of ketamine [32]. Ketamine administered through the epidural route in children has shown to produce fewer side effects due to Ketamine.

This also decreased the opioid consumption during the procedure [33]. The neurotoxicity caused due to Ketamine appears to be less in children than in adults. There are a few case reports of laryngospasm caused when Ketamine is given intramuscularly or in higher doses [33, 34]. One case report of a ketamine infusion for a child reports mycolonic movements in the child [35]. The report is unclear as to whether this was related to ketamine or the child's spinal cord tumour. There have been occasional incidences of reversible cystitis with chronic exposure to ketamine [36, 37].

The incidence of respiratory complications has been found to be higher with the use of intramuscular administration of Ketamine as compared to intravenous use. An increased incidence of laryngospasm has been reported especially due to the higher dose of ketamine required for effect as well as delayed absorption of intramuscularly administered drug. The incidence of respiratory adverse events was 2.4% with IM ketamine [34].

A retrospective study evaluated the usefulness of combining intranasal Dexmed (2 mcg/kg) and Ketamine (1 mg/kg) for procedural sedation found it to be useful in 93% of patients. The onset of sedation was 15 min and duration was found to be 62 min. Minor complications like nausea and vomiting only were observed in the study in 0.3% of the patients.

More than 11,000 cases have been reported of its use in children with no fatalities being described in the literature by Green et al. [5] the most frequently cited disadvantage is the emergence phenomenon, seen more commonly in adults where the incidence is 5–50% while in children it has been found to be 0–5%. Ketamine increases the salivary and tracheobronchial mucus gland secretions, and hence needs to be combined with an antisialagogue during GA. Emesis is the one of the most common side effect of ketamine. In a review by Green the incidence of vomiting was found to be 10% and more commonly seen in children undergoing dental procedures. Atropine has been found to decrease the emesis by reducing the salivary secretions. Laryngospasm was reported in 0.4% of cases. Laryngospasm was managed with 100% oxygen and positive pressure ventilation using bag and mask [38].

7. Ketamine in burns contracture release

In his study, Embu has described various techniques for burns contracture release. Some case were done with intermittent doses of Ketamine while patients were spontaneously breathing. Some patients were maintained on inhalational anaesthetic after Ketamine induction-either via face mask or LMA (laryngeal mask airway). After adequate surgical release, the patients were intubated by direct laryngoscopy. No airway complications were reported in the study. However, maintaining anaesthesia with an inhalation agent via facemask was found to be technically difficult owing to the proximity to the sterile surgical field [39].

Agarwal et al. have reported use of tumescent local anaesthesia for the release of neck contracture due to burns in 30 patients. 0.5–1.0 mg/kg of IV ketamine were used in these children at the start of the case. They were maintained on ketamine during the procedure also as intermittent IV boluses (dose has not been specified). No airway complications had been reported. All patients were maintained on spontaneous ventilation throughout the case [40].

8. Ketamine as an adjunct

Preservative-free ketamine added to caudal bupivacaine has been shown to improve the duration of analgesia, without affecting the analgesic intensity in a study done by Martindale et al. [41]. In a recent survey conducted among paediatric anaesthetists in UK by Sanders 32% had reported using epidural ketamine [42]. It is used in a dose of 0.25–1 mg/kg as an additive to bupivacaine or Ropivacaine.

9. Effects of use of ketamine on Perfusion Index (PI)

Children often are given regional anaesthesia for pain management following General anaesthesia (GA) in contrast to adult patients. Hence it is difficult to assess the usefulness of the regional technique except by use of surrogate indicators like tachycardia, hypertension. Perfusion Index is a newer technique to detect effectiveness of regional anaesthetic under GA.

Studies have demonstrated that PI can provide an early and reliable indication of the onset of epidural anaesthesia. Intravascular injection of epinephrine-containing local anaesthetic test dose can also be identified in the adult population [6, 8]. However, caudal blocks in paediatric patients are mostly performed under sedation or general anaesthesia, using ketamine or sevoflurane [9, 10]. Data has shown that ketamine itself can affect PI. Thus it is difficult to predict the onset of caudal block using PI in the paediatric patients who have been sedated using Ketamine. A previous study has shown that intravenous ketamine used in paediatric patients produced a fast and long-lasting decrease in peripheral PI. However the study also showed that caudal block reversed the decrease of PI measured in the toe, caused by ketamine anaesthesia in paediatric population. The PI was found to increase beyond the preinduction level. The study also showed that PI response criterion achieved 100% sensitivity and specificity in detecting the effects of caudal anaesthesia under IV ketamine anaesthesia in paediatric patients. However, neither HR nor MAP criteria were 100% reliable. Furthermore, the changes of PI caused by caudal block under ketamine anaesthesia were much earlier than those of HR and MAP.

Ketamine being a widely used intravenous anaesthetic in paediatric patients, it has been shown to produce an immediate and long-lasting decrease in peripheral PI due to its sympathomimetic effects through its effects on both central and peripheral mechanisms [17, 18]. In this study, a drop in PI was observed within one minute after the injection of ketamine (2.36 ± 0.79 to 1.58 ± 0.61) and after 30 min PI it had decreased to 0.80 ± 0.26, which was far below the baseline value of PI. The changes of MAP lasted about 15 min, and the changes of HR lasted about 5 min following ketamine injection. Caudal block not only reversed the decrease of PI on the toe caused by ketamine anaesthesia in paediatric patients, but also increased PI far beyond the preinduction PI value [43].

10. Use of ketamine in ICU

The sensory association areas of the cortex, components of the limbic system, and thalamus are directly depressed by ketamine. Consequently, higher central nervous system (CNS) centres are unable to receive or process sensory information and its emotional significance cannot be assessed. The result of ketamine administration is anaesthesia, analgesia, suppression of fear and anxiety, and amnesia, which appear to be ideal for the uncooperative child patient.

Ketamine is commonly used for sedation and analgesia during painful procedures because it maintains the cardiovascular and respiratory systems while providing effective sedation, analgesia, and amnesia. However Ketamine-induced emergence reactions like hallucinations, delusions, nightmares, and agitation are shown to be less in children [44]. Ketamine can be used prior to invasive procedures in the ICU like Lumbar puncture, central line insertions. It can be used in management of children with status asthamaticus.

Ketamine has many advantages due to which it is used for sedation in the paediatric population viz. a relatively short duration of action, multiple routes of administration, preservation of airway reflexes, and sympathomimetic properties including increase heart rates and blood pressure. Sedation can be achieved without much respiratory depression. However ketamine has various adverse effects too. These include hallucinations, emergence delirium, agitation, nausea and vomiting, hyper salivation, and laryngospasm. This can cause distress to both the child and parent. Reports of patients developing random movements of the extremities has been reported which renders this drug less than ideal for procedures where the patient must lie perfectly still like in the MRI suite. Thus, ketamine is used along with other sedative agents to counterbalance the side effects and enhance the beneficial effects for each drug rather than as a sole sedative agent for MRI. Ketamine can prevent the cardiorespiratory depression effect of propofol and prolonged recovery of dexmedetomidine by reducing the dose requirements of each drug when used for sedation in children in MRI suite [44–48].

Exposure to ketamine and other anaesthetic agents during early stages of postnatal brain development increases central nervous system neuronal apoptosis in animals receiving significantly larger and more prolonged doses than used for procedural sedation [49]. No evidence of neuronal injury after a single ketamine based sedation has been seen in small children but repeated use of ketamine for procedures may have detrimental effects. [50, 51].

11. Other uses of ketamine

Ketamine has been used as an induction agent in children with cyanotic congenital heart conditions like Tetralogy of Fallot. This is due to its effect in increasing the systematic vascular resistance and thus decreasing the incidence of righto left shunt. However it can increase the infundibular spasm. Thus it is combined with opioids or propofol. Another recently described alternative to this is Etomidate combined with Ketamine [52].

12. Conclusion

Recent studies have explored the use of Ketamine in other situations in adult population as well like prevention of postoperative sore throat, treatment of status epilepticus, alcohol withdrawal syndrome, status asthamaticus etc. There has been an increased usage of Ketamine in the acute pain setting to prevent excessive opioid use but these require further studies in the paediatric population. Thus Ketamine is a very useful drug in the paediatric age group which may be combined with other drugs to alleviate its side effects and achieve anaesthesia as well as analgesia.

Author details

Bhagyalakshmi Ramesh
Department of Anaesthesiology, Regional Cancer Centre, Thiruvananthapuram, Kerala, India

*Address all correspondence to: blakshmir71@gmail.com

References

[1] Baehner T, Kiefer N, Ghamari S, Graeff I, Huett C, Pflugradt S, et al. A National Survey: Current clinical practice in paediatric anaesthesia for congenital heart surgery. World Journal for Pediatric and Congenital Heart Surgery. 2020;**11**(3):257-264. DOI: 10.1177/2150135120902122

[2] Khurmi N, Patel P, Kraus M, Trentman T. Pharmacologic considerations for paediatric sedation and anaesthesia outside the operating room: A review for anaesthesia and non-anaesthesia providers. Paediatric Drugs. 2017;**19**(5):435-446. DOI: 10.1007/s40272-017-0241-5

[3] Owusu-Agyemang P, Grosshans D, Arunkumar R, Rebello E, Popovich S, Zavala A, et al. Non-invasive anaesthesia for children undergoing proton radiation therapy. Radiotherapy and Oncology. 2014;**111**(1):30-34

[4] Attri JP, Sharan R, Makkar V, Gupta KK, Khetarpal R, Kataria AP. Conscious sedation: Emerging trends in paediatric dentistry. Anaesthesia, Essays and Researches. 2017;**11**(2):277-281

[5] Green SM, Johnson NE. Ketamine sedation for paediatric procedures: Part 2. Review and implications. Annals of Emergency Medicine. 1990;**19**(9): 1033-1046

[6] Mazurek MS. Sedation and analgesia for procedures outside the operating room. Seminars in Pediatric Surgery. 2004;**13**(3):166-173

[7] Anderson BJ, Lerman J, Cote CJ. Pharmacokinetics and pharmacology of drugs used in children. In: Cote CJ, Lerman J, Anderson BJ, editors. Cote´ and Lerman's a Practice of Anaesthesia for Infants and Children. 5th ed. Philadelphia, PA: Elsevier; 2013. pp. 77-149

[8] Prescilla R, Mason KP. Recent advances and contributions to procedural sedation with considerations for the future. Minerva Anestesiologica. 2014;**80**(7):844-855

[9] McCarty EC, Mencio GA, Walker LA, Green NE. Ketamine sedation for the reduction of children's fractures in the emergency department. The Journal of Bone and Joint Surgery. 2000;**82-A**(7):912-918

[10] Mahmoud M, Mason KP. A forecast of relevant paediatric sedation trends. Current Opinion in Anaesthesiology. 2016;**29**(Suppl. 1):S56-S67

[11] Alletag MJ, Auerbach MA, Baum CR. Ketamine, propofol, and ketofol use for paediatric sedation. Pediatric Emergency Care. 2012;**28**(12):1391-1395

[12] Akin A, Esmaoglu A, Guler G, Demircioglu R, Narin N, Boyaci A. Propofol and propofol-ketamine in paediatric patients undergoing cardiac catheterization. Pediatric Cardiology. 2005;**26**(5):553-557

[13] Andolfatto G, Willman E. A prospective case series of single syringe ketamine-propofol (Ketofol) for emergency department procedural sedation and analgesia in adults. Academic Emergency Medicine. 2011;**18**(3):237-245

[14] Shah A, Mosdossy G, McLeod S, Lehnhardt K, Peddle M, Rieder M. A blinded, randomized controlled trial to evaluate ketamine/propofol versus ketamine alone for procedural sedation in children. Annals of Emergency Medicine. 2011;**57**(5):425-33 e2

[15] Ferguson I, Bell A, Treston G, New L, Ding M, Holdgate A. Propofol or ketofol for procedural sedation and analgesia in emergency medicine-the POKER study: A randomized double blind clinical trial. Annals of Emergency Medicine. 2016;**68**(5):574-82 e1

[16] Lo JN, Buckley JJ, Kim TH, Lopez R. Anaesthesia for high-dose total body irradiation in children. Anesthesiology. 1984;**61**(1):101-103

[17] Stokes MA, Soriano SG, Tarbell NJ, Loeffler JS, Alexander E 3rd, Black PM, et al. Anaesthesia for stereotactic radiosurgery in children. Journal of Neurosurgical Anesthesiology. 1995; 7(2):100-108

[18] Fortney JT, Halperin EC, Hertz CM, Schulman SR. Anaesthesia for paediatric external beam radiation therapy. International Journal of Radiation Oncology, Biology, Physics. 1999; **44**(3):587-591

[19] Anghelescu DL, Burgoyne LL, Liu W, Hankins GM, Cheng C, Beckham PA, et al. Safe anaesthesia for radiotherapy in paediatric oncology: St. Jude Children's Research Hospital Experience, 2004-2006. International Journal of Radiation Oncology, Biology, Physics. 2008;**71**(2):491-497

[20] Singh V, Gillespie TW, Harvey RD. Intranasal ketamine and its potential role in cancer-related pain. Pharmacotherapy. 2018;**38**(3):390-401. DOI: 10.1002/phar.2090

[21] White PF, Way WL, Trevor AJ. Ketamine: Its pharmacology and therapeutic uses. Anaesthesiology. 1982;**56**(2):119-136

[22] Malinovsky. Ketamine and nor ketamine plasma concentrations after i.v., nasal and rectal administration in children. British Journal of Anaesthesia. 1996;**77**(72):203-207

[23] Reich DL, Silvay G. Ketamine: An update on the first twenty -five years of clinical experience. Canadian Journal of Anaesthesia. 1989;**36**(2):186-197

[24] Schmid RL, Sandler AN, Katz J. Use and efficacy of low -dose ketamine in the management of acute postoperative pain: A review of current techniques and outcomes. Pain. 1999;**82**(2):111-125

[25] Swarm RA, Paice JA, Anghelescu DL, Are M, Bruce JY, Buga S, et al. Adult cancer pain, version 3.2019, NCCN clinical practice guidelines in oncology. Journal of the National Comprehensive Cancer Network. 1 Aug 2019;**17**(8):977-1007

[26] Yanagihara Y, Ohtani M, Kariya S, et al. Plasma concentration profiles of ketamine and nor ketamine after administration of various ketamine preparations to healthy Japanese volunteers. Biopharmaceutics & Drug Disposition. 2003;**24**(1):37-43

[27] Bredlau AL, Thakur R, Korones DN, Dworkin RH. Ketamine for pain in adults and children with cancer: A systematic review and synthesis of the literature. Pain Medicine. 2013;**14**(10):1505-1517. DOI: 10.1111/pme.12182

[28] Anderson BJ, Palmer GM. Recent developments in the pharmacological management of pain in children. Current Opinion in Anaesthesiology. 2006;**19**(3):285-292

[29] Bredlau AL, McDermott MP, Adam HR, et al. Oral ketamine for children with chronic pain: A pilot phase 1 study. The Journal of Pediatrics. 2013;**163**(1):194-200

[30] Ugur F, Gulcu N, Boyaci A. Oral ketamine for pain relief in a child with abdominal malignancy. Pain Medicine. 2009;**10**(1):120-121

[31] Finkel JC, Pestieau SR, Quezado ZM. Ketamine as an adjuvant for treatment of cancer pain in children and adolescents. The Journal of Pain. 2007;**8**(6):515-521

[32] Bergman SA. Ketamine: Review of its pharmacology and its use in paediatric anaesthesia. Anesthesia Progress. 1999;**46**(1):10-20

[33] Baduni N, Sanwal MK, Jain A, Kachru N. Recurrent episodes of intractable laryngospasm followed by laryngeal and pulmonary oedema during dissociative anaesthesia with intravenous ketamine. Indian Journal of Anaesthesia. 2010;**54**(4):364-365

[34] Melendez E, Bachur R. Serious adverse events during procedural sedation with ketamine. Pediatric Emergency Care. 2009;**25**(5):325-328

[35] Capape S, Mora E, Mintegui S, et al. Prolonged sedation and airway complications after administration of an inadvertent ketamine overdose in emergency department. European Journal of Emergency Medicine. 2008; **15**(2):92-94

[36] Klepstad P, Borchgrevink P, Hval B, Flaat S, Kaasa S. Long-term treatment with ketamine in a 12-year-old girl with severe neuropathic pain caused by a cervical spinal tumour. Journal of Pediatric Hematology/Oncology. 2001;**23**(9):616-619

[37] Shahani R, Streutker C, Dickson B, Stewart RJ. Ketamine-associated ulcerative cystitis: A new clinical entity. Urology. 2007;**69**(5):810-812

[38] Gregoire MC, MacLellan DL, Finley GA. A paediatric case of ketamine-associated cystitis (Letter-to-the Editor RE: Shahani R, Streutker C, Dickson B et al. Ketamine-associated ulcerative cystitis: A new clinical entity. Urology 69: 810-812, 2007). Urology. 2008;**71**(6):1232-12333

[39] Embu HY, Yiltok SJ, Isamade ES. Anaesthetic management of mentosternal contractures where resources are limited. Nigerian Journal of Medicine. 2008;**17**:143-145

[40] Agarwal P. Safe method for release of severe post burn neck contracture under tumescent local anaesthesia and ketamine. Indian Journal of Plastic Surgery. 2004;**37**:51-54

[41] Martindale SJ, Dix P, Stoddart PA. Double-blind randomized controlled trial of caudal versus intravenous S (+)-ketamine for supplementation of caudal analgesia in children. British Journal of Anaesthesia. 2004;**92**(3):344-347

[42] Sanders JC. Paediatric regional anaesthesia, a survey of practice in the United Kingdom. British Journal of Anaesthesia. 2002;**89**(5):707-710

[43] Xu Z, Zhang J, Shen H, Zheng J. Assessment of pulse oximeter perfusion index in paediatric caudal block under basal ketamine anaesthesia. ScientificWorldJournal. 2013;**2013**:183493

[44] Gupta A, Sen I, Bhardwaj N, Yaddanapudi S, Mathew PJ, Sahni N, et al. Prospective audit of sedation/anaesthesia practices for children undergoing computerized tomography in a tertiary care institute. Journal of Anaesthesiology Clinical Pharmacology. 2020;**36**(2):156-161

[45] Practice Guidelines for Moderate Procedural Sedation and Analgesia. A report by the American Society of Anaesthesiologists task force on moderate procedural sedation and analgesia, the American Association of Oral and Maxillofacial Surgeons, American College of Radiology, American Dental Association, American Society of Dentist Anaesthesiologists, and Society of Interventional Radiology. Anaesthesiology. 2018;**2018**(128): 437-479

[46] Kim JG, Lee HB, Jeon SB. Combination of dexmedetomidine and ketamine for magnetic resonance imaging sedation. Frontiers in Neurology. 2019;**10**:416

[47] Tomatir E, Atalay H, Gurses E, Erbay H, Bozkurt P. Effects of low dose ketamine before induction on propofol

anaesthesia for paediatric magnetic resonance imaging. Paediatric Anaesthesia. 2004;**14**(845):850

[48] Scheer I, Weiss M, Kellenberger C, O'Gorman Tuura R, Klaghofer R, Scheer I, et al. Sedation for magnetic resonance imaging using propofol with or without ketamine at induction in pediatrics: A prospective randomized double-blinded study. Paediatric Anaesthesia. 2018;**28**:264-274

[49] Yan J, Jiang H. Dual effects of ketamine: Neurotoxicity versus neuroprotection in anaesthesia for the developing brain. Journal of Neurosurgical Anesthesiology. 2014;**26**:155-160

[50] Yan J, Li Y, Zhang Y, et al. Repeated exposure to anaesthetic ketamine can negatively impact neurodevelopment in infants: A prospective preliminary clinical study. Journal of Child Neurology. 2014;**29**:1333-1338

[51] Roback MG, Wathen JE, MacKenzie T, Bajaj L. A randomized, controlled trial of i.v. versus i.m. ketamine for sedation of paediatric patients receiving emergency department orthopedic procedures. Annals of Emergency Medicine. 2006;**48**:605-612

[52] Dua N, Bhalotra AR. Induction of anaesthesia in cyanotic heart diseases: 'Ketomidate' to the rescue! Indian Journal of Anaesthesia. 2018;**62**(3):237

Chapter 15

Use of Oral Ketamine in Palliative Care

Mateja Lopuh

Abstract

Ketamine, an N-methyl-D-Aspartate receptor antagonist, has been used for more than 50 years. From its initial potential as an anesthetic drug, its use has increased in the fields of pain medicine, psychiatry, and palliative care. It is available in different formulations, of which oral use is promising due to its active metabolite, norketamine which reaches 2–3 times higher levels when administered orally in comparison with parenteral use. Oral use is also more feasible and easier to use in settings, where medical staff is not that present, such as home care or hospices. Oral solution of ketamine has not yet been officially licensed for use although there have been several reports which recommend its use in neuropathic pain, severe depression, airway obstruction, and anxiety. Palliative care is defined as total care for patients whose diseases do not respond to curative treatment. It encompasses good control of physical symptoms, and psychological, social and spiritual problems. Patients often experience pain, despite high doses of opioids, depression and anxiety, and dyspnea. Oral ketamine does not have the side effects of opioids therefore it represents a good alternative. It may also reduce the need for high opioid doses and be more suitable for patients who wish to avoid the necessary sedation.

Keywords: oral ketamine, neuropathic pain, opioids, symptom control, palliative care

1. Introduction

Ketamine is a potent noncompetitive NMDA receptor antagonist. It is primarily marketed as a general anesthetic, but it also shows analgesic properties at lower, subanesthetic doses [1]. It is used as a chlorhydrate in a slightly acid aqueous solution. It is a racemic mixture of two enantiomers of equal quantity of which only the S (+) enantiomer is active and is two times stronger than the racemic mixture and four times stronger than the R (−) enantiomer. In equianalgesic doses, the S-enantiomer is associated with lower levels of undesirable effects.

Ketamine metabolism is characterized by low binding to plasma proteins, about 10–30%. It is highly liposoluble and has therefore an extensive distribution. The central compartment volume is 70 liters and the distribution volume at steady state is around 200 liters. Oxidation is the primary process in the metabolism of ketamine, resulting in norketamine (80%), which is an active metabolite that itself is principally hydroxylated in 6-hydroxy-norketamine and finally excreted in bile and urine after glucuronoconjugation. Ketamine elimination clearance is dependent on the liver blood flow, half time is 2–3 hours, and it may be 20% higher in women than men [2].

IntechOpen

Ketamine is commonly administered via the intravenous, intramuscular, subcutaneous, or oral route. The subcutaneous route appears to be very practical because it avoids potential delays in treatment caused by the inability to establish intravenous access, has a rapid onset of action, and can be used by less skilled personnel, too [3].

The oral route availability of ketamine is incomplete and erratic. Only about 16–20% of an oral dose reaches systemic circulation due to extensive hepatic first-pass elimination. The bioavailability of intranasal ketamine was found to be 50%. Peak plasma concentrations are being reported within 30 minutes of oral administration. Norketamine as an active metabolite reaches 2- or 3-times higher levels when ketamine is administered orally than parenterally and the duration of action of oral ketamine is longer. To achieve a good analgesic effect, doses of oral ketamine can be one-third of the parenteral one, due to the active effect of norketamine [3]. In chronic use, norketamine may be the main analgesic agent. Because of norketamine accumulation the need for ketamine when given for a longer period of time, decreases over time. Norketamine is 33% as potent as the parent compound [4].

In palliative care patients often exhibit a variety of symptoms. They float between the desire to keep autonomy for as long as possible and the wish to avoid the unnecessary suffering, caused by poorly relieving symptoms. Many patients are afraid of opioids, especially morphine, and are reluctant to use them. Some physicians still believe that morphine accelerates death, and they would only use it when patients already entered the dying phase. Ketamine with its analgesic properties may be a good option to keep the opioid levels low as long as possible.

Ketamine has not yet been widely used in palliative care probably because it has always been marketed as an anesthetic drug and therefore reserved for use in the operating theaters. Even its use has not been very prominent due to the psychomimetic side effects when used in anesthetic dosage. Its domains of use expanded in pain medicine, where the doses can be lower, but it was used parenterally, therefore intravenous or subcutaneous access was needed. Longer subcutaneous use often resulted in necrosis of subcutaneous tissue and reduced flow from elastomeric pumps.

Oral and nasal use of ketamine has not been officially licensed although several papers have already been published which suggest that both routes are safe and feasible. These two routes seem to offer advantages over the intravenous and subcutaneous approaches as they allow the patient to be self-sufficient and autonomous in drug administration.

Some pharmacokinetics data are summarized in **Table 1**.

Palliative care may expand over the whole trajectory of the incurable disease. Ketamine is used as a co-analgesic in poorly controlled pain, especially neuropathic pain, to reduce the dose of opioids, to relieve anxiety and depression, severe epileptic seizures, and as bronchodilator. The long-term use of ketamine has not been studied extensively. In palliative care, the studies are limited because symptoms accumulate in the course of the disease and that makes the observation of side effects more difficult.

	Bioavailability (%)	Onset of action (min)	Duration of action (h)	Elimination half time (h)
Parenteral route	100	0.5	0.5–2	2
Oral route	17–25	30	4–6	
Nasal route	50	20	Up to 3	2

Table 1.
Pharmacokinetics of ketamine.

Symptom	Suggested mechanism
Pain control	Antagonism at NMDA receptor complex – inhibition of 'wind-up' pain and hyperalgesia Reduction of opioid tolerance Enhancement of endogenous pain inhibition Antiinflammatory effects Central plasticity
Anxiety and depression	Antagonism at NMDA receptor complex Interaction with calcium and sodium channels Cholinergic transmission Noradrenergic and serotonergic reuptake inhibition Glutamate transmission Synapse formation
Bronchodilatation	inhibition of inflammatory cascade reduction in markers of inflammation
Epileptic status	reduces the NMDA receptor-induced neurotoxicity

Table 2.
Suggested useful mechanisms of ketamine action.

This chapter focuses on the oral/nasal route of ketamine administration in patients with palliative diseases, its useful properties in clinical practice, and its side-effects. Some suggestions are given about the formulation of the drug and the dosage regimens.

2. Clinical uses of ketamine

Ketamine is approved as a general anesthetic agent. At subanesthetic doses, it can be considered for use in a palliative care setting for pain refractory to opioids and as an adjuvant analgesic. Ketamine was approved by FDA for antidepressant use in 2019 as a nasal spray. Ketamine has no reversal agent [5].

Ketamine can be used in the intensive care units as a sedative and analgesic drug. It can be safely used in patients with traumatic brain injury as it does not raise the intracranial blood pressure, caution is needed when used with raised intraocular pressure. When used as an analgesic drug, it may reduce pain scores, opioid consumption, and postoperative nausea and vomiting.

In chronic, non-cancer pain, ketamine can be used as add-on therapy when other therapeutic options have failed. The long-term effects remain controversial.

In cancer pain, ketamine is considered an essential adjuvant drug but the evidence for its efficiency is low [6, 7].

Ketamine has proven to be efficient in treating major depression, bipolar disorders, and suicidal behavior. It acts very fast, and relieves depression in less than 2 hours. In the approved nasal spray only the S (+) enantiomer is used [8, 9].

Other uses of ketamine with the low level of evidence are alcohol withdrawal, status epilepticus, and persistent bronchospasm in critical care settings [8].

Suggested mechanisms of ketamine action are summarized in **Table 2**.

3. Oral formulations

Ketamine is not licensed for oral use. Physicians should properly inform the patients about the advantages and possible side-effects of the drug and the route of administration.

A parenteral formulation is utilized for oral formulations of ketamine. Use generic ketamine 50 mg/ml 10 ml vials and purified water. Alternatively, one can use flavored syrup instead of water, but most patients find it too sweet.

To prepare 100 ml of oral solution with a concentration of 50 mg/ 5 ml use two 10 ml vials of ketamine 50 mg/ml for injections and 80 ml of purified water. The solution can be refrigerated with an expiry date of 1 week from manufacture [1].

It is useful to provide the patient with a syringe to ease the administration of ketamine.

4. Nasal route

Ketamine is not licensed for nasal use. Physicians should properly inform the patients about the advantages and possible side-effects of the drug and the route of administration.

The nasal route appears very promising as it allows the patient to self-administer the drug when needed due to the rapid onset of action which is similar to intramuscular injection. As the capacity of the human nostrils is 0.2 ml, a greater volume may be swallowed or may run out of the nose. Ketamine may be administered via MAD which delivers a mist of atomized medication or via metered-dose nasal spray. The concentration of ketamine, commercially available is 100 mg per ml or 10 m per ml. Up to 40 mg can be reliably delivered intranasally. Higher doses are ingested [10].

Patients can be prescribed oral ketamine basal treatment and use nasal formulation for treating breakthrough pain.

5. Regimens for switching from parenteral to oral administration

Ketamine has been predominantly used parenterally as a co-analgesic in addition to opioids and co-adjuvant drugs. Oral use has obvious advantages: it is not necessary to carry the pump around, which needs frequent refilling and it avoids inflammation on the site of subcutaneous administration. It has been proven in studies that a 1:1 dose ratio is safe and effective in switching from parenteral to oral administration [11]. Another report suggested switching to one-third of the parenteral dose as a result of the effect of norketamine. Oral ketamine may in fact be a more potent analgesic and produce adverse effects less frequently than parenteral ketamine. After oral administration of 0.5 mg/kg ketamine approximately 20% is absorbed and its analgesic action seems to be mediated by its first metabolite norketamine, which has a half-life of 12 hours [12].

A good therapeutic response to parenteral ketamine suggests a greater likelihood of benefit from oral dosing. Patients who could benefit from switching to oral use of ketamine are those whose pain has been stable for 48 hours after subcutaneous infusion of ketamine, patients who wanted to be discharged home and had good pain control with ketamine, patients with a life expectancy longer than 2 weeks, and patients who could swallow or had a possibility to be tube fed.

When switching from parenteral to the oral route, benzodiazepines are discontinued [12].

The usual starting dose is 10–25 mg three or four times daily plus when needed. The dose can be increased in steps of 10–25 mg up to 100 mg three times daily [13].

Authors of the so far published studies differ in their recommendations about oral ketamine initiation. Some recommend one should always begin first with parenteral application and then switch to oral ketamine. The parenteral route could be either intravenous or subcutaneous. When used as an adjuvant to oral morphine, patients begin as well with oral ketamine [14, 15]. For the patient, who are, due to advanced disease, unable to swallow, the nasal route is more suitable [10].

6. Useful properties in the palliative care setting

6.1 Analgesic properties

Ketamine is considered one of the World Health Organization's essential drugs for the management of refractory pain and is associated with reduced opioid consumption and reduced opioid tolerance. It can be used in the treatment of acute and chronic pain as a co-analgesic and for alleviating the breakthrough pain episodes. Prescribing subanesthetic doses of ketamine can reduce postoperative morphine necessity and so diminish the side-effects of morphine.

The use of ketamine in the treatment of pain as an adjuvant analgesic is not licensed but the evidence for its efficiency is considerable. Its use has been recommended in the Scottish Palliative Care Guidelines and the Palliative Care Formulary. When used, a prescribing physician should notify the patient.

Ketamine is indicated for the treatment of neuropathic pain which has not responded to other medications, including strong opioids, anticonvulsants (gabapentin), and tricyclic antidepressants, including a trial of high dose dexamethasone.

Experimental data provide evidence that norketamine is effective in preventing central sensitization and in reversing an established hyperalgesia.

Although clinical evidence has been adding up, there are just a few comparative studies, and the majority of evidence is in the form of case reports [16–18].

A usual starting dose of oral ketamine is 10 mg four times daily initially, increasing to a maximum of 100 mg four times daily according to the response. Frail patients may be started at a lower oral dose: 25–30 mg over 24 hours. The maximum reported dose is 200 mg three times daily. It is possible to withdraw ketamine for several weeks after good pain control is achieved and restart the regimen when the pain returns.

Occasionally oral ketamine or sublingual/buccal ketamine is used as required. Usual dose is 2.5–5 mg (using 50 mg/5 ml solution). This dose is an individual decision.

There is no time limit to the treatment, but the success of pain relief should be regularly assessed, and the dose adjusted when needed [19–21].

6.2 Antidepressant and anxiolytic actions

Ketamine can produce rapid relief of major depression, bipolar disorders, and suicidal ideation. The mechanism for this effect is not yet fully understood but the major depressive disorder is associated with synaptic downregulation in the prefrontal cortex and hippocampus and it is believed that ketamine causes a glutamate surge that leads to a series of events resulting in synaptogenesis and reversal of the negative effect of depression and chronic stress. It appears that ketamine normalizes depression-related prefrontal dysconnectivity.

The rapid effect of ketamine on stress, anxiety, and depression may be of huge importance for the treatment of psychiatric conditions of patients in palliative care. Anxiety and depression are related to lower quality of life [22–24].

The positive psychological effect of ketamine is attributed to an induction of neuroplasticity which reverses the negative effect of stress and depression on neural cells and synapses [25].

There are various dosage regimens described in studies, in one case report patients received a bolus of one single dose of ketamine racemate (0.5 mg/kg). The reduction in anxiety was more pronounced in the first 4 days. After daily oral administration over 28 days of ketamine racemate, a significant effect was sustained with a large effect size for anxiety and depression. There was a significant response after the first 3 days [25, 26].

FDA-approved nasal spray formulation for the treatment of anxiety and depression [27, 28].

6.3 Bronchodilatatory effects

Ketamine produces bronchodilation, allowing secure induction of anesthesia in a patient with a life-threatening asthma and intense acute bronchial constriction. It is reported that ketamine doses of 0.1–0.2 mg/kg followed by 0.15–2.5 mg/kg/h can be used in patients with refractory bronchospasm and intensive status of asthma. The proposed mechanism of action is inhibition of inflammatory cascade and reduction in markers of inflammation and bronchodilation [29].

6.4 Topical ketamine in the treatment of mucositis pain

Ketamine oral rinse significantly reduced radiation-induced mucositis pain and hyperalgesia in a patient with head and neck cancer and so preserved the possibility of oral intake. It is speculated that the analgesia could be produced locally and systemically due to the absorption across the oral mucosa. The possibility of systemic absorption may result in psychomimetic and sedative effects. In the published paper the dose of 20 mg was arbitrarily chosen, being twice as the usual empiric starting dose for sublingual administration. As the literature is scarce on data for the topical use of ketamine further studies are needed before its use can be routinely recommended [30].

6.5 Refractory status epilepticus

Evidence suggests that the activity as well as the number of NMDA receptors is increased in refractory status epilepticus. Ketamine reduces the NMDA receptor-induced neurotoxicity and also has a neuroprotective role. On the other hand, evidence also shows that ketamine, at usual doses, has an epileptogenic potential and should be avoided in patients with epilepsy. From the so far published studies, no conclusive results can be drawn and further clinical trials are needed to assess the safety and efficiency of ketamine in both adult and pediatric populations [31].

7. Side effects of ketamine use

Side effects of ketamine use are dose-dependent. They are more common when ketamine is used as an anesthetic. Very common side effects are vivid dreams, hallucinations, dysphoria, and sedation. Incidence of psychotic effects can be reduced by using haloperidol or benzodiazepines. Sometimes can be enough just to reduce the dose of ketamine. Among less common side effects are cardiovascular side effects which are normally not serious. An increase in blood pressure and heart rate may occur. There are several reports about urinary tract symptoms that might require discontinuation of ketamine infusion. The bladder is most severely affected. There is a strong correlation between higher age (older than 30 yrs), longer duration of use (more than 24 months), and co-use of illicit drugs.

Other side effects include increased muscle tone, involuntary movements, dizziness and nausea, liver toxicity, and neuropsychiatric toxicities [32, 33].

8. Recommendations for use of ketamine in palliative care

Palliative care aims to relieve symptoms of the advanced incurable disease and improve the quality of life throughout illness and in the bereavement period so that the patients and families can realize their full potential to live even the life is approaching its end.

Patients in palliative care may report a variety of symptoms among which poor pain control merits full attention. The concept of total pain is applicable as pain may occur on a physical, psychological, social, and spiritual level. Physical pain and psychological distress are connected. About two-thirds of patients with advanced cancer suffer from pain and more than half of those experience moderate to severe pain. Following the WHO cancer pain relief guidelines, one can achieve acceptable pain relief in over 50% of treated patients. About 50% of the patient may have poor pain control.

Many of the symptoms in palliative care require a pharmacological approach and drug prescription. Most strong analgesics have a strong sedative effect and therefore impact patients' cognition. Many patients, who list as their value being able to think clearly, are reluctant to use them. Some are also afraid of the addiction potential of these drugs.

Having in mind that many patients in palliative care have psychiatric symptoms and sometimes they cannot wait for the classic antidepressant drugs to act, ketamine is promising due to its rapid action. Up to 42% of hospice patients have symptoms of depression and up to 70% have symptoms of anxiety. Untreated psychiatric symptoms are associated with significant morbidity and mortality, when left untreated, these symptoms can also interfere with their ability to make decisions and make realistic goals.

Oral ketamine may prove particularly useful for hospice patients who wish to remain home instead of receiving treatment in the hospital. To fasten the onset of oral ketamine, it was suggested to start patients on parenteral dosing before switching to oral administration. Another alternative to oral ketamine is an intranasal spray, which has been approved for the treatment of depression, but it might be more difficult to use [33–36].

9. Summary

Although ketamine has been in clinical practice for many years, it has been predominantly used as an anesthetic drug. Newer insight into its action shows its effectiveness in treating pain, anxiety, depression, bronchial spasm, refractory status epilepticus, and radio-induced mucositis.

This is especially important in the palliative setting, where patients commonly have pain combined with some other symptoms. They usually become refractors to high doses of opioids, with a detrimental quality of life.

Ketamine has a sparing effect on opioid consumption which may prolong their analgesic effect, reduce their dose and make pain treatment effective again. It can be used as an adjuvant as a baseline treatment or/and s a breakthrough medication.

Besides it, rapid relief of anxiety with just a single dose of ketamine is promising as well as the fact that the effect is sustainable.

Oral and nasal routes appear to be a good alternative for patients who are not institutionalized and who wish to avoid painful injections. Further studies are needed to define a suitable dosing protocol for ketamine.

Author details

Mateja Lopuh
Center for Interdisciplinary Pain Treatment and Palliative Care, Mobile Palliative Care Unit, General Hospital Jesenice, Slovenia

*Address all correspondence to: mateja.lopuh@gmail.com

References

[1] Quibell R, Prommer E, Mihalyo E, Twycross R, Wilcock A. Therapeutic reviews ketamine. Journal of Pain and Symptom Management. 2011;**41**(3): 640-649

[2] Mion G, Villevieille T. Ketamine pharmacology: An update (pharmacodynamics and molecular aspects, recent findings). CNS Neuroscience and Therapeutics. 2013;**19**:370-380

[3] Legge J, Ball N, Elliott DP. The potential role of ketamine in hospice analgesia: A literature review. The Consultant Pharmacist. 2006;**21**(1): 51-57

[4] Mion G, Villevieille T. Ketamine pharmacology. An Update (Pharmacodynamics and Molecular aspects, recent finding). CNS Neuroscience & Therapeutics. 2013;**19**:370-380

[5] Dulin JD, Hardcopf J, Coyne PJ. Iatrogenice oral ketamine overdose in palliative care. Journal of Palliative Care. 2020;**20**:1-3

[6] Kumar A, Kohli A. Comeback of ketamine: Resurfacing facts and dispelling myths. Korean Journal of Anaesthesiology. 2021;**74**(2):103-114

[7] Bell RF, Eccleston C, Klasso EA. Ketamine as an adjuvant to opioids for cancer pain. Cochrane Database of Systematic Reviews. 2012;**11**:CD003351

[8] Abdollahpour A, Saffarieh E, Zoroufchi BH. A review on the recent application of ketamine in the management of anesthesia, pain and health care. 2020;**9**:1317-1324

[9] Hashimoto K. Rapid acting antidepressant ketamine: Its metabolites and other candidate. A historical overiew and future perspective. Psychiatry and Clinical Neurosciences. 2019;**73**:613-627

[10] Singh V, Gillespie TW, Harvey D. Intranasal ketamine and its potential role in cancer related pain. Pharmacotherapy. 2018;**38**(3):390-340

[11] Benitez-Rosario M, Salinas-Martin A, Gonzales-Guillermo T, Feria M. A strategy for conversion from subcutaneous to oral ketamine in cancer pain patients: Effects of a 1:1 ratio. Journal of Pain and Symptom Management. 2011;**41**(6): 1098-1104

[12] Soto E, Stewart DR, Mannes AJ, Ruppert SL, Baker K, Zlotte D, et al. Oral ketamine in palliative care setting; a review of the literature and case report of a patient with neurofibromatosis type 1 and glomus tumor associated complex regional pain syndrome. The American Journal of Hospice & Palliative Care. 2012;**29**(4):308-317

[13] Shared Care Guideline for the Use of Ketamine in Palliative Care Initiated by Palliative Care Specialists. 2020. Available from: http://www.northoftyneapc.nhs.uk/wp-content/uploads/sites/6/2020/07/Ketamine-in-Palliative-Care-pain-2020

[14] Kannan TR, Saxena A, Bhatnagar S, Barry A. Oral ketamine as an adjuvant to oral morphine or neuropathic pain in cancer patients. Journal of Pain and Symptom Management. 2002;**23**(1): 60-65

[15] Grant IS, Nimmo WS, Clements JA. Pharmacokinetics and analgesic effects of IM and oral ketamine. British Journal of Anaesthesia. 1981;**53**:805-810

[16] Culp C, Hee Kee K, Abdi S. Ketamine use for cancer and chronic pain management. Frontiers in Pharmacology. 2021;**11**:599721

[17] Hocking G, Cousins MJ. Ketamine in chronic pain management: An evidence-based review. Anesthesia and Analgesia. 2003;**97**:1730-1739

[18] Fitzgibbon EJ, Hall P, Schroder C, et al. Low dose ketamine as an analgesic adjuvant in difficult pain syndromes: A strategy for conversion from parenteral to oral ketamine. Journal of Pain and Symptom Management. 2002; **23**:165-175

[19] Benitez-Rosario MA, Feria M, Salinas-Martin A, Martinez-Castillo LP, Martin-Ortega JJ. A retrospective comparison of the dose ration between subcutaneous and oral ketamine. Journal of Pain and Symptom Management. 2003;**25**:400-402

[20] Prommer E. Ketamine to control pain. Journal of Palliative Medicine. 2003;**6**:443-446

[21] Fine PG. Low-dose ketamine in the management of opioid nonresponsive terminal cancer pain. Journal of Pain and Symptom Management. 1999;**17**:296-300

[22] Irwin SA, Iglewicz A. Oral ketamine for the rapid treatment of depression and anxiety in patients receiving hospice care. Journal of Palliative Medicine. 2010;**13**:903-908

[23] Irwin SA, Iglewicz A, Nelesen R, Lo JY, Carr CH, Romero SD, et al. Daily oral ketamine for the treatment of depression and anxiety in patients receiving hospice care: A 28-day open-label proof-of-concept trial. Journal of Palliative Medicine. 2013;**16**:958-965

[24] Duman RS, Li N, Liu R-J, Durc V, Aghajanien G. Signaling pathways underlying the rapid antidepressant actions of ketamine. Neuropharmacology. 2012;**102**:72-79

[25] Falk E, Schlieper D, Van Caster P, Lutterbeck MJ, Schwartz J, Cordes J, et al. A rapid positive influence of S-ketamine in anxiety of patients in palliative care: A retrospective pilot study. BMC Palliative Care. 2020;**19**:1

[26] Delgado-Guay M, Parsons HA, Li Z, Palmer JL, Bruera E. Symptom distress in advanced cancer patient with anxiety and depression in the palliative care setting. Support Care Cancer. 2009;**17**(5):573-579

[27] Iqbal SZ, Mathew SJ. Ketamine for depression clinical issues. Advances in Pharmacology. 2020;**89**:131-162

[28] Kurdi MS, Theerth KA, Deva RS. Ketamine. Current applications in anesthesia, pain and critical care. Anesthesia, Essays and Researches. 2014;**8**:283-290

[29] Natoli S. The multiple faces of ketamine in anesthesia and analgesia. Drugs. Context. 2021;**10** 2020-2112-8

[30] Slatkin NE, Hiner M. Topical ketamine in the treatment of mucositis pain. Case report. Pain Medicine. 2003;**4**(3):298-303

[31] Rosati A, De Masi S, Guerrini R. Ketamine for refractory status epilepticus: A systematic eeview. CNS Drugs. 2018;**32**(11):997-1009

[32] Bell RF, Kalso EA. Ketamine for pain management. Pain Report. 2018;**3**: e674

[33] Storr TM, Quibell R. Can ketamine be prescribed for pain cause damage to urinary tract? Palliative Medicine. 2009;**23**:670-672

[34] Dulin DJ, Hardcopf J, Coyne PJ. Iatrogenic oral ketamine overdose in palliative care. Journal of Palliative Medicine. 2021;**24**(1):148-151

[35] Baumrucker SJ. Ketamine and problems with advanced palliative care in the community setting. American

Journal of Hospice and Palliative Care. 2000;**17**:369-370

[36] Goldman N, Frankenthaler M, Klepacz L. The efficacy of ketamine in the palliative care setting: A comprehensive review of the literature. Journal of Palliative Medicine. 2019;**22**:1154-1161

Chapter 16

The Role of Ketamine in Trauma

Mihai Octavian Botea and Erika Bimbo-Szuhai

> *"I would especially commend the physician who, in acute diseases, by which the bulk of mankind are cutoff, conducts the treatment better than others."*
>
> *Hippocrates*

Abstract

Early and effective pain control in trauma patients improves outcomes and limits disability, but analgesia is often missed in the unstable patient, or hemodynamically depressing medications are avoided for fear of losing stability. This chapter outlines the role of ketamine in managing traumatic emergencies in both out-of-hospital and hospital environment, and beyond. Low-dose ketamine also called a sub-dissociative dose is safe, efficient and effective analgesic that can be considered for trauma patients, pediatric or adults, as an alternative to opioids or in combination with opioids for on additive or synergistic effect, with minimal impact on hemodynamic stability. Ketamine at higher doses is also an excellent drug for induction of anesthesia in rapid sequence induction (RSI), post-intubation sedation maintenance or procedural sedation in the trauma patient. Also, can be used for acute agitation and excited delirium. In this chapter, we are describing this drug focusing on a deeper understanding of the safety and efficacy of this agent and, if supported, to encourage physicians to consider ketamine for pain control in trauma and beyond. Also, we are presenting the current literature surrounding ketamine's evidences in the trauma condition to establish its utility and profile of safety for these patients.

Keywords: ketamine, analgesia, anesthesia, shock, trauma

1. Introduction

Trauma is one of the leading causes of death worldwide [1] with 5.8 million lives lost each year as a direct result of injury [2], and it is a major economic burden to society in both Europe and United States [1, 3]. Trauma management is demanding for clinicians, often a life-threatening and most of the time a painful condition. Early and effective pain control in trauma is essential not only for acute status control, but has also been associated with a lesser incidence of chronic pain, as well as a shorter period of recovery [1, 2]. Many factors influence the selection of analgesics, and we have available a generous options of pain killers, but in reality, an adequate pain control is often difficult to achieve. According to many reports, trauma patient analgesia is remaining an undermanaged condition [3–5]. Opioid analgesics are often appropriate first-line pain killers for acute pain but come with hemodynamic and respiratory depression, as well as concerns about the addiction risks. Ketamine is a dissociative and analgesic drug that can be used alone or in combination with other analgesic medication. The terms low-dose, analgesic, pain control and sub-dissociative dose can be used interchangeably.

2. Pharmacologic properties

Ketamine is an agent with attractive pharmacological and pharmacokinetic characteristics. Ketamine is a potent dissociative agent with an evolving role in the management of both pediatric and adult trauma patients due to its sedative, analgesic and anesthetic properties, beside its sympathomimetic effect. Ketamine is a derivate of phenylcyclidine with a hallucinogenic property, beside its primarily antagonist activity on N-methyl-D-aspartate receptors although it also acts on opioid (μ), and muscarinic receptors, and sodium channels. Its action is targeting the central nervous system *via* the thalamo-cortical tracts. This drug inhibits presynaptic reuptake of catecholamines, with an onset time of 30 s. For being highly lipophilic, ketamine has a distribution half-life of 10 min, for a short duration of action after an initial bolus. Ketamine is the least protein bound from the i.v. anesthetics (25%) suffering a liver metabolization, generating active compounds (norketamine and hydroxynorketamine), and is eliminated mainly in the urine with an elimination half-life of 1.5–3 h.

The sedative and analgesic effects of this drug begin to wear off in 10–15 min.

For many years, ketamine was considered to be a harmful drug to use for airway management or in multiple trauma conditions, especially where a traumatic brain injury component was involved, due to fears of increasing intracranial pressure (ICP) [6]. But recent studies show which can be a real helpful drug, in certain conditions like the combative trauma patient who needs airway management or other situations like improving pain control or anesthesia induction in a hemodynamically unstable trauma patient [6]. Recent experiences show that do not raise intracranial pressure as was once assumed and does raise blood pressure improving cardiovascular stability, unlike most sedating drugs [6]. Also, a drug should be considered extremely helpful for acute invasive procedures that need to be performed under sedation [7, 8], offering a great advantage of analgesia and respiratory stability at the same time. Ketamine is known an optimal drug in various emergency settings. Also, away from the emergency room, studies have been performed to assess the safety and efficacy of ketamine for trauma patients, showing that ICU patients with a sub-dissociative ketamine infusion needed fewer opioid analgesics and had a better hemodynamic stability [9]. In this chapter, we present the current literature surrounding the safety and efficacy of ketamine in the trauma condition to establish its utility for these patients.

3. Systemic effects

Ketamine has minimal effects on the respiratory drive and protective reflexes of the protective airway reflexes are maintained, thus allowing to keep spontaneous ventilation. However, administering high doses that would be used for anesthetic effect there is a risk of respiratory depression [5, 9]. Ketamine is also responsible for bronchodilation, increased salivation, pulmonary vasodilation and increased cardiac output, through increasing mean arterial pressure and heart rate. Its profile on hemodynamics is favorable, making this agent a unique drug, a considerable option especially in approaching a shocked trauma patient. Also, its depressant effects on the gastrointestinal system are very minimal. Ketamine could have an antiplatelets action by inhibiting phosphoinositide breakdown and mobilization of Ca^{2+} in those platelets stimulated by collagen [10].

4. Cerebral effects

The physiological mechanisms lead to neuroprotection, vasodilation and increased cerebral blood flow.

In particular, new clinical data and case studies support a therapeutic effect of ketamine in suppression of spreading depolarization (SD) following traumatic brain injury (TBI). This is fundamental as SD has been suggested as an important mechanism for secondary brain injury and delayed cerebral ischemia [10].

Ketamine has been recently discovered to be a "glutamate modulator." Its action is exerted at two levels: (a) presynaptic, inhibiting the release of glutamate and (b) post-synaptic, performing as a competitive blocker of NMDA receptors, also inhibiting calcium entrance into cells and the production of nitric oxide and oxygen-free radicals, modulating glucose metabolism and the generation of mitochondrial ATP, and also, inhibiting the apoptotic phenomenon. Furthermore, it inhibits the production and release of cytokines not only by the microglia but also by interleukin-8, tumor necrosis factor, Ca++, K+, oxygen-free radicals, adenosine triphosphate.

The cerebral metabolic rate of oxygen is increased, although in a heterogeneous action, more in insula and the frontal lobes, while decreasing in the temporal lobes, pons and cerebellum. Cerebral blood flow does not follow the same pattern. Probably, a dose-dependent uncoupling mechanism is implied. Intracranial pressure remains unaffected or even sometime decreased, being associated with increases in cerebral perfusion pressure.

Cerebral oxygenation remains unchanged. Moreover, ketamine does not compromise the autoregulatory mechanisms or the carbon dioxide (CO_2) reactivity of the cerebral vasculature [10, 11].

It is important to promote recent findings that NMDA receptors have different protein subpopulations in their composition, capable of triggering various pathways that stimulate proliferation, synaptogenesis or neuronal regeneration, depending on which protein is activated [12].

Extensive studies have shown that after stroke or traumatic brain injury, NMDA receptors remain hypofunctional, which could be responsible for cognitive impairments. Activating and stimulating these receptors by alternative pathways (glycine/serine) is a promising strategy [12].

5. Summary of evidence

5.1 What is the efficacy of ketamine for analgesia?

There are convincing evidences demonstrating the efficacy and safety of ketamine as an analgesic for trauma patients.

In a very recent meta-analysis published in 2020, where controlled human studies were included, Mahmoud Yousefifard performed extensive search conducted in electronic databases gathering data to the end of 2018. The efficacy and side effects of ketamine administration in prehospital pain management were compared with those of opioid analgesics. Data from seven articles were included in the present meta-analysis. Ketamine administration was not much more effective than administrating morphine or fentanyl in prehospital pain management of trauma patients.

However, co-administration of ketamine + morphine was considerably more effective than ketamine alone, in alleviating pain in prehospital settings. Finally, it was concluded that ketamine alone had less side effects than morphine alone. However, co-administration of ketamine + morphine increases the risk of side effects compared with when morphine is prescribed alone [13].

In 2020, Gaël de Rocquigny published a systemic review in regarding the use of ketamine for prehospital pain control on the battlefield [14]. This included a database searching for studies on ketamine use in combating prehospital settings, at the point of injury or during evacuation. Eight studies were included with 2029 casualties receiving ketamine. Ketamine use increased from 3.9% during the period preceding its addition to the Tactical Combat Casualty Care guidelines in 2012 to 19.8% after this guidelines release. It was the analgesic of choice (up to 52% of casualties) in one of the studies. Ketamine has been preferred to be given during tactical medical evacuation when no analgesic was administered at the point of injury. Pain score decreased from moderate or severe to mild or none, often after only one dose. In one study, ketamine administration during tactical evacuation was associated with increased systolic blood pressure as opposed to those situations when morphine was given. Incoherent speech, hallucinations and extremity movements were the most seen adverse events reported. However, all studies tend to strengthen the belief in the efficacy and safety of ketamine when given at 50-mg to 100-mg intravenous for prehospital analgesia in combat casualties. So, from these army studies, we can easily extrapolate these findings and apply to the civil medicine.

In 2018, Mary K. Walters published a study on the ketamine as an analgesic adjuvant in a trauma patient with rib fractures. This was a retrospective study, based on case-control chart review assessing ICU adult patients with a diagnosis of ≥1 rib fracture and an Injury Severity Score > 15. Patients received standard-of-care analgesia with the physician's choice medication with or without ketamine as a continuous, fixed, intravenous infusion at 0.1 mg/kg/h. The authors pointed out that low-dose ketamine appears to be a safe and effective adjuvant option to reduce pain and decrease opioid use in rib fracture [15].

In 2019, Thomas Carver published a prospective, randomized, double-blind placebo-controlled trial on ketamine infusion for pain control in multiple rib fractures. This level II of evidence study included adult patients with three or more rib fractures admitted to a Level I Trauma Center. Other exclusion criteria were Glasgow Coma Scale score less than 13 and chronic opiate use. The experimental arm received low-dose ketamine (LDK) at 2.5 μg/kg/min, while the placebo cohort received an equivalent rate of 0.9% normal saline. The primary outcome was reduction in numeric pain score (NPS) during the first 24 h. From the secondary outcomes studied, oral morphine equivalent (OME) utilization was included. The average Injury Severity Score (ISS) was 14. Low-dose ketamine failed to decrease NPS or OME within the overall cohort, but a decrease in OME was observed among patients with an ISS greater than 15. This study authors also conclude that confirmatory studies are necessary to determine whether LDK is a useful adjunct among severely injured patients [16].

In 2017, Babak Mahshidfar conducted a randomized double-blinded clinical trial to compare low-dose ketamine (LDK) with morphine for pain relief in trauma patients. He enrolled 300 trauma patients from the emergency room of two university hospitals. The patients were randomly divided into two groups. The first group was administered i.v. 0.2 mg/kg of ketamine, while the second group received 0.1 mg/kg of i.v. morphine. The results of this study suggest that LDK, at a dose of 0.2 mg/kg, in the earlier minutes leads to significant reduction of pain when compared with that of intravenous morphine. It also created fewer complications than morphine [17].

In 2014, Joshua P Miller performed an institutional review board-approved, randomized, prospective, double-blinded trial at a tertiary, Level 1 Trauma Center. The study was focused on low-dose ketamine vs. morphine for acute pain control in the ED. They enrolled adult patients with acute abdominal, flank, low back or extremity pain. Subjects were consented and randomized to intravenous LDK (0.3 mg/kg) or intravenous MOR (0.1 mg/kg). The primary outcome was the maximum change in NRS scores. Low-dose ketamine compared with MOR for acute pain did not produce a greater reduction in NRS pain. But it is assumed that LDK induced a significant analgesic effect within 5 min and provided a moderate reduction in pain for 2 h. The time to achieve maximum reduction in NRS pain scores was at 5 min for LDK and 100 min for MOR. Vital signs, adverse events, clinician and nurse satisfaction scores were similar between groups [18].

In 2012, Paul A. Jennings proved that intravenous morphine plus ketamine provides analgesia superior to that of intravenous morphine alone. This is a prehospital study, randomized, prospective and controlled study. Patients with traumatic condition and a verbal pain score of greater than 5 after 5 mg of i.v. morphine were eligible for enrollment. Patients included in the ketamine group were administered a bolus of 10 or 20 mg, followed by 10 mg every 3 min. The second group patients received just morphine 5 mg i.v. every 5 min until pain free. Pain scores were regularly assessed until hospital arrival. The study conclusion was intravenous morphine plus ketamine for out-of-hospital adult trauma patients providing analgesia superior to that of intravenous morphine alone but was associated with an increase in the rate of minor adverse effects [19].

In 2017, Benov and colleagues published a review of data cases from 17 years of time frame from the military prehospital trauma registry of the Israeli Defense Forces. This included data from 141 solders patients, victims of explosion, who had received ketamine for analgesia. This review made a relatively conclusive statement: “Ketamine in subanesthetic doses is almost an ideal analgesic exhibited through its profound pain relief, its margin of safety, and its role in potentiation of opioids and prevention of opioid hyperalgesia” [20].

In 2007, Michel Galinski investigated the morphine consumption associated with ketamine for severe acute pain in emergency setting, where patients with a visual analog scale (VAS) score of minimum 60/100 were included. The K group patients received 0.2 mg/kg of i.v. ketamine over 10 min, while the P group patients received sodium chloride, as the control group. The patients from both groups were given an initial intravenous morphine dose of 0.1 mg/kg, plus as required doses were supplemented with 3 mg every 5 min. Efficient analgesia was defined as a VAS score not exceeding 30/100. The goals of this study were to assess morphine consumption and VAS at 30 min. They concluded that morphine consumption was much less in the K group vs. the P group. The VAS score at T30 did not differ significantly between the two groups [21]. We could assume the fact that the VAS score at T30 was similar for the two groups due to the fact that the time action for the ketamine dose is roughly around 10–15 min, and the K group received just an initial dose. So probably I would have been better also to have a VAS score at T15, for example, for more realistic and objective findings.

In 2019, Sheila C. Takieddine investigated whether ketamine administered *via* patient-controlled analgesia (PCA) provides adequate analgesia while reducing opioid consumption in the traumatically injured patient. Non-intubated trauma patients in intensive care, who were receiving PCA, were randomized to ketamine or hydromorphone PCA plus opioid analgesics for breakthrough pain. They concluded that ketamine PCA led to lower cumulative opioid consumption and lower oxygen supplementation requirements, though hallucinations occurred more frequently with the use of ketamine. They also concluded that additional studies are needed to investigate the tolerability of ketamine as an alternative to traditional opioid-based PCA [22].

In 2017, Kaitlin A. Pruskowski conducted a study to investigate the efficiency of the initiation of a ketamine continuous infusion in critically ill trauma patients for sedation and analgesic purposes. The secondary goals were to find out the patient population in which ketamine was administered, assess the time patients reached their goal level of sedation and find out the dosing required as adjunctive sedative agents. This retrospective chart review was investigated for 19-month period. This study was focused on the critically ill mechanically ventilated trauma patients. The study concluded that the use of ketamine in critically ill mechanically ventilated adult trauma patients was associated with decreased opioid use but it was also associated with the increased use of dexmedetomidine and ziprasidone to achieve and maintain sedation [23].

In 2014, Kim Phung Tran published a prospective study aiming to compare the analgesic effects and side effects of ketamine and morphine in out-of-hospital environment. The conclusion of this research was that ketamine had a pain control effect similar to morphine, and also accompanied by a lower risk of airway patency issues. The side effects as agitation and hallucinations were higher in incidence in the ketamine group. These conclusions are to be well appreciated as utility and application, particularly in rough and low-resource environments [24].

Bredmose PP conducted in 2009 another prospective study in the field of prehospital care investigating ketamine for analgesia and procedural sedation. This study evaluated the role of ketamine for analgesia and sedation in 1030 trauma patients in a prehospital trauma service led by physicians. Ketamine administration was the first choice in awake non-trapped victims with blunt trauma for analgesia and procedural sedation. This study data interpretation did not point out concerns for loss of airway, oxygen desaturation or clinically significant emergence reactions associated with ketamine use. Ketamine could be considered relatively safe when administered by physicians in out-of-hospital trauma care [25].

Still remaining in the prehospital field, it is advocated that there are many features of ketamine that seem to make it an ideal drug for prehospital use, including disaster surgery where extra personnel and advanced monitoring are not available.

In light of these premises, James E. Svenson performed a retrospective study of all patients transported by a regional aeromedical program. Data were collected from 40 patients, where ketamine was used. The study included pediatric and adult patients with age between 2 months and 75 years old. The indications for administration varied, from trauma to medical conditions. Shock status with need for analgesia, combativeness or agitation, intact airway concerns, or pain unresponsive to opioid drugs were the most common indications for use. Ketamine was administered either intravenously or intramuscularly (when no intravenous access was available). Minimal or no adverse effects [26] were reported.

In 2019, Kugler, Nathan published a level I of evidence study, randomized, double-blind placebo-controlled prospective trial enrolling elderly patients (age, ≥65 years) with three or more rib fractures presented to a Level I trauma center. The exclusion criteria were Glasgow Coma Scale score less than 14 and/or chronic opiate medication. Patients were randomized in two groups, either low-dose ketamine (LDK) at 2 μg/kg/min or an equivalent rate of 0.9% natrium chloride. This study conclusion is that low-dose ketamine failed to affect NPS or OME within the overall cohort, but a decrease in OME was observed in those with an Injury Severity Score greater than 15. Also, in this view, it is recommended that additional studies are necessary to confirm whether LDK benefits severely injured elderly patients [27].

5.2 What is the clinical evidence of ketamine in RSI and sedation?

One of other benefits of using ketamine in trauma is that could be an option for rapid sequence intubation (RSI) induction and maintaining sedation. Ketamine has emerged as an alternative for RSI induction, because the conventional propofol makes hemodynamics vulnerable and induction doses of etomidate during rapid sequence intubation cause transient adrenal dysfunction, where clinical significance on trauma patients is uncertain.

Cameron P. Upchurch in 2017 published the four-year retrospective study comparing etomidate and ketamine for induction during rapid sequence intubation of adult trauma patients. In this analysis spanning an institutional protocol switch from etomidate to ketamine as the standard rapid sequence intubation induction agent for adult trauma patients, patient-centered outcomes were similar for patients who received etomidate and ketamine [28].

In 2019, Josefine Baekgaard investigated whether ketamine should be preferred over other induction agents for RSI in trauma patients. Library was systematically searched for studies reporting RSI of adult trauma patients with ketamine compared with another induction agent (etomidate, propofol, thiopental or midazolam). Extremely few studies have compared induction agents for RSI in trauma patients. Only four studies were included. The review conclusion was that no significant differences have been found in mortality, length of hospital stay or a number of blood transfusions after induction with ketamine compared with other induction agents, but a clinically relevant benefit or harm cannot be excluded [29].

In 2021, Lucy Stanke aiming to bring more evidences in the prehospital field of RSI drug comparison published a retrospective study to evaluated adult patients undergoing prehospital RSI over 13 months within a regional emergency transport medicine service. The purpose of this study was to evaluate hemodynamic changes after the administration of ketamine versus etomidate in prehospital RSI. The analysis emphasized that no cardiovascular differences were reported between patients who received ketamine versus etomidate for out-of-hospital RSI. None of these two drugs was associated with an increased requirement for additional hypnotics, and neither drug was associated with an increased first-attempt tracheal intubation success rate. This study also concluded that more studies, on larger cohorts and prospective designs, are needed to identify patients who may benefit from either ketamine or etomidate [30].

During emergency situations where RSI of anesthesia is required like in shocked or hypotensive patients (e.g., massive hemorrhage due to ruptured major vessels, pelvic fracture or other polytrauma conditions), prior resuscitation is often suboptimal and comorbidities (particularly cardiovascular) may be extensive, making challenges even worst. The induction drugs with the most favorable pharmacological properties offering a hemodynamic stability appear to be etomidate and ketamine. However, etomidate has been withdrawn from use in some countries and is known to impair steroidogenesis. Ketamine has been traditionally contra-indicated in the presence of head trauma, but we argue in this article that any adverse effects of the drug on intracranial pressure or cerebral blood flow are in fact attenuated or reversed by a better cardiovascular stability, sedation and controlled ventilation conferred by the drug. Ketamine represents a very rational option for RSI in hemodynamically compromised patients [31].

5.3 What is the clinical evidence of ketamine in traumatic brain injury?

For many years, the use of ketamine was restricted in TBI patients based on evidence from the 70s that suggested its detrimental effect on intracranial pressure. New research in healthy volunteers or in patients without neurological comorbidities scheduled for general surgery demonstrated that intracranial pressure, cerebral blood flow and cerebral perfusion pressure increase during anesthesia with variable doses of ketamine and no neurological side effects or sequels were noticed [32, 33]. Other series of studies with small numbers of patients with different central nervous system pathologies that had in common abnormal cerebral spinal fluid circulation reported similar findings, emphasizing the absence of side effects [34–39]. Other recent systematic studies with various degrees and types of limitations reported that in heterogeneous acute brain populations (subarachnoid hemorrhage, tumors, TBI), ketamine induces only temporary variations in intracranial pressure without modifying cerebral perfusion pressure and has no detrimental effect on outcome, intensive care unit stay or mortality [36–38]. When assessing populations of severe acute bran injury, ketamine was not associated with an increase of intracranial pressure in sedated and normocapnic mechanically ventilated patients; furthermore, ketamine may decrease intracranial pressure in some individualized situations [39]. Other recent updates of ketamine administration in TBI led to similar findings [40].

As regards the ketamine use in acute phase of severe traumatic brain injury (TBI), in 2021, Daniel Agustin Godoy stated that ketamine is "an old drug for new uses," having more and more evidences of its benefits even in this condition. In the acute phase of severe acute brain injury, it is paramount to prevent and avoid secondary insults that can further complicate a primary brain injury [41]. Managing a goal-driven sedation and optimal pain control is a cornerstone of improving patient survival, satisfaction and minimizing distress. Without an optimal sedation, there are rising consequences including delayed recovery, difficult weaning from mechanical ventilation, higher complication rate and prolonged hospital staying [42].

Several different classes of hypnotic drugs are used in the management of patients with TBI [43–45]. These drugs are used at induction of anesthesia, to provide and keep sedation, to reduce elevated intracranial pressure, to control seizures and facilitate mechanical ventilation [46, 47]. To date, it is unclear which agent or combination of drugs is the most effective in achieving these goals. Ketamine is a versatile agent with attractive pharmacological and pharmacokinetic properties.

Controversies concerning the optimal sedation management persist, especially in critically TBI, who were systematically excluded from large randomized studies [44]. Different from other agents, ketamine does not depress respiratory activity or airway reflexes (except at very high doses) and may have potential neuroprotective effects, as well as a potential in decreasing seizures and non-convulsive epileptic activity [48, 49]. These properties make from ketamine a realistic choice when profound analgesia and sedation are required.

But there are still some restrictions in severe traumatic brain injury, and certain conditions would contraindicate ketamine administration, such as loss of cerebral autoregulation, hydrocephalus or the concomitant presence of untreated brain aneurysms [40, 50, 51].

5.4 What is the ketamine evidence in eye pathology?

Ketamine induces intraocular pressure (IOP) changes bur, which are mild and without clinical significance [52, 53]. The current guidelines do not limit the use of ketamine in known or suspected open globe injuries [54].

Ketamine is not recommended to be used for procedural sedation in eye examination as one of the known side effects of this drug is nystagmus.

6. When not to use ketamine?

An absolute contraindication is hypersensitivity to this drug [40]. Due to hepatic metabolism and mainly kidney elimination, it should not be administrated in the context of liver failure and/or renal failure [40, 50, 51]. Other relative contraindications are those conditions where high blood pressure triggers potentially dangerous complications such as diastolic cardiac dysfunction, coronary ischemia or aortic dissection [40, 55]. In severe alcoholism, toxicity of ketamine has been described [40]. Use of ketamine in pediatrics is restricted to children younger than 3 months of age. There was reported higher incidence of airway complications like laryngospasm in very young patients [52].

Concerning the TBI, there are only a few contraindications nowadays. These were presented in a previous section.

Nevertheless, ketamine attributes to psychotomimetic effects, which could be the main reserve for not being a first choice when sedation is required [48, 49].

7. When to use ketamine?

In this section, indications for ketamine use will be divided in four general situations: analgesia, procedural sedation, induction of anesthesia/RSI and acute agitation/excited delirium [56].

Analgesia

- Ketamine's analgesic effect is comparable to opioids but with a lesser impact on hemodynamics or respiratory system.
- Ketamine could be an optimal analgesic in a trauma condition with moderate to severe pain, in or at risk for developing hemorrhagic shock or respiratory failure [57].
- Ketamine potentiates the analgesic effect of opioids and could be given to trauma patients with insufficient pain control after receiving opioids or when a top-up of opioids may be risky or harmful.
- Ketamine may be given to the trauma condition, as an alternative to opioids or other non-opioids medication.
- Ketamine could be an adequate option for the trauma patient receiving buprenorphine/naloxone for opioid misuse.

Procedural sedation

- Ketamine is optimal choice as a procedural sedation agent in patients with or at risk for respiratory failure or hemorrhagic shock.
- For short sedation procedures as in burns debridement or musculoskeletal injuries maneuvers.

Induction of anesthesia/rapid sequence intubation

- Is an optimal choice in shocked trauma patients for RSI due to its analgesic and sedative features and also for its cardiovascular stability?

Acute agitation/excited delirium

- Ketamine may be used in trauma conditions when fast control of agitation is required such as in patients with delirium or when rapid control is essential to diminish the risk of injury to staff, family or the patients themselves.

8. Dosing

The dose considerations of ketamine in adults can be either body weight-based or non-weight-based. For a better accuracy in dose calculations in pediatrics, the dose should always be weight or length based using a standardized measuring tape.

There are no standard recommendations for the ketamine dose. What follows are dose recommendations based on literature review and expert opinion.

Analgesia dosing recommendations

Intermittent dose:

- 0.1–0.3 mg/kg (maximum 30 mg) i.v. every 20 min as required for a maximum of three doses.
- This can be given by slow i.v. push or as an i.v. bag over 10–15 min (associated with side effects such as feelings of unreality and oversedation with no difference in analgesic efficacy) [58].
- 0.5–1.0 mg/kg intranasal (i.n.)

Adult continuous infusion dose:

- 0.1–0.4 mg/kg/hour i.v.

Adult non-weight-based analgesic dosing:

50 mg i.m., repeat as required every 30–60 min for pain control or until nystagmus develops indicating approach of the dissociative state.

20 mg slow i.v./i.o. push over 1 min, repeat as required every 20 min for desired analgesia or until nystagmus appears indicating reaching the dissociative state.

Procedural sedation

- 1 mg/kg i.v. (maximum 100 mg per dose)

Induction of anesthesia/RSI

- 2 mg/kg i.v. (maximum 200 mg)

Acute agitation/excited delirium

- 3–5 mg/kg i.m.
- 1–2 mg/kg i.v.

Other observations

- i.v. access in the acutely agitated patient or the patient with excited delirium might be too risky and difficult; so, it is not advisable due to the increased risk to the practitioner of occupational needle stick injury.
- High-dose (5 mg/kg) prehospital i.m. ketamine administration is associated with an increased intubation rate upon arrival to the hospital [59–61]. Clinicians giving high-dose ketamine should be prepared to control the airway.

- In some expert's opinion doses between 0.5 and 0.9 mg/kg i.v. are not efficacious for sedation and could trigger a sense of unreality that can lead to issues in patient management.

9. Safety profile

Ketamine can induce a transient apnea in high doses or with fast administration. These conditions are associated with higher intubation rate. Patients given ketamine should be kept under observation for the risk of respiratory failure, and clinicians using ketamine, especially in high doses, should be ready to take over airway control.

There is a lack of safety data to support recommendations in what concerning the use of ketamine in pregnancy and during breast feeding [62].

Another previous controversy, but recently cleared, ketamine use can be considered in trauma patients with schizophrenia as there does not seems to be a higher incidence of psychosis in these kinds of conditions [63, 64].

10. Complications and side effects

Fast IV administration can trigger transient apnea. Ketamine should be given in a slow bolus, over 1 min or more unless being used in RSI where it is followed shortly by a muscle relaxing drug and intubation. Transient apnea following i.m. administration appears to be extremely rare [43].

Reported side effects are laryngospasm, hypersalivation, nausea, dizziness, nystagmus, dysphoria and emergence agitation. Most of the time, these side effects are transient and self-limited and do not require any intervention or rescue. If laryngospasm occurs, it can be managed with repositioning or jaw thrust and positive pressure ventilation. In rare instances, intubation may be necessary.

Emergence reactions are notable to be rare. When appears, these can be safely managed with benzodiazepine use. Pre-medicating with benzodiazepines is not recommended.

11. Co-administration with other drugs

When used in concomitantly, ketamine increases the pain control effects of opioids. The administration of ketamine and opioids in combination improves analgesia with lesser doses of opioids thus decreasing the chance of opioid-induced adverse effects on cardiovascular and respiratory system [65].

Combining ketamine with opioid medication has been reported to block opioid-induced hyperalgesia and acute opioid tolerance.

When used in concomitantly, ketamine increases the sedative effects of benzodiazepines with its risk for respiratory depression. Extra caution should be sought, and airway monitoring should be considered.

Benzodiazepines should not be used prophylactically to prevent emergence reactions and should only be considered to manage an emergence reaction if the patient is a danger to themselves or staff. Suboptimal sedation requesting additional ketamine versus a true emergence reaction should be taken into consideration before the benzodiazepine administration.

12. Considerations with non-prescribed drugs

Ketamine increases the sedative effects of alcohol, and it is essential to anticipate the risks of respiratory decompensation when ketamine is administered to an acutely intoxicated patient [57].

Ketamine should be excluded if cocaine use is suspected as ketamine's sympathomimetic effects could superimpose over the cardiovascular toxicity of cocaine [18].

13. Geriatrics

In the literature, there are not sufficient data in what concerning the use of ketamine in the geriatrics. It is advisable to decrease the dose when using ketamine in the elderly since NMDA receptor binding is slowed with age.

14. Pediatrics

Ketamine is an alternative option to opioids and benzodiazepines for analgesia and sedation in the pediatric trauma patient over the age of 3 months.

Because of possible negative consequences on the developing brain in kids who have received repeated or prolonged exposure to drugs that block NMDA receptors, the use of ketamine in infants less than 3 years of age should be assessed within the context of the benefits and risks of the procedure [19].

Before ketamine use, it is first to take into account the adjunct measures for analgesia such as fractures immobilization or dislocations reductions.

Precautions should be taken when using ketamine out of hospital in the head-injured child. Adverse effects of ketamine in the children with head injuries have not been reported in the literature, though evidence on this topic is limited [66].

15. Conclusion

Analgesia and sedation are dynamic processes that must meet specific goals, be controlled and be easily modified according to the progress of patient's condition. Knowledge of drug pharmacology and its safety margin and profile are paramount to limit their side effects. Setting a goal-directed strategy, establishing local protocols of administration and monitoring treatment are the cornerstone of an efficient analgesia and sedation strategy. These qualities contribute to fulfilling an optimal and safe level of sedation, looking to balance the deleterious effects of under or over sedation [12].

Further studies on the use of ketamine in the adult and pediatric trauma patient population are required.

Author details

Mihai Octavian Botea* and Erika Bimbo-Szuhai
Pelican Clinic Hospital, University of Oradea, Oradea, Romania

*Address all correspondence to: drmob78@yahoo.com

References

[1] Finkelstein EA, Corso PS, Miller TR. The Incidence and Economic Burden of Injuries in the United States. New York, NY: Oxford University Press; 2006. Available from: http://www.oxfordscholarship.com/view/10.1093/acprof:oso/9780195179484.001.0001/acprof-9780195179484

[2] GBD 2013 Mortality and Causes of Death Collaborators. Global, regional, and national age-sex specific all-cause and cause-specific mortality for 240 causes of death, 1990-2013: A systematic analysis for the Global Burden of Disease Study 2013. Lancet. 2015;**385**:117-171

[3] Scholten AC, Haagsma JA, Panneman MJM, van Beeck EF, Polinder S. Traumatic brain injury in the Netherlands: Incidence, costs and disability-adjusted life years. PLoS One. 2014;**9**:e110905

[4] McGreevy K, Bottros M, Raja S. Preventing chronic pain following acute pain: Risk factors, preventive strategies, and their efficacy. European Journal of Pain Supplements. 2011;**5**(2):365-372. DOI: 10.1016/j.eujps.2011.08.013

[5] Peters M, Sommer M, et al. Somatic and psychologic predictors of long-term unfavorable outcome after surgical intervention. Annals of Surgery. 2007;**245**(3):487-494. DOI: 10.1097/01.sla.0000245495.79781.65

[6] Epps C, Ware L, Packard A. Ethnic wait time differences in analgesic administration in the emergency department. Pain Management Nursing. 2008;**9**(1):26-32. DOI: 10.1016/j.pmn.2007.07.005

[7] Anantha R, Stewart T, Rajagopalan A, Walsh J, Merritt N. Analgesia in the management of paediatric and adolescent trauma during the resuscitative phase: The role of the pediatric trauma centre. Injury. 2014;**45**(5):845-849. DOI: 10.1016/j.injury.2013.10.048

[8] Aminiahidashti H, Shafiee S, Hosseininejad S, et al. Propofol-fentanyl versus propofol-ketamine for procedural sedation and analgesia in patients with trauma. The American Journal of Emergency Medicine. 2018;**36**(10):1766-1770. DOI: 10.1016/j.ajem.2018.01.080

[9] Silka P, Roth M, Geiderman J. Patterns of analgesic use in trauma patients in the ED. The American Journal of Emergency Medicine. 2002;**20**(4):298-302. DOI: 10.1053/ajem.2002.34195

[10] Hartings JA et al. Prognostic value of spreading depolarizations in patients with severe traumatic brain injury. JAMA Neurology. 2020;**77**:489-499. DOI: 10.1001/jamaneurol.2019.4476

[11] Slupe AM, Kirsch JR. Effects of anesthesia on cerebral blood flow, metabolism, and neuroprotection. Journal of Cerebral Blood Flow and Metabolism. 2018;**38**:2192-2208

[12] Godoy DA, Badenes R, Pelosi P, et al. Ketamine in acute phase of severe traumatic brain injury "an old drug for new uses?". Critical Care. 2021;**25**:19. DOI: 10.1186/s13054-020-03452-x

[13] Yousefifard M, Askarian-Amiri S, Alavi SNR, Sadeghi M, Saberian P, Baratloo A, et al. The efficacy of ketamine administration in prehospital pain management of trauma patients; a systematic review and meta-analysis. Archives of Academic Emergency Medicine. 2020;**8**(1):e1

[14] Bakes KM, Buchanan JA, Moreira ME, Byyny R, Pons PT. Emergency Medicine Secrets. 5th ed. Maryland Heights, Missouri, United States: Elsevier Mosby; 2011. p. 563

[15] Walters M, Farhat J, Bischoff J, Foss M, Evans C. Ketamine as an

analgesic adjuvant in adult trauma intensive care unit patients with rib fracture. The Annals of Pharmacotherapy. 2018;**52**(9):849-854. DOI: 10.1177/1060028018768451

[16] Carver TW, Kugler NW, Juul J, Peppard WJ, Drescher KM, Somberg LB, et al. Ketamine infusion for pain control in adult patients with multiple rib fractures: Results of a randomized control trial. Journal of Trauma and Acute Care Surgery 2019. 2019;**86**(2):181-188. DOI: 10.1097/TA.0000000000002103

[17] Mahshidfar B, Mofidi M, Fattahi M. Acute pain management in emergency department, low dose ketamine versus morphine, a randomized clinical trial. Anesthesiology and Pain Medicine. 2017;**7**(6):e60561. DOI: 10.5812/aapm.60561

[18] Miller JP, Schauer SG, Ganem VJ, Bebarta VS. Low-dose ketamine vs morphine for acute pain in the ED: A randomized controlled trial. The American Journal of Emergency Medicine. 2015;**33**(3):402-408. DOI: 10.1016/j.ajem.2014.12.058

[19] Jennings PA, Cameron P, Bernard S, Walker T, Jolley D, Fitzgerald M, et al. Morphine and ketamine is superior to morphine alone for out-of-hospital trauma analgesia: A randomized controlled trial. Annals of Emergency Medicine. 2012;**59**(6):497-503. DOI: 10.1016/j.annemergmed.2011.11.012

[20] Benov A, Salas M, Nakar H, et al. Battlefield pain management: A view of 17 years in Israel Defense Forces. Journal of Trauma and Acute Care Surgery. 2017;**83**(1 Suppl 1):S150-S155. DOI: 10.1097/TA.0000000000001481

[21] Galinski M, Dolveck F, Combes X, et al. Management of severe acute pain in emergency settings: Ketamine reduces morphine consumption. The American Journal of Emergency Medicine. 2007;**25**(4):385-390. DOI: 10.1016/j.ajem.2006.11.016

[22] Takieddine SC, Droege CA, Ernst N, Droege ME, Webb M, Branson RD, et al. Ketamine versus hydromorphone patient-controlled analgesia for acute pain in trauma patients. Journal of Surgical Research. 2018;**225**:6-14. DOI: 10.1016/j.jss.2017.12.019

[23] Pruskowski KA, Harbourt K, Pajoumand M, Chui SHJ, Reynolds HN. Impact of ketamine use on adjunctive analgesic and sedative medications in critically ill trauma patients. Pharmacotherapy: The Journal of Human Pharmacology and Drug Therapy. 2017;**37**(12):1537-1544. DOI: 10.1002/phar.2042

[24] Tran KP, Nguyen Q, Truong XN, Le V, Le VP, Mai N, et al. A comparison of ketamine and morphine analgesia in prehospital trauma care: A cluster randomized clinical trial in rural Quang Tri Province, Vietnam. Prehospital Emergency Care. 2014;**18**(2):257-264. DOI: 10.3109/10903127.2013.851307

[25] Bredmose PP, Lockey DJ, Grier G, et al. Pre-hospital use of ketamine for analgesia and procedural sedation. Emergency Medicine Journal. 2009;**26**:62-64

[26] Svenson JE, Abernathy MK. Ketamine for prehospital use: New look at an old drug. The American Journal of Emergency Medicine. 2007;**25**(8):977-980. DOI: 10.1016/j.ajem.2007.02.040

[27] Kugler NW, Carver TW, Juul J, Peppard WJ, Boyle K, Drescher KM, et al. Ketamine infusion for pain control in elderly patients with multiple rib fractures: Results of a randomized controlled trial. Journal of Trauma and Acute Care Surgery. 2019;**87**(5):1181-1188. DOI: 10.1097/TA.0000000000002479

[28] Upchurch CP, Grijalva CG, Russ S, Collins SP, Semler MW, Rice TW, et al. Comparison of etomidate and ketamine for induction during rapid sequence intubation of adult trauma patients. Annals of Emergency Medicine. 2017;**69**(1):24-33. DOI: 10.1016/j.annemergmed.2016.08.009. ISSN 0196-0644

[29] Baekgaard JS, Eskesen TG, Sillesen M, Rasmussen LS, Steinmetz J. Ketamine as a rapid sequence induction agent in the trauma population: A systematic review. Anesthesia & Analgesia. 2019;**128**(3):504-510. DOI: 10.1213/ANE.0000000000003568

[30] Stanke L, Nakajima S, Zimmerman LH, Collopy K, Fales C, Powers W IV. Hemodynamic effects of ketamine versus etomidate for prehospital rapid sequence intubation. Air Medical Journal. 2021;**40**(5):312-316. DOI: 10.1016/j.amj.2021.05.009

[31] Morris C, Perris A, Klein J, Mahoney P. Anaesthesia in haemodynamically compromised emergency patients: Does ketamine represent the best choice of induction agent? Anaesthesia. 2009;**64**(5):532-539. DOI: 10.1111/j.1365-2044.2008.05835

[32] Sari A, Okuda Y, Takeshita H. The effect of ketamine on cerebrospinal fluid pressure. Anesthesia and Analgesia. 1972;**51**:560-565

[33] Gardner AE, Olson BE, Lichtiger M. Cerebrospinal-fluid pressure during dissociative anesthesia with ketamine. Anesthesiology. 1971;**35**:226-228

[34] Tjaden RJ, Ethier R, Gilbert RG, et al. The use of CI-581 (Ketalar) for pediatric pneumoencephalography. Journal of the Canadian Association of Radiologists. 1969;**20**:155-156

[35] Evans J, Rosen M, Weeks RD, et al. Ketamine in neurosurgical procedures [letter]. Lancet. 1971;**1**:40

[36] Gibbs JM. The effect of intravenous ketamine on cerebrospinal fluid pressure. British Journal of Anaesthesia. 1972;**44**:1298-1302

[37] List WF, Crumrine RS, Cascorbi HF, et al. Increased cerebrospinal fluid pressure after ketamine. Anesthesiology. 1972;**36**:98-99

[38] Lockhart CH, Jenkins JJ. Ketamine induced apnea in patients with increased intracranial pressure. Anesthesiology. 1972;**37**:92-93

[39] Shapiro HM, Wyte SR, Harris AB. Ketamine anaesthesia in patients with intracranial pathology. British Journal of Anaesthesia. 1972;**44**:1200-1204

[40] Gregers MCT, Mikkelsen S, Lindvig KP, Brøchner AC. Ketamine as an anesthetic for patients with acute brain injury: A systematic review [published online ahead of print, 2020 Apr 23]. Neurocritical Care. 2020. DOI: 10.1007/s12028-020-00975-7

[41] Maas AI, Stocchetti N, Bullock R. Moderate and severe traumatic brain injury in adults. Lancet Neurology. 2008;**7**:728-741

[42] Petrica A, Ionac M, Brinzeu C, Brinzeu A. Surgical site infections surveillance in neurosurgery patients. Timisoara Medical Journal. 2009;**59**(3):339-343

[43] Godoy DA, Lubillo S, Rabinstein AA. Pathophysiology and management of intracranial hypertension and tissular brain hypoxia after severe traumatic brain injury: An integrative approach. Neurosurgery Clinics of North America. 2018;**29**:195-212

[44] Devlin JW, Skrobik Y, Gélinas C, et al. Clinical practice guidelines for the prevention and management of pain, agitation/sedation, delirium, immobility, and sleep disruption in

adult patients in the ICU. Critical Care Medicine. 2018;**46**:e825-e873

[45] Ciobanu D, Banicioiu-Covei M, Rotaru LT, Nica S, Petrica A, Puticiu M. Theoretical docking studies of anesthetic drugs interactions used in emergency departments. Journal of Science and Arts. 2020;**20**(2):419-424

[46] Dejeu IL, Vicaş LG, Jurca T, Fritea L, Svera P, Gabor GA, et al. Liposomes with caffeic acid: Morphological and structural characterisation, their properties and stability in time. PRO. 2021;**9**:912. DOI: 10.3390/pr9060912

[47] Huniadi A, Sorian A, Iuhas C, Bodog A, Sandor MI. The effect of cannabis in the treatment of Hodgkin's lymphoma in a pregnant patient—Extensive case report and literature review. Journal of BUON. 2021;**26**(1): 11-16

[48] Takeshita H, Okuda Y, Sari A. The effects of ketamine on cerebral circulation and metabolism in man. Anesthesiology. 1972;**36**:69-75

[49] Kolenda H, Gremmelt A, Rading S, Braun U, Markakis E. Ketamine for analgosedative therapy in intensive care treatment of head-injured patients. Acta Neurochirurgica (Wien). 1996;**138**:1193-1199

[50] Himmelseher S, Durieux ME. Revising a dogma: Ketamine for patients with neurological injury? Anesthesia and Analgesia. 2005;**101**:524-534

[51] Hurth KP, Jaworski A, Thomas KB, Kirsch WB, Rudoni MA, Wohlfarth KM. The reemergence of ketamine for treatment in critically ill adults. Critical Care Medicine. 2020;**48**:899-911

[52] Halstead SM, Deakyne SJ, Bajaj L, Enzenauer R, Roosevelt GE. The effect of ketamine on intraocular pressure in pediatric patients during procedural sedation. Academic Emergency Medicine. 2012;**19**(10):1145-1150. DOI: 10.1111/j.1553-2712.2012.01450.x

[53] Drayna PC, Estrada C, Wang W, Saville BR, Arnold DH. Ketamine sedation is not associated with clinically meaningful elevation of intraocular pressure. The American Journal of Emergency Medicine. 2012;**30**(7):1215-1218. DOI: 10.1016/j.ajem.2011.06.001

[54] Tactical Combat Casualty Care. TCCC Guidelines for Medical Personnel; 2019. Available from: https://www.naemt.org/docs/default-source/education-documents/tccc/tccc-mp-updates-190801/tccc-guidelines-for-medical-personnel-190801.pdf?sfvrsn=cc99d692_2 [Accessed: July 16, 2020]

[55] Green SM, Andolfatto G, Krauss BS. Ketamine and intracranial pressure: No contraindication except hydrocephalus. Annals of Emergency Medicine. 2015;**65**:52-54

[56] Morgan MM, Perina DG, Acquisto NM, Fallat ME, Gallagher JM, Brown KM, et al. Ketamine use in prehospital and hospital treatment of the acute trauma patient: A joint position statement. Prehospital Emergency Care. 2021;**25**(4):588-592. DOI: 10.1080/10903127.2020.1801920

[57] Butler FK, Kotwal RS, Buckenmaier CC, Edgar EP, O'Connor KC, Montgomery HR, et al. A triple-option analgesia plan for tactical combat casualty care: TCCC Guidelines Change 13-04. Journal of Special Operations Medicine. 2014;**14**(1):13-25

[58] Motov S, Mai M, Pushkar I, Likourezos A, Drapkin J, Yasavolian M, et al. A prospective randomized, double-dummy trial comparing IV push low dose ketamine to short infusion of low dose ketamine for treatment of pain in the ED. The American Journal of Emergency Medicine. 2017;**35**(8):1095-1100. DOI: 10.1016/j.ajem.2017.03.004

[59] Burnett AM, Peterson BK, Stellpflug SJ, Engebretsen KM, Glasrud KJ, Marks J, et al. The association between ketamine given for prehospital chemical restraint with intubation and hospital admission. The American Journal of Emergency Medicine. 2015;**33**(1):76-79. DOI: 10.1016/j.ajem.2014.10.016

[60] Hollis GJ, Keene TM, Ardlie RM, Caldicott DG, Stapleton SG. Prehospital ketamine use by paramedics in the Australian Capital Territory: A 12 month retrospective analysis. Emergency Medicine Australasia. 2017;**29**(1):89-95. DOI: 10.1111/1742-6723.12685

[61] Guldner GT, Petinaux B, Clemens P, Foster S, Antoine S. Ketamine for procedural sedation and analgesia by nonanesthesiologists in the field: A review for military health care providers. Military Medicine. 2006;**171**(6):484-490. DOI: 10.7205/milmed.171.6.484

[62] Bumbu A, Nacer K, Bratu O, Berechet M, Bumbu G, Bumbu B. Ureteral lesions in gynecological pathology. In: Proceedings of the 14th National Congress of Urogynecology and the National Conference of the Romanian Association for the Study of Pain, Bucharest, Romania. 2017. pp. 26-27

[63] Lebin JA, Akhavan AR, Hippe DS, Gittinger MH, Pasic J, McCoy AM, et al. Psychiatric outcomes of patients with severe agitation following administration of prehospital ketamine. Academic Emergency Medicine. 2019;**26**(8):889-896

[64] Kudoh A, Katagai H, Takazawa T. Anesthesia with ketamine, propofol, and fentanyl decreases the frequency of postoperative psychosis emergence and confusion in schizophrenic patients. Journal of Clinical Anesthesia. 2002;**14**(2):107-110. DOI: 10.1016/S0952-8180(01)00363-4

[65] Botea M. In: Waisundara VY, Banjari I, Balkić J, editors. Analgesics, Pain Management—Practices, Novel Therapies and Bioactives. London: IntechOpen; 2020. DOI: 10.5772/intechopen.94319. Available from: https://www.intechopen.com/chapters/73965

[66] De Rocquigny G, Dubecq C, Martinez T, Peffer J, Cauet A, Travers S, et al. Use of ketamine for prehospital pain control on the battlefield: A systematic review. Journal of Trauma and Acute Care Surgery. 2020;**88**(1):180-185. DOI: 10.1097/TA.0000000000002522

Chapter 17

Ketamine and Low-Resource Countries

Chimaobi Tim Nnaji

Abstract

Safe anaesthesia and surgery are piloted to reduce the morbidity and mortality associated with anaesthesia and surgery, and improve surgical outcomes. This goal is far-fetched in developing countries as a result of limited manpower, poor operation theatre infrastructure, unavailability of equipment, life-saving drugs, and anaesthetic agents. Postoperative pain is also widely undertreated in this environment, mostly due to financial constraints patients and their relatives face and the unavailability of analgesics. Sometimes the physicians face problems associated with their resource-limited working environment, such as unreliable electricity, unavailability of compressed oxygen and other gases, sophisticated machines, and modern drugs. Thus, easy adaptability and proper utilisation of available resources have been described as a resounding quality required of anaesthetists working in developing countries, to thrive and provide anaesthetic services. Ketamine is readily available in resource-limited environments, and adaptability to the use of this drug has made it possible for the anaesthetist to provide anaesthesia, pain care services, sedation, and save lives.

Keywords: anaesthesia, low-resource country, ketamine anaesthesia

1. Introduction

Anaesthesia practice remains a challenge in the developing and low-resource or income countries of the world, particularly in Sub-Saharan Africa where the growing population and the need for surgical and anaesthesia intervention are overwhelming the insufficient number of trained anaesthesia personnel and available resources [1]. This has been described by some clinicians as problems associated with human, technical, investment, and educational resources [1, 2]. Anaesthesia service delivery has also been negatively affected by poor operation theatre infrastructure, unavailability of equipment, lifesaving drugs, and anaesthetic agents, inadequate clean water supply, transportation, electricity, oxygen, and blood banks services [2]. Thus, easy adaptability and proper utilisation of the available resource remains the keyway to delivering safe anaesthesia services in the low-resource countries. The regular use of a cheap, safe, and accessible drug called "ketamine" in clinical practice in the resource-limited countries has become overwhelming, as a result of the unavailability of anaesthesia equipment, oxygen, lifesaving drugs, and anaesthetic agents. A drug that is frequently described as a "unique drug" because it shows hypnotic, analgesic, and anterograde amnesic effects [3].

Ketamine is used in the operating room during induction and maintenance of hypnosis, with its analgesic property being beneficial for intraoperative and early

IntechOpen

postoperative analgesia. Its place in procedural sedation and total intravenous anaesthesia is insurmountable. Ketamine is used as an adjuvant together with other drugs during peripheral nerve blocks and neuraxial blocks to prolong the duration of analgesia provided by these techniques of anaesthesia [3].

Developing countries and low-income/resource countries are often used interchangeably. A developing country is a nation with a less developed industrial base and a low Human Development Index (HDI) relative to other countries. The term low-income country is often used to refer only to the economy of the country. The World Bank classifies the world's economies into four groups, based on Gross National Income (GNI) per capita, and these are high, upper-middle, lower-middle, and low-incomes countries. Low-income countries have a GNI per capita of less than 1026 United State dollars [4, 5]. More than 2 billion of the world's population reside in low- and middle-income countries. In most of these areas, the healthcare systems suffer from issues that involve institutional, human resources, financial, technical, and political developments. The provision of emergency, essential surgical care, and anaesthesia are quite limited. This area of the world has not been able to meet up with the World Health Organization (WHO) 2007 proposed framework of healthcare systems. World Health Organization proposed that, for a country to have an effective healthcare structure, components, such as service delivery, healthcare workforce, healthcare information systems, medicines and technologies, financing, and leadership/governance must be met. Poor governance, funding, and human resource challenges are linked to ineffective integration of services in resource-limited nations [6].

The clinical role of ketamine in providing anaesthesia in low-income countries with inadequate healthcare infrastructure and equipment has been demonstrated. Despite health care being identified as a strategic priority, relatively little information has been established about the capacity of the health system in low-income countries to deliver essential and safe surgical and anaesthesia services. In many rural hospitals in developing countries, patients undergo surgical procedures on room air or rarely with the delivery of oxygen from the oxygen concentrator. The anaesthesia providers keep the patients' airway open by simply positioning, chin lift, and jaw thrust. The airway is suctioned by the use of mucus extractors, rubber bulb suction devices, and rarely with foot-pedal manually operated suction machines as a result of lack of electricity. An improvised precordial stethoscope becomes vital in monitoring a patient's breath sounds, heart rate, and volume. Many of these hospitals do not have anaesthesia machines and the ability to provide inhaled anaesthesia, thus, in such situations, ketamine becomes a lifesaver [3, 7, 8].

2. Anaesthesia practice in low-resource countries

In the years 2000 and 2007, Hodges and co-workers described the state of anaesthesia delivery in low-resource and Sub-Saharan African countries as inadequate, with emphasis that in the twenty-first century, millions of people in this area of the world may not have access to safe anaesthesia and pain relief during surgery and childbirth, which are considered as a basic human right. This is not different from another report by Adamu and co-workers in 2010, which noted the increasing difficulty with the preparation of patients for emergency surgery and getting them to surgical theatre within an acceptable time in limited-resource countries. The delays were related to the constraints in poor health institutional organisation and the socio-economic status of the patients. Thus, a significant portion of the patients waits too long for emergency surgery at the expense of perioperative morbidity and mortality [1, 9, 10].

An estimation of 234 million surgeries is performed every year to alleviate some disabilities and reduce the risk of death from some common medical conditions, and this is achieved with the help of anaesthesia. However, access to safe surgery has been suggested to be 3.5% in the world third poorest countries. An epidemiological study reported that 30% of the world's population lack access to safe surgery, as well as safe anaesthesia. In most areas of Sub-Saharan Africa, government hospitals provide few supplies for resuscitation, anaesthesia, and surgery, making patients pay out of their pockets or provide materials for their surgical and anaesthesia care. Sometimes, delays in the procurement of these resources and materials often lead to delayed surgical and anaesthesia intervention, with the poor perioperative outcome. Ketamine has been shown to be safe and effective for a wide range of surgical procedures and its suitable in many clinical situations because of its safety profile [8, 11, 12].

The quality and type of anaesthesia services provided during surgery are highly related to perioperative outcomes. Nevertheless, this can be affected by the level of training of the medical personnel, the availability of surgical theatre infrastructure and resources, anaesthesia drugs, unreliable electricity, unavailability of compressed oxygen and other gases, anaesthesia machines, and modern drugs—a problem common with low-income countries. Thus, physician anaesthetists in this environment have learned to adapt and utilise any available resources to provide safe anaesthetic services and save lives. The use of ketamine as the sole anaesthetic agent has been in clinical use for a long period of time and it has been found to be beneficial and cost-effective. Ketamine has a place in the management of acute pain through intraoperative low-dose infusion, even in opioid-tolerant patients. It has likewise been used in low-resource countries after surgery with minimal psycho-mimetic effects [3, 8].

3. Ketamine anaesthesia in low-resource countries

Ketamine has gained lots of credit in surgical practice in low-resource countries. It has also been demonstrated to be vital in global healthcare practice too. Limited resource countries rely heavily on ketamine as a sole anaesthetic agent in the face of the growing need for surgical services. The global burden of diseases preventable by surgery is on the rise and is expected to surpass those of human immunodeficiency virus, tuberculosis, and malaria by 2026. Ketamine has been shown to be the most widely used and safest anaesthetic drug, as reflected by being 'always available' according to 92% of anaesthetists surveyed in Uganda [1, 13].

The clinical administration of ketamine has been shown to be very effective in a wide range of surgical procedures, even amongst all age groups. Ketamine can be administered conveniently through different routes. The intravenous route offers the optimal channel of administration, but sometimes it's difficult to achieve in emergencies, children, and obese patients. Ketamine can be administered efficiently through the intraosseous and intramuscular routes. The intramuscular administration of ketamine during anaesthesia, is associated with a longer recovery time. The oral administration of ketamine has also been documented, even with its mixture with soda to enhance the oral administration, however, this route has a reduced bioavailability [14–16].

Ketamine anaesthesia provides analgesia, amnesia, immobility, and loss of consciousness. It has been found to have a wide margin of safety when compared with other general anaesthetic agents. In addition, its sympathomimetic effects provide hemodynamic stability, which is beneficial in critically ill and hemodynamically unstable patients. Furthermore, the use of ketamine in pain medicine (multimodal analgesia, chronic pain, and palliative care), critical care (status epilepticus), emergency medicine, and psychiatry (depression) in developing countries with a shortage of trained personnel could not be overemphasised [3, 7, 8]. Nevertheless, the administration of ketamine is associated with some side effects. It causes dissociative anaesthesia, which alters the sensory perceptions of the patients. It can increase the incidence of postoperative nausea and vomiting, cause transient apnoea especially when administered rapidly, and increases salivary secretions, which may increase the incidence of laryngospasm. The increased salivation can be minimised by co-administration of atropine. Ketamine has been found to provoke imaginative, dissociative states and psychotic symptoms due to its NMDA-antagonistic action, as well as severely impair semantic and episodic memory. It

Author	Objective	Country	Variables	Discussion	Conclusion
Hodges et al. [1]	Assessment of anaesthesia facilities in different units.	Uganda	Availability of ketamine	Ketamine is always available in 92% of the period	Identification of shortages of personnel, drugs, equipment, and anaesthesia training in Uganda
Vo et al. [13]	Use of ketamine as an anaesthetic compared with basic anaesthetic infrastructure and equipment at facilities in 22 low- and middle-income countries.	Low- and middle-income countries	Ketamine anaesthesia	Current ketamine use exceeds the availability of other anaesthetic options.	Restrictions on ketamine need to consider the larger impact on the global burden of surgical diseases where ketamine is vital in the care of surgical patients.
Olasinde et al. [19]	To highlight the experience from a specialist hospital in south-western Nigeria	Nigeria (South-West)	Ketamine anaesthesia	52% ketamine utilisation	Ketamine and local infiltration with lidocaine are commonly used in this environment.
Ikechebelu et al. [20]	A retrospective review of 295 cases of laparoscopy over 28 months in a fertility unit.	Nigeria (South-East)	Ketamine is used by an untrained healthcare personnel	Ketamine uses for laparoscopic procedures	Ketamine produces a safe, effective and simple general anaesthesia and is recommended for use in day-case laparoscopy
Elusoji et al. [21]	To evaluate the efficacy and safety of ketamine hydrochloride anaesthesia without endotracheal intubation in thyroidectomy.	Nigeria	Ketamine anaesthesia	Ketamine uses for thyroidectomy	Ketamine anaesthesia is safe and economical for thyroidectomy.

Author	Objective	Country	Variables	Discussion	Conclusion
Lonnée et al. [22]	To assess the type of anaesthesia used for caesarean delivery, the level of training of anaesthesia providers, and to document the availability of essential aesthetic drugs and equipment.	Zimbabwe	Rural setting	100% ketamine utilisation. Shortage of essential drugs for anaesthesia, inconsistent use of recovery area, and insufficient blood supplies.	Training of medical officers and nurse anaesthetists should be strengthened in leadership, teamwork, and management of complications.
Nuhu et al. [23]	Evaluation of workforce situation and availability of anaesthetic drugs/ equipment in public secondary health facilities.	Nigeria (North-Central)	Ketamine anaesthesia	100% utilisation	There is a dearth of aesthetic and surgical workforce and basic infrastructure in public hospitals.
Masaki et al. [24]	To assess the feasibility and safety of ketamine in support of obstetric and gynaecologic surgeries in severely resource-scarce settings when there is no available anaesthetist.	Kenya	Ketamine anaesthesia	Improved provider's competency due to ketamine raining	Ketamine is safe for use in support of emergency and essential obstetric and gynaecologic surgeries in extremely resource-limited settings when no anaesthetist is available.
Makin et al. [25]	To gain surgeons' perceptions on performing operations supported by ketamine and to recommend best practices and techniques.	Low-income countries.	Ketamine is used amongst surgeons	Global standards on ketamine training and use should be established.	Ketamine is safe, can provide increased access to emergency and essential surgery, and requires few operative technical changes.
Koka et al. [26]	To describe the anaesthesia practice at two tertiary hospitals	Sierra Leone	Ketamine anaesthesia	Utilisation rate of 44.7%	Gaps in the application of internationally recommended anaesthesia practices at both hospitals are caused by a lack of resources.

Table 1.
Summary of ketamine in low-resource countries.

can also cause various emergent phenomena when the patient is awakening from anaesthesia. This has been described as a floating sensation, vivid pleasant dreams, nightmares, hallucinations, and delirium [17, 18].

Most clinicians and nurses involved in anaesthesia service providers understand that they must add benzodiazepines, such as diazepam or midazolam, to combat the hallucinatory effects of ketamine and the emergence phenomenon. Nevertheless, diazepam is readily available and cheap in low-resource countries, thus, ketamine in combination with atropine and diazepam forms a reliable regimen for the conduct of total intravenous general anaesthesia for different modalities of surgery, with room air and minimal equipment [1, 17].

The use of intravenous ketamine at the induction dose of 2 mg/kg in adults or 1 mg/kg in children, followed by an increment of 1–1.5 mg/kg for maintenance of the anaesthesia. While the patients were pre-medicated with intravenous atropine 0.6 mg in adults and 0.3 mg in children plus diazepam 10 mg in adults and 0.45 mg/kg in children was documented in a study conducted in Nigeria, that had the incidence of general anaesthesia with intravenous ketamine of 58.4%. This study involved different varieties of surgeries, such as intra-abdominal operations (herniorrhaphies and herniotomies), perineal, pelvic, and genital surgeries, as well as extremities, chest, head, and neck surgeries. A retrospective study reviewed 295 cases of laparoscopy that were performed over the period of 28 months at a fertility healthcare facility in Nigeria that does not have an anaesthesia machine or trained anaesthesia personnel. They showed that the regimen of atropine-ketamine-diazepam general anaesthesia was safely used for all the patients that had day-case laparoscopy. Elusoji and colleagues also reported the safety of using ketamine anaesthesia in combination with diazepam in 55 patients that had a thyroidectomy in a low-resource country. They reported complications, such as hallucination and postoperative restlessness, which were managed with intravenous diazepam, chlorpromazine, or paraldehyde (**Table 1**) [19–21].

4. Anaesthesia service adaptations

4.1 Anaesthesia providers

Anaesthesia is an essential part of healthcare services. In developed countries and some of developing countries, anaesthesia is not merely limited to the operating room, but the services also involve the emergency room, intensive care unit, angiography-catheterisation laboratory, magnetic resonance imaging suite, pain clinics, resuscitative rooms, electroconvulsive therapy room, and other life-saving hospital services. These services require the skill of trained anaesthesia providers, however, in most low-resource countries, there are still no strategic measures for assessing the safe anaesthesia services, particularly in rural areas because of the shortage of anaesthesia personnel. In most of these areas, the health care system is usually overburdened by patients load with limited or no anaesthesia provider.

The number of physician anaesthetists in most low-resource countries is below what is needed to provide a safe and quality anaesthesia service. A study conducted by Davies and co-workers recommended a minimum of four physician anaesthetists per 100,000 population for the provision of reasonable, safe, and standard anaesthesia care for surgical interventions. However, this figure is far-fetched in developing countries with steaming and growing populations [27]. World Federation Societies of Anaesthesiologists (WFSA) workforce survey that was based on the 2015 world population estimated that to achieve a minimum density of 1 per 100,000 physician anaesthetists in all countries, over 8000 additional physician anaesthetists would be required. While over 136,000 additional physician anaesthetists would be required worldwide to achieve 5 per 100,000. Nevertheless, the majority of the countries in Sub-Saharan Africa and some in Asia have a physician anaesthetists density of <1 per 100,000 population [28].

Anaesthesia professionals, especially in Sub-Saharan Africa, are often poorly remunerated, supported and undervalued. The recruitment process of healthcare personnel often neglects the anaesthesia providers, thus resulting in shortages of anaesthesia physician and their allied personnel, such as nurse anaesthetist, anaesthesia technicians, and anaesthesia attendants. In some low-resource countries, some of the anaesthesia physician support staff are not included and are sometimes poorly placed in the civil service, making it difficult for them to be remunerated. Ho et al. reported in 2019 that 30.4% of the 344 medical facilities they surveyed had no anaesthesia provider at any level (physicians, nurses, or technicians) accessible for patient care [29]. In most low-income countries, anaesthesia services are often provided by unqualified physician personnel, nurse anaesthetists, or anaesthesia technicians who are trained by physician anaesthetists, to use anaesthesia resources to provide safe anaesthesia services. This day-to-day reality of shortage of physician anaesthetists in the operating room coupled with a lack of resources, persuades the available anaesthesia providers to use simple and effective techniques that are not too expensive and readily available.

The properties of ketamine anaesthesia, such as analgesia, amnesia, immobility, and loss of consciousness make it the technique of choice, alongside local and spinal anaesthesia in low-resource countries. In a study reported in the Democratic Republic of Congo, 771 patients had general anaesthesia with ketamine in an operating room that had no physician or nurse anaesthetist, but untrained personnel. They reported that most of their patients were females (85.86%) and 97.4% of the patients who had surgery were classified as ASA II and the intermediate surgical risk was more represented in 82.9%. The adverse event they noted were arterial hypertension (10.2%), salivation (5.5%), respiratory distress (4.8%), agitation on awakening (30.8%), and hallucinations (22.6%), respectively. They did not record any mortality. Indicating ketamine is safe and effective, even in regions where anaesthesia is conducted by untrained anaesthesia personnel [30].

Anaesthesia in Zambia, a low-resource country, is under-developed and under-resourced. The anaesthesia specialty is focused almost exclusively on intraoperative patient care. In small hospitals and hospitals in rural areas, there is lack adequate staffing. A study conducted in this country showed that 80% of anaesthesia cases were performed by non-physicians with little or no formal training in anaesthesia. The reliance of the anaesthesia providers on ketamine is a result of inadequate training, inexperience with, and access to, more advanced equipment like laryngoscope and materials like endotracheal tubes. A limited number of anaesthetists have almost no involvement in emergency medicine and pain therapy [31].

4.2 Shortage of modern drugs and anaesthesia agents

In most areas of developing countries, a shortage of essential drugs used in anaesthesia practice is a common problem. Thus, the anaesthesia providers engage in the use of simple and effective techniques that are not expensive, but readily available. The properties of ketamine make the drug a product of choice, for simplified general anaesthesia like total intravenous anaesthesia, alongside its use as an additive to prolong the analgesic effect of local and neuraxial anaesthesia. In well-equipped health institutions with trained anaesthesia personnel, inhalation anaesthesia is normally the first choice of maintaining hypnosis during anaesthesia; however, ketamine has proved to be useful in settings without recovery facilities, as well as trained anaesthesia providers and in areas where patients need to wake up in their own beds in the various wards, especially in low-income and middle-income countries, and in emergency situations [1, 32]. Ketamine anaesthesia was found to predominate other techniques or modes of anaesthesia in most hospitals evaluated (72.9%), whereas inhalational anaesthesia was only available in 56.2% of the hospitals. Also, techniques of anaesthesia like regional and spinal anaesthesia, were available in 58.9 and 65.9% of hospitals, respectively studied [28].

A study published in Uganda in 2007 stated that drugs used for the conduct of anaesthesia are usually limited in supply. The availability of narcotics is 45%, nondepolarizing muscle relaxants 15%, inhalational agents 38%, and intravenous induction agents 59% [1]. In another study done by Khan in Pakistan, he reported that there is a non-availability of some essential drugs, such as narcotics, inhalational agents, induction agents, and some vasoactive drugs in Pakistan [33].

There are several factors that contribute to the anaesthesia drug shortages, some of them are common in both high-income and low-income countries. For example, regulatory issues, manufacturing problems, raw material acquisition problems, business decisions based upon the profitability of some drugs, and disturbances or faults in the supply chain. The factors that affect low-income countries alone include issues of licensing by healthcare regulatory authorities, imports from abroad, shortage of ingredients for local manufacture, government policies, and drug smuggling to other countries. The implication of anaesthesia drug shortage is that it can result in the cancellation of surgery which may be psychologically traumatic to both patients and their families. The economic implication for both patients and hospitals are incurred from prolongation of hospital stay and higher risk of exposure to hospital-acquired infections [34, 35].

4.3 Shortage of anaesthesia vapours and compressed gases

The anaesthesia gas supply system is designed to provide a safe, cost-effective and convenient system for the delivery of medical gases at the point of use in the hospital. The medical gases used in anaesthesia and intensive care medicine are oxygen, nitrous oxide, medical air, Entonox, carbon dioxide, and heliox. Oxygen is one of the most widely used gases for life-support and respiratory therapy besides anaesthetic procedures. There is a lack of adequate supply of oxygen in most of low-resource countries. In a recent survey of anaesthetic care in 22 low- and middle-income countries, uninterrupted access to oxygen was available in only 46% of the healthcare facilities, while 35% reported no access to oxygen. Ketamine can be administered through various routes and it does not require the availability of oxygen, electricity, anaesthetic equipment, or trained anaesthesia providers, all of which remain scarce in low-resource countries. Hence, ketamine is the most widely used and safest anaesthetic drug in resource-limited environments [13].

5. Conclusion

Ketamine is an example of how an old drug can still be renowned in the practice of medicine. It has been recognised as the sole anaesthetic/analgesic of choice in areas with low resources. Ketamine administration does not require costly equipment or appropriately trained physician anaesthetists, and it is cheap, readily available, and safe, Ketamine is effective in a wide range of surgical procedures, including short painful, long complex, and day-case procedures. The use of ketamine in low-resource countries has enhanced safe anaesthesia and surgical care, thus reducing perioperative morbidity and mortality, as well as improving surgical outcomes. The regular use of this cheap, safe, and accessible drug called "ketamine" in clinical practice in resource-limited countries has become overwhelming, despite the dwindling number of trained anaesthesia providers.

Acknowledgements

I want to express my gratitude to God Almighty, for granting me the knowledge and wisdom to contribute a chapter to this book. Also, for helping me to find my ground in human capacity building in Anaesthesia.

Conflict of interest

The author declares no conflict of interest.

Author details

Chimaobi Tim Nnaji
Department of Anaesthesia, Federal Medical Centre Owerri,
Owerri, Imo State, Nigeria

*Address all correspondence to: chymaoby@yahoo.com

References

[1] Hodges SC, Mijumbi C, Okello M, et al. Anaesthesia services in developing countries: Defining the problems. Anesthesia. 2007;**62**:4-11

[2] Nnaji CT, Chikwe K. Anesthesia for abdominal myomectomy: A five years audit of a Federal Medical Centre in Owerri, Nigeria. Journal of Anesthesia. 2017;**1**(1):16-19

[3] Mei Gao M, Rejaei D, Liu H. Ketamine use in current clinical practice. Acta Pharmacologica Sinica. 2016;**37**:865-872

[4] O'Sullivan A, Sheffrin SM. Economics: Principles in Action. Upper Saddle River: Pearson Prentice Hall; 2003. p. 471

[5] World Economic Outlook (PDF). 2018. pp. 134-135 [Retrieved: 31 October 2018]

[6] WHO. Everybody's Business: Strengthening Health Systems to Improve Health Outcomes. WHO's Framework for Action. Geneva: World Health Organization; 2007

[7] Aroni F, Iacovidou N, Dontas I, Pourzitaki C, Xanthos T. Pharmacological aspects and potential new clinical applications of ketamine: Reevaluation of an old drug. Journal of Clinical Pharmacology. 2009;**49**: 957-964

[8] Joshi GP, Onajin-Obembe B. The role of ketamine in low- and middle-income countries: What would happen if ketamine becomes a scheduled drug? Anesthesia & Analgesia. 2016;**122**(3):908-910

[9] Hodges SC, Hodges AM. A protocol for safe anaesthesia for cleft lip and palate surgery in developing countries. Anaesthesia. 2000;**55**:436-441

[10] Adamu A, Maigatari M, Lawal K, Iliyasu M. Waiting time for emergency abdominal surgery in Zaria, Nigeria. African Health Sciences. 2010;**10**(1):46-53

[11] Weiser TG, Regenbogen SE, Thompson KD, Haynes AB, Lipsitz SR, Berry WR, et al. An estimation of the global volume of surgery: A modelling strategy based on available data. The Lancet. 2008;**372**(9633):139-144

[12] Funk LM, Weiser TG, Berry WR, Lipsitz SR, Merry AF, Enright AC, et al. Global operating theatre distribution and pulse oximetry supply: An estimation from reported data. The Lancet. 2010;**376**(9746):1055-1061

[13] Vo D, Cherian MN, Bianchi S, et al. Anesthesia capacity in 22 low- and middle-income countries. Journal of Anesthesia and Clinical Research. 2012;**3**:207

[14] Helm M, Hossfeld B, Schlechtriemen T, Braun J, Lampl L, Bernhard M. Use of intraosseous infusion in the German air rescue service: Nationwide analysis in the time period 2005 to 2009. Anaesthesist. 2011;**60**:1119-1125

[15] Green SM, Roback MG, Kennedy RM, Krauss B. Clinical practice guideline for emergency department ketamine dissociative sedation: 2011 update. Annals of Emergency Medicine. 2011;**57**:449-461

[16] Heidari SM, Saghaei M, Hashemi SJ, Parvazinia P. Effect of oral ketamine on the postoperative pain and analgesic requirement following orthopedic surgery. Acta Anaesthesiologica Taiwanica. 2006;**44**:211-215

[17] Ogboli-Nwasor E, Amaefule KE, Audu SS. Use of oral ketamine for analgesia during reduction/

manipulation of fracture/dislocation in the emergency room: An initial experience in a low-resource setting. Pain Studies and Treatment. 2014;**2**:17-20

[18] Song JW, Shim JK, Song Y, Yang SY, Park SJ, Kwak YL. Effect of ketamine as an adjunct to intravenous patient-controlled analgesia, in patients at high risk of postoperative nausea and vomiting undergoing lumbar spinal surgery. British Journal of Anaesthesia. 2013;**111**:630-635

[19] Olasinde AA, Oluwadiya KS. Anaesthesia practice in a hospital, developing countries: An 18 month's experience. Internet Journal of Third World Medicine. 2005;**3**:1-4

[20] Ikechebelu JI, Udigwe GO, Obi RA, Joe-Ikechebelu NN, Okoye IC. The use of simple ketamine anaesthesia for day-case diagnostic laparoscopy. Journal of Obstetrics and Gynaecology. 2003;**23**:650-652

[21] Elusoji SO, Iribhogbe PE, Osime OC. Thyroidectomy under ketamine anaesthesia in a semi urban hospital in Nigeria. Pakistan Journal of Medical Sciences. 2009;**25**(4):695-697

[22] Lonnée HA, Madzimbamuto F, Erlandsen ORM, Vassenden A, et al. Anesthesia for cesarean delivery: A cross-sectional survey of provincial, district, and mission hospitals in Zimbabwe. Anesthesia & Analgesia. 2018;**126**(6):2056-2064. DOI: 10.1213/ANE.0000000000002733

[23] Nuhu SI, Embu HY, Onoja AA, Dung D. Anaesthesia workforce and infrastructure in a north central state of Nigeria: A survey. Highland Medical Research Journal. 2017;**17**(1):50-54

[24] Masaki CO, Makin J, Suarez S, Wuyke G, et al. Feasibility of a ketamine anesthesia package in support of obstetric and gynecologic procedures in Kenya when no anesthetist is available. African Journal of Reproductive Health. 2019;**23**(1):37-45

[25] Makin J, Suarez-Rebling D, Suarez S, et al. Operations supported by ketamine anesthesia in resource-limited settings: Surgeons' perceptions and recommendations e qualitative study. International Journal of Surgery Open. 2021;**29**:1-8

[26] Koka R, Chima AM, Sampson JB, et al. Anesthesia practice and perioperative outcomes at two tertiary care hospitals in Freetown, Sierra Leone. Anesthesia & Analgesia. 2016;**123**:213-227

[27] Davies JI, Vreede E, Onajin-Obembe B, et al. What is the minimum number of specialist anaesthetists needed in low-income and middle-income countries? BMJ Global Health. 2018;**3**:e001005

[28] Kempthorne P, Morriss WW, Mellin-Olsen J, et al. The WFSA global anesthesia workforce survey. Anesthesia & Analgesia. 2017;**125**:981-990

[29] Ho M, Livingston P, Bould MD, et al. Barriers and facilitators to implementing a regional anesthesia service in a low-income country: A qualitative study. The Pan African Medical Journal. 2019;**32**:152. DOI: 10.11604/pamj.2019.32.152.17246

[30] Ketha JK, Ilumbulumbu MK, Valimungighe MM, Nzanzu BPF, Bekaert P, et al. Use of ketamine in rural area at the East of the Democratic Republic of the Congo (DRC). Journal of Anesthesia and Clinical Research. 2019;**10**(6):1000895

[31] Jochberger S, Ismailova F, Lederer W, Mayr VD, Luckner G, Wenzel V, et al. "Helfen Berührt" Study Team. Anesthesia and its allied disciplines in the developing world: A nationwide survey of the Republic of Zambia. Anesthesia & Analgesia. 2008;**106**:942-948

[32] Dobson M, Blockmans D, King M, Joy JS. Anaesthesia at rural hospital, office of studies and research for health promotion, mediaspaul, Kinshasa. 2010. p. 192

[33] Khan TH. Availability of essential drugs in Pakistan (Editorial). Anaesthesia, Pain & Intensive Care. 2009;**13**:1-3

[34] ASHP Expert Panel on Drug Product Shortages, Fox ER, Birt A, James KB, Kokko H, Salverson S, et al. ASHP guidelines on managing drug product shortages in hospitals and health. American Journal of Health-System Pharmacy. 2009;**66**:1399-1406

[35] Atif M, Malik I, Mushtaq I, Asghar S. Medicine shortages in Pakistan. A qualitative study to explore current situation, reasons and possible solutions to overcome the barriers. BMJ Open. 2019;**9**:e027028

Chapter 18

An Update of Ketamine Illicit Use

Patrycja Kleczkowska and Malgorzata Zaremba

Abstract

Ketamine is a derivative of phencyclidine with unique anesthetic, analgesic, as well as antidepressant pharmacological properties. Despite its clinical use, ketamine is classified on the list with new psychoactive substances having psychedelic properties. The abuse trend of ketamine increasing globally, and it became a common club drug over the past few decades. Of note, recreational use of ketamine may pose a threat to public health, leading to numerous physical, as well as psychiatric negative effects. In addition, simultaneously or sequentially ketamine use with other drugs, resulting in serious health consequences. Currently, there are no specific treatment options for managing compulsive drug-seeking behavior in patients with ketamine use disorder, while the pharmacotherapy of side effects is limited and mostly symptomatic. In this chapter, we discuss ketamine abuse history. Further, we proposed the mechanisms of neural disinhibition underlying addiction development in ketamine-dependent patients. We have also included details of possible negative consequences focusing on long-term and recreational ketamine use for both, central and peripheral systems. Finally, we provide an overview of ketamine concomitant use and corresponding adverse interactions.

Keywords: ketamine, abuse, club drug, k-hole, k-cramps, ketamine bladder

1. Introduction

Ketamine has long been known as a potent anesthetic drug with analgesic properties, however, it quickly evolved into a recreational drug in the early 1980s [1]. The first use of ketamine as a drug was recorded in 1965 [2]. Widespread, nonmedical uses of ketamine expanded through that time due to sub-cultures began experimented with the drug for mind exploration the inner psyche, and New Age spiritualism.

Ketamine is also known as the 'club drug' and since the mid-1980s, it has been linked to a variety of dance cultures, because of its trance-like state potency. That also explained why teenagers and young adults (16 to 25 years) are the people who are most susceptible to ketamine abuse. Ketamine is known by various names, by clubbers usually called "K", "vitamin K", "super K", or "special K" [3, 4]. In the United States of America as well as in the United Kingdom ketamine was used as an adulterant in methylenedioxy-methamphetamine (MDMA) under the name of "horse pill" [5].

The typical ketamine users are regular visitors of the electronic dance music scene [6]; psychonauts; injecting heroin users, and the 'gay' club/party scene [7]. In addition, according to the data from the Crime Survey for England and Wales (CSEW) for 2012/2013, it is usually single male, aged 20–24, unemployed or studying, and from Chinese or mixed-race ethnic roots [8].

The most important reasons for ketamine's recreational use are as follows: short time to effect; duration of action (up to 3 h), as well as low cost. Ketamine was gained popularity as a party drug due to the appearance of powerful psychoactive effects even at low, subanesthetic (0.1–0.5 mg/kg) doses [9]. As a dissociative anesthetic, ketamine and other drugs such as phencyclidine (PCP) or dextromethorphan (DXM), distort the user's perception of sight and sound, while producing illusions of detachment from the environment or body, known as a „falling into a K-hole" (near-death experience). This state is also associated with the lack of the ability to speak and move around easily, not accompanied by actual loss of consciousness [10]. It is considered that; ketamine had the highest degree of out-of-body experiences among any other drugs, like a bad LSD trip. While not all ketamine users had out-of-body experiences, less than 10% of subjects experience this phenomenon regularly [11]. Of note, these symptoms can be prolonged and even create psychosis associated with schizophrenic and other psychotic disorders. In fact, ketamine has been used experimentally to develop a 'ketamine model' of psychosis [12, 13].

Additionally, hallucinations, emotional withdrawal, and "melting into the surrounding" may occur. It is also very likely for users (at very high doses of ketamine or those combining ketamine with alcohol or other drugs) to experience numbness, amnesia, more intense dissociations, and delirium [14].

Ketamine's ability to induce confusion, amnesia and alter some of the perceptual effects make this drug a so-called "date rape drug". For this reason, ketamine was included in the Drug-Induced Rape Prevention Act of 1966 [15]. Unfortunately, some of the symptoms and side-effects are long-lasting (i.e., impairment to episodic and possibly attentional functioning). Although semantic memory impairments are thought to be reversible as a consequence of ketamine cessation or substantial reduction of its use [9, 16].

2. Epidemiology of ketamine illicit use

The recreational use of ketamine has climbed over decades in the UK [17, 18], Australia [7], Southeast Asian countries such as Taiwan, Malaysia, and China, particularly such phenomenon was reported among the youth and adolescents [19–22]. It could be, in part, due to ketamine's lower status in regulatory systems and lower price, compared to still expensive "ecstasy" or methamphetamine. In Hong Kong, where ketamine was classified as a Schedule I drug since 2000, ketamine became the most commonly misused drug in the early 2000s [21].

The abuse of ketamine has been declining over the past years but is still relatively common. According to the national survey-based 'Monitoring the Future Study' in the United States ketamine ingestion decreased between 2002 and 2012 from 2.5% to 1.5%, and from 1.3% to 0.4%, among 12th graders and college students, respectively [23].

The decreasing ketamine popularity was also noticed in the United Kingdom (UK), where it has been classified on the list as a Class C drug since 2006 [21], and then was reclassified as a Class B drug from 10 June 2014 [24]. The World Health Organization fact file has demonstrated the ketamine usage in the UK decreased from 0.6% to 0.4% and from 1.8% to 0.8%, respectively, between 2011 and 2013 [23]. Similarly, in another study the level was continued to fall in 2013 to 50.6% and 31.5%, but these were still higher than for US respondents (26.3% and 15.4%, respectively) [25].

Before the COVID-19 pandemic global last year use rates of ketamine were 6.72% in 2016, 8.6% in 2017 and 6.5% in 2018; lifetime rates for 2017 and 2018 were 11.7% and 10.4%, respectively [26, 27]. During the COVID-19 pandemic state, a reduction in 'party drugs'-like ketamine consumption was expected. As the limited access to pubs, clubs, and festivals cancelation were the primary reasons for decreases in the recreational use of illicit drugs which are typically linked to the nightlife and party scenes. In fact, in Australia, the use of ecstasy/MDMA and related drugs (e.g., cocaine, ketamine) had fallen compared to the pre-pandemic level [28, 29]. The less interest in club drugs like ketamine was also noticed by Neutravel, an Italian non-governmental organization (NGO) [30].

Surprisingly, in the U.S. according to the national survey-based 'Monitoring the Future Study', it has been demonstrated the ketamine use raised between 2019 and 2020 from 0.7 to 1.3% respectively among 12th graders [31]. Some individuals paradoxically start to use ketamine due to anxiety caused by the pandemic time, while others increased its consumption during lockdown spent at home [32].

3. Ketamine status in the regulatory systems

In 1999, ketamine including its salts, isomers, become a Schedule II non-narcotic substance under the Federal Controlled Substances Act in the U.S. This means that the drug does have lower misuse potential but is still approved for use in hospitals and other medical settings as an anesthetic. Because of this, it is illegal to possess ketamine without a medical reason, prescription, or as a part of the research. Thus, the illicit use of ketamine appears to be from illegal diversion from legal prescription, but analogs which usually contain a range of undeclared psychoactive substances (i.e., amphetamine, benzocaine, cocaine, MDMA, methoxetamine, paracetamol, piperazines, and synthetic cathinones) may also be found on the streets [33].

Nowadays, in the U.S., ketamine is classified as a schedule III drug under the DEA Controlled Substances Act. Medications in this category are often used for pain control, or anesthesia, or appetite suppression. It means that ketamine has less potential for abuse than Schedule I (heroin) or Schedule II (cocaine) drug, and it is not as tightly regulated as most opioids. However, abuse of Schedule III substances may lead to moderate or low physical dependence but more commonly leads to high psychological dependence. This means that for users outside the approved limits, its adverse mental and physical health effects can be hazardous [34].

Ketamine has been revived a couple of times in 2003, 2006, and 2012 by The Expert Committee on Drug Dependence of the World Health Organization (WHO), and finally, it has remained on the list as an essential medicine. The experts considered that the international control is not appropriate in this case, as new facts about ketamine were not sufficient to warrant scheduling. In the recent World Drug Report by United Nations Office on Drugs Control 2019 (UNOD 2019) [35], ketamine is classified under new psychoactive substances (NPSs), which are not under the control of international drug conventions, but which may pose a threat to public health. Since 2000, in the European Union, ketamine is not under the control, however further monitoring of drug use is recommended by the European Commission. Despite the increasing trends of abuse, dependence, and dying from ketamine recreational use, its status did not change significantly over time. It seems to be still relatively low, especially when compared with other Novel Psychoactive Substances (i.e., synthetic cannabinoids and cathinones or 'designer benzos'). This raises important concerns about the underestimation of ketamine.

4. Methods of ketamine abuse

The route of ketamine administration is crucial for the type and the intensity of the experience the effect. Ketamine has a dose–response curve with variable effects

Dose range [mg]	Related effects
Low: 10–75	mild euphoria, feeling of well-being, feelings of calmness and relaxation, empathy, smell, and tastes muted, visual hallucinations, enhanced color vision, sense of touch deterioration
Medium: 60–125	slow motion, auditory hallucinations (ringing in the ears), detached feeling from the body, loss of coordination, diminished reflexes
High: 100–250	felling light, timelessness, body dysmorphia, 'K-hole' out-of-body experiences

Table 1.
The common effects of ketamine in snorted doses.

Single dose [mg]*	Route	Onset of action [min]	Duration of action [min]
75–125	i.m.	1–5	30–45
60–250	i.n.	5–10	45–60
50–100	i.v.	seconds	30–45
200–300	p.o.	15–20	60–120

Abbreviations: intramuscular (i.m.); insufflation, intranasal or "snorting" (i.n.); intravenously (i.v.), per os, orally "by mouth" (p.o). *Typical recreational dose is 10–25% of the effective general anesthetic dose [37].*

Table 2.
Ketamine recreational dose ranges, the routes of administration, onset and duration of action ([36] with some modifications).

(**Table 1**). However, unlike other psychedelic drugs like LSD, ketamine triggers a short trip, lasting no more than 1.5 hours. The illicit product mostly involves evaporating the liquid from the diverted injectable solution to produce a dry powder that is formed into tablets or sold as a powder. The most common method of ketamine abuse is "snorting" and 96% of ketamine users choose such a way for its usefulness and rapid action noticed in roughly 5 to 10 minutes [33]. In comparison, oral consumption requires between 15 and 20 minutes (**Table 2**) [25]. For nonmedical use, a typical intranasal dose is 50 mg and the oral dose is 100 mg [38, 39], but the usual recreational dose range between 60 and 250 mg of ketamine [40]. Ketamine abusers will often self-administer several sequential doses of the drug to maintain psychotropic effects over time. However, an injection results in the most rapid effect (within seconds to minutes), though such a way of administration is quite difficult especially in clubs. Interestingly, a recent animal study has revealed that a high IV ketamine dose caused the complete cessation of cortical EEG activity for several minutes, similarly to the 'K-hole' in humans [41]. Recently, online user fora, as well as research findings, also support vaping as a possible route of ketamine administration [42, 43].

5. The central and peripheral consequences of long-term and recreational ketamine misuse

There are no medical uses in which ketamine is provided chronically. The majority of reported long-term effects of ketamine are those which have developed in chronic recreational users or animals during preclinical studies. Although controlled human studies of repeated doses of ketamine are prohibited because it would be unethical to give an anesthetic with pronounced adverse effects more often. In clinical settings, ketamine is rather well tolerated. Although the pattern of adverse effects of non-medical ketamine use may differ from that expected from prescribed medical use. In individuals who misuse ketamine, serious sequelae, including prolonged neuro-, urological-, and gastro-toxicity may occur. The residual effects which may persist beyond acute ketamine dosing and its long-term consequences have been compiled and presented in the following subsections below.

5.1 Psychosis

Evidence of the psychotogenic potency of ketamine initially emerged from general anesthetic use where clinicians noted drug- related post-anesthetic reactions (i.e., confusion, vivid dreams, and hallucinations) leading to a reduction in the clinical drug utility [9, 44, 45].

There are some evidences that infrequent and frequent ketamine users exhibited higher levels of schizophrenia-like, dissociative, and depressive symptoms [13]. Hansen et al. [46] described the most common subjective effects of ketamine in recreational users including the sensation of light through the body; novel experiences concerning "body consistency" (e.g., being made of wood, rubber, or plastic); unreal shape or size of body parts; a sensation of floating or hovering in a weightless condition; timeless; sudden insight into the self; the experience of being at one with the universe; an experience of leaving the body; visions and hallucinations).

Subanesthetic doses of ketamine in healthy volunteers also trigger positive and negative schizophrenic-like symptoms as well as perceptual alterations similar to dissociative states with altered body perception, depersonalization, derealization, and distorted sensory perception. Of note, ketamine had the highest degree of out-of-body experiences compared to the other drugs as was mentioned in the previous section. While it is given to chronic, stable schizophrenics, ketamine has been shown to cause a re-emergence of the acute phase of the illness [47].

Ketamine exerts its unique behavioral effects mostly by blocking the NMDA receptors [48, 49]. Although phencyclidine (PCP; "angel dust") has a 10-fold greater affinity for the NMDA receptor and is more excitotoxic than ketamine. Over the past several decades many animal models have been developed using drug mimics endogenous deficits in NMDA receptor function to study the mechanism of schizophrenia [48]. The cumulative effect of repeatedly using ketamine and/or a residual effect has occurred 3 days after abusers took this drug [50]. More importantly, even strong schizophrenic-type symptoms and perceptual distortions may persist after cessation of ketamine use [17, 36].

One of the explanations of such effect is NMDA receptor dysfunction even several days after acute use. Second, a residual effect may also be psychological in that ketamine produces an intensely subjective experience that could affect users' perceptions of the world for several days after it is taken [13, 50].

5.2 Cognitive deficits

There is increasing evidence that regular and long-lasting ketamine use can induce central nervous system depression and impair cognition, in particular visual and verbal memory as well as executive function [50–52]. The frequent ketamine users with increasing drug doses were more likely to have cognitive deficits, especially with short- and long-term spatial working memory and pattern recognition memory tasks [53]. Short-term memory and visual memory deficits occur usually in users who abused the drug at least 4 days per week. Similarly, according to findings from animal studies, ketamine seems to deteriorate memory at relatively high doses. Short-term memory and spatial memory were impaired in rats administered 30 mg/kg i.p.

and were revealed by the delayed spatial alternation task and finding to the hidden platform in the Morris water maze test [54, 55].

Interestingly, ketamine appears to have greater potency to reduce cognition than other drugs of abuse [13]. These cognitive deficits may affect functioning in the abuser's daily life due to difficulty in remembering conversations and other people's names [13]. It has been also found that men to be more affected by these effects than women [56]. In addition, cognitive deficits are also related to the impairment of the psychomotor performance, such as coordination, balance, and hand-eye movements. This lack of coordination may cause the inability to drive or operate machinery, thereby increasing accidental injury or even mortality from motor vehicle collisions. Data from an epidemiological study involving drug-related motor vehicle collision fatalities found 9% related to ketamine use, representing a disproportionate number of fatalities compared to alcohol and opioid misuse [57].

In 2007, according to data from a single trauma centre in Hong Kong roughly 4.5% of drivers involved in non-fatal crashes tested positive for ketamine [58].

In addition, ketamine may gradually change the brain's chemical system affecting opioids, dopamine (it activates dopamine systems), serotonin, noradrenaline, nitric oxide, sigma, GABA (gamma amino-butyric acid), and acetylcholine, among others [59, 60].

Ketamine has been also induced electrophysiological dissociation between the thalamo-neocortical and limbic systems and potentiated the synaptic inhibition of GABA [36, 61, 62]. However, the key pharmacological mechanisms underlying ketamine-related cognitive deficits are mediated via an NMDA glutamate receptors hypofunction [4]. There have been also shown that NMDA antagonists' potency induced degeneration in a subset of limbic structures like those which are altered in patients with psychoses [63]. Animal studies revealed that direct apoptotic neurodegeneration was induced by NMDA-R antagonists, including ketamine, in the developing rodent brain. However, this ketamine effect was more evident in older rats [64]. According to other findings from animal studies the racemic ketamine (with its preservative benzethonium chloride) and S-ketamine have been associated with neuronal apoptosis and sensorineural consequence following high dose and/or long-term i.v. administration [65–68]. However, translatability to humans is questioned and the impact of lower subanesthetic doses is uncertain.

In this way, ketamine abuse may display structural damage in multiple brain areas, such as the frontal, occipital, parietal, limbic, and corpus striatum [69, 70].

There have been shown that such detrimental effect is related to time and the dose of ketamine abuse [69]. Data have also revealed that the brain atrophies may occur within 1 year of ketamine intensive use with expected further progression in the following years [70]. In fact, ketamine dose reduction may restore cognition, but we cannot rule out irreversible and residual effects [17, 50].

As data have demonstrated NMDA receptors must be blocked for at least 24 hours to produce irreversible effect or death in the cells, but ketamine has a short half-life (about 20 minutes in rats) thus many injections are needed, over a prolonged period, to produce persistent change [71].

Although we have still limited data regarding cognitive ability from the ketamine ex-user population to provide straightforward conclusions for these findings. To date, there is no specific pharmacotherapy to avoid cognitive deficits in long-term ketamine use. The management of these problems is largely supportive and symptomatic. The cognitive enhancers are taken into consideration, such as modafinil, commonly used in stimulant addiction, as well as cholinesterase inhibitors (i.e., rivastigmine, donepezil, galantamine) usually recommended in other disorders with cognitive impairments (i.e., Alzheimer's disease, Parkinson's disease, traumatic brain injury, and schizophrenia), among others [51, 72].

5.3 Pro-depressant effect

Compared to growing evidence available for the anti-depressant effect of ketamine, there is still less for its pro-depressant potency [73]. Ironically, an intranasal ketamine formulation was recently approved in the USA, and Europe to treat intractable depression and acute suicidal ideation [74]. The depressive potency of ketamine seems to be dose and time-related. Insights from the animal study indicate that the antidepressant action at a dose of 10 mg/kg was not observed in rats receiving a higher dose of ketamine (80 mg/kg) [75]. Likewise, the anti-depressive effects linked to the subanesthetic ketamine dose (0.5 mg/kg) might not correspond to the same effect at the dosages range, preferred by recreational users. It was suggested that an opposite pro-depressant effect may be linked to certain neuroadaptation changes [76]. In fact, some studies demonstrated that chronic use of ketamine causes more lasting depressive effects [4, 36, 53]. There have been shown that ketamine abusers reported depressive symptoms quite common, roughly 72.5%–77.5% of them were diagnosed with moderate to severe depression based on the Beck Depression Inventory scores [77, 78].

According to the results from various studies, the prevalence of major depressive disorder (MDD) in outpatient settings fluctuating between 7.8–18.5%, in comparison to inpatient populations with nearly one-fourth (23.3%) ketamine-dependent MDD comorbidity [79–81]. Though, according to certain authors, the mood measures revealed little and clinically insignificant difference between groups with slightly higher scores in the ketamine users [50].

Interestingly, increased depression scores have been found in both daily users and ex-users in a longitudinal study, although not more infrequent users [53]. The mechanism of the acute antidepressant and chronic depressant effects may be linked, but it is unclear exactly how this opposite effect is mediated. Why abstinent ketamine users were more depressed is also less clear but may be linked with a change in their lifestyle. In fact, the frequent ketamine users had experienced more negative life events over the 12 months, due probably to their chaotic lifestyles, which may also trigger depressive symptoms [82].

In addition, previous evidence indicates that the depressive symptoms in ketamine users may persist even for 1 year after abstinence [53]. Furthermore, increased depression in frequent users could also reflect their increased dependency on ketamine, as depression is also commonly comorbid in opiate- and alcohol-dependent populations [83, 84]. Recent data imply that depression might be associated with craving (stronger propensity to administer more ketamine). There have been shown that patients with higher craving intensity demonstrated a greater severity of depression, longer history of ketamine administration, and greater use frequency than those with lower craving intensity [81].

5.4 Tolerance

Ketamine-induced tolerance may be considered in many aspects, although it is exceptionally mentioned in psychopharmacological clinical studies.

Firstly, ketamine is known as an effective anesthetic drug widely used in the clinic, however, as with many drugs, this effectiveness is often compromised due to tolerance to ketamine's anesthetic effects, which might be of great importance especially when the patient has a history of drug abuse. Similarly, there are several papers indicating tolerance to the antidepressive effects of ketamine during repeated administrations [85]. Nonetheless, tolerance to ketamine can develop rapidly in all species, including after one large dose [86, 87], or even in patients with major depressive disorder. A great example derived from the case study of

Bonnet [85] provided evidence that a continuous antidepressant response to daily ketamine injections can be followed by a swift return of a major depressive episode after cessation of ketamine. Other papers demonstrate animals chronically given ketamine that required increased doses of ketamine to reach the target anesthetic plane. Moreover, animals had a shorter duration of anesthesia [86, 88]. Surprisingly, rats pretreated with intraperitoneal morphine at a dose of 5.6 mg/kg demonstrated cross-tolerance to ketamine's anesthetic effects [88].

5.5 Withdrawal

Ketamine, being a drug easily abused, may induce several uncomfortable adverse reactions as a consequence of its cessation. There is increasing evidence that ketamine causes psychological but not physical dependence. Withdrawal symptoms are usually like withdrawal from cocaine with very strong cravings. Symptoms of acute withdrawal may be short-lived and not identified as such [89]. However, the withdrawal from ketamine may paradoxically cause depression [90]. Other withdrawal symptoms after ketamine discontinuation include dysphoria, shaking, sweating, palpitations, tiredness, low appetite, low mood, chills, autonomic arousal, lacrimation, restlessness, anxiety, nightmares, paranoia, delusions, and hallucinations [81, 91, 92]. Noteworthy, these withdrawal symptoms typically begin within 24 h of discontinuation and last approximately 3 days, although in some cases, they may persist for 2 weeks and thereafter stabilize [93].

Apart from the abovementioned, there several reports are indicating that due to ketamine discontinuing mild forms of schizophrenic-like symptoms occur [17].

5.6 Ketamine-induced uropathy: "the ketamine bladder"

Recreational abuse of ketamine has been associated with bladder pain syndrome; ulcerative cystitis also known as 'ketamine bladder'. Up to a quarter of ketamine, abusers may experience such problems. According to the European Medicines Agency (EMA) and the UK Yellow Card Scheme pharmacovigilance database about 23% and 17% of ketamine-related adverse drug reactions (ADR) respectively referred to renal/urinary disorders. Interestingly, such issues being more common among women than men [94]. In general, urological problems occur within 1 month-1 year time frame following the start of ketamine use, but recent pharmacovigilance data revealed that even an acute ketamine administration may be associated with urological risks, as in some cases the risk was noticed within 48 hours of treatment [94].

Initially, ketamine associate bladder disturbance may mimic common conditions such as urine infections and it may be difficult to diagnose, but further urinary symptoms may substantially disturb the quality of the abuser's life thus extreme individuals have difficulty with passing urine. There are reports of needing to pass urine up to 20 times an hour, leading to hydronephrosis and finally kidney failure [4].

Damage to the urinary barrier initiates bladder pain and, in ketamine-induced cystitis, loss of urothelium from large areas of the bladder wall was reported [95]. Ketamine abuse also induces small bladder volume, bladder wall thickening, and mucosal enhancement. The most common ketamine bladder symptoms reported in the 2018 Global Drug Survey were as follows: urine frequency 38%; pain in the abdomen 25%; burning when urinating 18%; incontinence 7%; and blood 3% [96].

The first report of the urological syndrome was published in 2007 by Shahani and colleagues [97]. The cause of urinary toxicity appears to be multifactorial and not fully explained. It is postulated that the direct toxic effect of ketamine or its active metabolite (norketamine) on the urinary tract may play a crucial role [98]. It is also pointed out, that the urinary toxicity seems to be unrelated to ketamine interaction with NMDA receptors (NMDAR). Thus, in vitro studies revealed that normally human urothelial cells were unresponsive to NMDAR agonists or antagonists, and no expression of NMDAR transcript was detected [95].

A recent study offers new evidence for a mechanism of direct toxicity of ketamine to the urothelial by activating the intrinsic apoptotic pathway. In fact, exposure to ketamine in noncytotoxic concentrations initiates the transient release of calcium Ca(2+) from the endoplasmic reticulum into the cytosol. However, ketamine concentrations >1 mmol/L become cytotoxic and provokes a larger-amplitude increase in cytosolic Ca(2+) concentration. Consequently, sustained elevation in Ca(2+) leads to pathological mitochondrial oxygen consumption and ATP deficiency, and it initiates damage to the urinary barrier [95].

The chronic immune response of the bladder interstitial cells may be another possible underlying mechanism of toxicity [99, 100]. Biopsies have also revealed epithelial denudation, eosinophilic, as well as mast cell infiltration [97, 101]. Ketamine may also trigger interstitial fibrosis by damaging the papillary medullary interstitial cells [98]. There are also reports of metaplasia in the intestine related to ketamine abuse [102]. Furthermore, ketamine through its central action may disturb the contractile response of smooth muscle from appropriate stimuli [103].

In addition, ketamine may induce highly destructive microvascular changes causing epithelial-to-mesenchymal transition, which finally contributes to bladder or kidney fibrogenesis [100, 104].

Compared to the urinary tract, renal damage and bilateral hydronephrosis are less frequent but may also occur. Chronic kidney failure may develop as the final consequence of a long-term sequel [105].

Of note, there a no specific and casual pharmacotherapy for ketamine-related urinary tract disorder. The symptomatic treatment with antibiotics, anti-inflammatory agents, steroids, and anticholinergics in most cases has failed [106]. In such a scenario, the second line of alternative treatment with intravesical agents such as hyaluronic acid, and injections of Botulinum toxin-A should be considered. Preclinical studies have also suggested a future therapy with combined intravesical liposomal onabotulinum toxin-A instillation and mesenchymal stem cells placed directly into the bladder submucosal layer [107]. However, the urinary problems may improve and became reversible if ketamine use is reduced/withdrawn, thus ketamine abstinence should be the first step in ketamine-induced uropathy treatment. The abstinence greater than 3 months is related to some improvement and less severe symptoms. Of note, in some cases, urological issues may persist for up to 1 year after ketamine abstinence [108]. More invasive methods, such as a catheter (tube into the bladder), urinary diversion, and nephrectomy may be required in the prolonged ketamine abuse and irreversible renal damage which may produce a burden to healthcare resources [100, 102, 103].

5.7 Gastrointestinal pathology: 'K cramps'

Regular and long-term ketamine use is associated with gastric pathology of unknown etiology, colloquially termed 'KCramps' [37, 98].

In line with the 2010 *Mixmag* Survey, 'K cramps' occurred in 30% of ketamine users and was a more common issue among women [109]. The persistent epigastric pain is classified as the commonest upper GI symptoms as was presented in 73% of abusers after a higher dose, daily ketamine use [110]. Among symptoms that were also frequently diagnosed in ketamine users are cystic dilatations of the common bile duct, in association with abnormal liver function tests [111–113].

In a retrospective study of GI symptoms followed by inhalational ketamine use, 28/37 of the subjects experienced upper GI symptoms. The mean time of ketamine use was 4 years before admission. Exclusion criteria included potential risk factors and a history of GI disorder. The most common finding was epigastric pain only, which occurred in 23 (62.2%) users. Four users had epigastric pain with vomiting. In sporadic cases, gastroduodenitis, and intestinal metaplasia have occurred. More importantly, all symptoms relief with abstinence from ketamine use [110]. Of note, pains symptomatology related to GI in ketamine users may resemble irritable bowel syndrome as in some parts tend to be triggered by psychological changes [37, 114].

There has been shown that gastric pathology among ketamine users correlated with the duration of drug use [111, 115]. The exact mechanism by which ketamine produces cholestasis and biliary dilation is unclear but is a possible direct link to NMDA receptor blockade in smooth muscle. In addition, ketamine may also act through the dorsal motor nucleus of the vagus, projecting to the gall bladder [116].

Effective treatment of GI toxicity includes discontinuation of ketamine use which can lead to the relief of symptoms, otherwise, treatment options are nonspecific [110].

Of note, there are certain cases of evidence of causal risk between chronic ketamine use and GI toxicity as dilated common bile duct regressed with abstinence but recurred following a return to ketamine use [111].

6. Ketamine and other substances/drugs adverse reactions

The phenomenon of interaction is used in clinical practice as multi-drug therapy. Its aim is to increase the pharmacological potency and obtain desired therapeutic effect while reducing doses of individual drugs. Such steps reduce the likelihood of side effects and are beneficial for the patient. However, the problem arises when unwanted drug interactions occur, and this includes i) pharmaceutical interactions, i.e. incompatibilities arising outside the patient's body; ii) pharmacokinetic interactions related to the fate of the drug in the body at the stage of its absorption, distribution, metabolism and excretion; and finally iii) pharmacodynamic interactions, where one drug modifies the action of another drug.

All these benefits as well as undesired interactions are true for ketamine and other substances. Use with multiple drugs has been fatal.

Firstly, ketamine (both its R(−)- and S(+)-enantiomers) undergoes hepatic biotransformation through the cytochrome P450 (CYP450), particularly with the involvement of CYP2B6 and CYP3A4, to form norketamine. Therefore, an alteration of CYP450 metabolism results in clinically significant drug–drug interactions that can further cause unanticipated adverse reactions and/or therapeutic failures. For instance, drugs that induce both these cytochrome isoforms may reduce exposure to ketamine. In contrast, substances inhibiting CYP enzymes can lead to an increase the exposure to the drug. As a great example is the treatment with diazepam, being a substrate of CYP3A4, which increases ketamine plasma half-life, thus its sedative effects [117, 118]. On the other hand, ketamine can also influence diazepam metabolism as its decreases CYP3A4 enzyme activity [119].

Apart from the involvement of CYP 450 isoforms in the metabolism of ketamine, also another hepatic phase II enzymes may be taken under consideration. Indeed, ketamine has been shown to inhibit UGT2B7 and thus the metabolism of morphine both in vitro and in vivo [120, 121], therefore increases the liver concentration of the opioid. Intriguingly, also the brain concentration of morphine is found to increased (three- to five-fold 90 min after administration). However, such drug concentration changes in the brain are not because of changes at the blood–brain barrier as it was compared with oxycodone mainly metabolized by cytochrome P450 (CYP) enzymes [122]. Also, when considered oppositely, morphine, but not oxycodone, pretreatment increased the brain and serum concentrations of ketamine [123].

CYP3A4 enzyme is known to be affected by compounds derived from grapefruit juice or whole fruit (i.e., furanocoumarins and, to a lesser extent, flavonoids) [124]. Therefore, in the case of ketamine given orally, a significant increase in plasma concentration can be found in healthy volunteers [125].

Unfortunately, drug metabolism via CYP450 enzymes exhibits also genetic variability (polymorphism), thus in this case also some variations in the exposure to ketamine are obvious. Poor metabolizers of enzymes metabolizing ketamine are extremely rare. However, the paper of Rao et al. [126] provided with information that CYP2B6*6 polymorphism variant did not affect single, low-dose ketamine metabolism, clearance, and pharmacokinetics in healthy human volunteers, though diminished ketamine metabolism in vitro.

Concerning pharmacodynamic interaction once should be said that the nature of ketamine-drug interactions together with the observable effect is highly dependent on the drug type and thus the molecular target (i.e., opioidergic system, dopaminergic, serotoninergic, etc.) as well as from the dose used. There is a great several papers characterizing possible pharmacodynamics interactions between ketamine and different drugs both natural and synthetic. For instance, estrogen together with progesterone potentiated ketamine-induced antidepressant effect [127], while BNN27, a synthetic derivative of dehydroepiandrosterone reduced ketamine-induced ataxia [128]. Ketamine was found to produce additive effects when combined with gamma-aminobutyric acid (GABA) activity. This was found true for barbiturates such as thiopental at a hypnotic endpoint [129], but not with a benzodiazepine - midazolam [130]. Also, for anesthesia induction, the combination of ketamine and midazolam was found additive rather than synergistic at the endpoint of loss of response to verbal command [130]. When introduced with other benzodiazepines (i.e., clonazepam, alprazolam, lorazepam), specifically for the treatment of long-lasting depression, as well as considering that both types of drugs act on interneurons, ketamine antidepressant efficacy was mute [131, 132]. This finding suggested that benzodiazepines inhibitory activity towards ketamine's antidepressant effect may be related to attenuation of neuroplastic processes, emerging subsequently after the acute effect and after ketamine and its active metabolites are eliminated from the blood since benzodiazepines occurred ineffective in the first 24 h post-concomitant administration of both drugs [131].

Analyzing other effects mediated by simultaneous ketamine and benzodiazepines, the following can be mentioned: (1) inhibition of ketamine-induced hyperlocomotion by diazepam [133]; (2) ketamine's emotional stress reduction by a sub-hypnotic lorazepam [134]; (3) lorazepam intensification of ketamine sedative effects [134]; (4) potentiation of ketamine amnestic action by diazepam and lorazepam [134, 135]; (5) antagonism of the cardiovascular effects of ketamine by diazepam [136], or (6) ketamine-induced emergence delirium prevented by midazolam [137]. Whereas concerning antipsychotics such as haloperidol it has been shown that it can reduce ketamine-induced cognitive impairment. In addition, haloperidol was found to attenuate the increase of locomotor activity and stereotyped behavior, reversed the motor incoordination, and blocked the hypermobility induced by acute administration of ketamine in rodents [138].

Yet another possible interaction occurs between ketamine and the opioid system, as ketamine (in particular (S)-ketamine) was characterized as a drug that partially interacts with the opioid system, particularly mu-opioid receptors [139]. Indeed, as already mentioned, ketamine enhances levels of morphine, which may explain the long-lasting morphine-induced antinociception [120]. Importantly, the enhanced level of morphine is strictly associated with ketamine inhibitory activity towards morphine tolerance, which is mainly by N-methyl-d-aspartate (NMDA) receptor antagonism [121, 140]. On the other hand, it has long been suggested that opioids may enhance the antidepressant effect induced by ketamine, as naltrexone attenuated this activity [141]. However, currently, the involvement of the opioid system in this specific action is unclear since partial agonists (i.e., methadone and buprenorphine) did not influence ketamine's antidepressant effect [142].

Opioids are well known for their great ability to induce respiratory depression, especially when overdosed. Intriguingly, also in this aspect, an interaction between ketamine and opioids exists. In fact, intraperitoneal (i.p.) administration of ketamine has led to significant respiratory depression in mice, but not in mu-opioid receptor knock-out mice [143].

As with other CNS medications, it should be mentioned that ketamine is capable of modifying effects mediated by alcohol consumption and illicit drugs. In the first case, it has been revealed that subjects simultaneously taking alcohol and ketamine are more vulnerable to suffer from the urinary tract and gastrointestinal problems such as pain with urination, increased frequency of urination, or even lower abdominal pain [144]. Of note, individuals with a family history of alcoholism with altered NMDA activity may have a blunted effect on the negative psychological reactions to ketamine. Whereas, as a great example of a drug of abuse, apart from the aforementioned opioids, for which a concomitant use with ketamine may result in unpredictable and extremely dangerous side effects is a so-called "liquid Extasy" [92, 145]. This compound is a gamma-hydroxybutyric acid (GHB), being a naturally occurring analog of gamma-aminobutyric acid (GABA), with esthetic and euphoric properties. Concerning ketamine, it has been shown that this drug together with GHB, in particularly high doses, results in an increased risk of respiratory depression and fatality. In addition, ketamine produced and enhanced GHB-mediated cataleptic effects in mice [146]. Also, can lead to a significant increase in sleep time.

Dangerous interactions were also noted for ketamine and methamphetamine both in vitro and in vivo. In fact, the co-exposure of these two drugs resulted in significant cytotoxicity and synergy on oxidative stress in HepG2 cells [147]. While in mice treated with a low dose of methamphetamine and ketamine, the stress-related depressive and anxiety-related behavioral alterations caused by the psychostimulant were antagonized consistently by both high and low doses of ketamine [148]. Furthermore, a combined repeated administration of both drugs was reported to increase significantly the risk of psychological dependence as shown in a rat conditioned place preference test [149]. In turn, in methamphetamine-dependent humans, a very high prevalence of psychotic disorders was suggested for those who occasionally or continuously use ketamine [150]. Moreover, when used with other stimulant drugs such as ecstasy, high blood pressure may appear [50]. Ketamine may be also toxic when is combined with caffeine. Theoretically, this may be a concern in people who have consumed energy drinks, especially at nightclubs where ketamine may be abused.

Ketamine is also a very popular drug taken together with cocaine. Unfortunately, such a combination occurred to result in a potentiation of cocaine-induced hepatotoxicity associated with sub-massive hepatic necrosis. These observations were indicated for rats pretreated with ketamine for three consecutive days at a dose of 100 mg/kg with a single dose of cocaine (5 mg/kg, i.v.) [151]. This information is especially intriguing when compared with recent data demonstrated that a single ketamine infusion in cocaine abusers, coupled with a mindfulness behavioral modification program, seems to be a promise to achieve both the abstinence and reduction of the risk of relapse [152].

Ketamine is known to be related to several molecular targets, either directly or indirectly. Indeed, due to its interactions with sodium channels (local anesthetic properties), i.e. L-type calcium channels and potassium channels [153], ketamine when administered with grapefruit juice may cause harmful effects ranging from relatively mild hypotension and dizziness. Furthermore, ketamine being an antagonist towards acetylcholinergic receptors produces various effects while interacting with cholinesterase and anticholinesterase agents. One great example is the interaction with atropine which was found to slightly increase the ketamine-induced time of immobility in rats [154]. On the other hand, ketamine blocked the EEG and the behavioral toxic effects of neostigmine and physostigmine. While physostigmine can reverse the central anticholinergic effects and also antagonize ketamine hypnotic effects [155]. However, in the aspect of somnolence reverse, there are contradictory results. In fact, while Balmer [156] found physostigmine effective in reversing ketamine-induced somnolence. Drummond et al. [157] indicated physostigmine as ineffective in producing a rapid patient awaking or even in reducing hallucinatory behavior.

Another possible cellular target of ketamine includes the monoaminergic system, particularly noradrenergic and serotonergic. Alpha2 agonists such as xylazine or medetomidine as well as dexmedetomidine were found safe when combining with ketamine [158]. Both these drugs were shown to reduce the dosage of ketamine and the occurrence of psychomotor symptoms after ketamine. As for compounds actin at serotonergic receptors of various types or being selective serotonin reuptake inhibitors (SSRIs) it can be provided that repeated subanaesthetic doses of ketamine can redeem the time lag for the antidepressant-like effects of citalopram [159]. Also, such a combination given to rats resulted in a decrease in the immobility time and increase in struggle time in the Forced Swim Test (FST) and Tail Suspension Test (TST) as compared to control group [160].

Beneficial effects were also observed for other serotonergic agents. For instance, intravenous ketamine emetic properties were inhibited by ondasteron in children [161]. Moreover, ketamine was reported to potentiate the anxiolytic effects of SSRIs such as fluoxetine [162].

Apart from the above-mentioned, also cannabinoids were indicated to be vulnerable to interact with ketamine. These includes delta 9-tetrahydrocannabinol being the major psychoactive molecule among synthetic cannabinoid ligands that act at cannabinoid 1 receptor (CB1), as well as cannabidiol (CBD) displaying potency as an antagonist of CB1 and CB1 receptor agonist, respetively. Indeed, Frizza et al. [163] reported 9-tetrahydrocannabinol to prolong the anesthesia induced by ketamine in mice. Whereas CBD was found reduced depersonalization when administered with ketamine, as measured by the Clinical Administered Dissociative State Scale in healthy humans [164].

Overall, it can be noted that ketamine, possibly due to the complex mechanism of action, may interact with various molecular targets resulting in both critical and beneficial effects. Therefore, there is no unequivocal opinion as to whether ketamine should be used with caution or not; this depends strictly on the type of the second drug used as well as on other physiological and pathophysiological factors, including age, genetic polymorphism, and occurrence of diseases and disorders.

7. Conclusions

Non-medical, recreational use of ketamine has increased in certain populations/sub-groups with geographical variations in its use patterns. Ketamine abuse seems to be an important public health challenge due to its association with multiple physical and psychological harms. Noteworthy, the psychedelic effect may have a therapeutic value in some points and be harmful in others. Long term users may develop different neurobiological alterations, psychological dependency, withdrawal, tolerance, schizophrenia-type symptoms, poor psychological well-being, memory difficulties, and finally worse quality of daily life. In the long-term use, there is also evidence of deleterious effects for the peripheral system, associated with serious lower urinary tract symptoms, and gastrointestinal pathology. In addition, polysubstance consumption is inherently risky and can lead to serious adverse consequences, especially when abusers mixing ketamine with eighter depressants or stimulants. Although of concern did not cause any significant changes in ketamine's legal status over the years. There are numerous studies revealed the effects of a single administration of ketamine, thus the effects following repeated use and long-term consequences are still less known and underestimated. More study is needed to better elucidate the real ketamine safety profile regarding both its long-term recreational use and its clinically use as an antidepressant agent.

Acknowledgements

There is no funding information.

Conflict of interest

The authors declare no conflict of interest.

Author details

Patrycja Kleczkowska[1,2*] and Malgorzata Zaremba[2,3]

1 Analytical Group, Department of Analytical Chemistry and Biomaterials, Faculty of Pharmacy with Laboratory Medicine Division, Medical University of Warsaw, Warsaw, Poland

2 Military Institute of Hygiene and Epidemiology, Warsaw, Poland

3 Department of Experimental and Clinical Pharmacology, Centre for Preclinical Research (CBP), Medical University of Warsaw, Warsaw, Poland

*Address all correspondence to: hazufiel@wp.pl

References

[1] Collier BB. Ketamine and the conscious mind. Anaesthesia, 1972;27:120-134. DOI: 10.1111/j.1365-2044.1972.tb08186.x

[2] WFSA Resources. Update in Anesthesia, Jan 2005; 20:25-29. Available from: https://resources.wfsahq.org/wp-content/uploads/uia20-KETAMINE-A-REVIEW.pdf [Accessed: 2021-08-21]

[3] Darke S, Lappin J, Farrell M. The clinician's guide to illicit drugs and health. London, United Kingdom: Silverback Publishing; 2019. ISBN: 9781912141128

[4] Morgan CJ, Curran HV, Independent Scientific Committee on Drugs. Ketamine use: a review. Addiction, 2012;107:27-38. DOI: 10.1111/j.1360-0443.2011.03576.x.

[5] Pal HR, Berry N, Kumar R, Ray R. Ketamine dependence. Anaesth. Intensive Care, 2002;30:382-384. DOI: 10.1177/0310057X0203000323.

[6] Palamar JJ, Salomone A, Rutherford C, Keyes KM. Extensive underreported exposure to ketamine among electronic dance music party attendees. J. Gen. Intern. Med., 2021;36:235-237. DOI: 10.1007/s11606-020-05672-x.

[7] Dillon P, Copeland J, Jansen K. Patterns of use and harms associated with non-medical ketamine use. Drug Alcohol Depend., 2003;69:23-28. DOI: 10.1016/s0376-8716(02)00243-0.

[8] Drug Misuse: Findings from the 2012/13 Crime Survey for England and Wales. London: Home Office; 2013 Available from: https://assets.publishing.service.gov.uk/government/uploads/system/uploads/attachment_data/file/225122/Drugs_Misuse201213.pdf [Accessed: 2021-08-03]

[9] Krystal JH, Karper LP, Seibyl JP, Freeman GK, Delaney R, Bremner JD, Heninger GR, Bowers MB Jr, Charney DS. Subanesthetic effects of the noncompetitive NMDA antagonist, ketamine, in humans. Psychotomimetic, perceptual, cognitive, and neuroendocrine responses. Arch. Gen. Psychiatry, 1994;51:199-214. DOI: 10.1001/archpsyc.1994.03950030035004.

[10] Bonta IL. Schizophrenia, dissociative anaesthesia and near-death experience; three events meeting at the NMDA receptor. Med. Hypotheses, 2004;62:23-28. DOI: 10.1016/s0306-9877(03)00307-4.

[11] Stirling J, McCoy L. Quantifying the psychological effects of ketamine: from euphoria to the K-hole. Subst. Use Misuse, 2010;45:2428-2443. DOI: 10.3109/10826081003793912.

[12] Fletcher PC, Honey GD. Schizophrenia, ketamine and cannabis: evidence of overlapping memory deficits. Trends Cogn. Sci., 2006;10:167-174. DOI: 10.1016/j.tics.2006.02.008.

[13] Morgan CJ, Muetzelfeldt L, Curran HV. Ketamine use, cognition and psychological wellbeing: a comparison of frequent, infrequent and ex-users with polydrug and non-using controls. Addiction, 2009;104:77-87. DOI: 10.1111/j.1360-0443.2008.02394.x.

[14] Félix L, Antunes L, Campos S, Venâncio C, Coimbra AM. Recreational use of ketamine and its interaction with NMDA receptors. In: Preedy VR, editor. Neuropathology of drug addictions and substance misuse, vol. 2. Cambridge: Academic Press; 2016. p. 672-680. DOI: https://doi.org/10.1016/C2013-0-14225-0.

[15] Lockwood B. Ketamine: dangerous hallucinogen. New York: Rosen

Publishing Group; 2007. ISBN: 9781404209114

[16] Morgan CJ, Mofeez A, Brandner B, Bromley L, Curran HV. Acute effects of ketamine on memory systems and psychotic symptoms in healthy volunteers. Neuropsychopharmacol., 2004;29:208-218. DOI: 10.1038/sj.npp.1300342.

[17] Morgan CJ, Monaghan L, Curran HV. Beyond the K-hole: a 3-year longitudinal investigation of the cognitive and subjective effects of ketamine in recreational users who have substantially reduced their use of the drug. Addiction, 2004;99:1450-1461. DOI: 10.1111/j.1360-0443.2004.00879.x.

[18] Muetzelfeldt L, Kamboj SK, Rees H, Taylor J, Morgan CJ, Curran HV. Journey through the K-hole: phenomenological aspects of ketamine use. Drug Alcohol Depend., 2008;95:219-229. DOI: 10.1016/j.drugalcdep.2008.01.024.

[19] Chen WJ, Fu TC, Ting TT, Huang WL, Tang GM, Hsiao CK, Chen CY. Use of ecstasy and other psychoactive substances among school-attending adolescents in Taiwan: national surveys 2004-2006. BMC Public Health, 2009;9:27. DOI: 10.1186/1471-2458-9-27.

[20] Lua AC, Lin HR, Tseng YT, Hu AR, Yeh PC. Profiles of urine samples from participants at rave party in Taiwan: prevalence of ketamine and MDMA abuse. Forensic Sci. Int., 2003;136: 47-51. DOI: 10.1016/S0379-0738(03)00261-5.

[21] Li N, Liu RJ, Dwyer JM, Banasr M, Lee B, Son H, Li XY, Aghajanian G, Duman RS. Glutamate N-methyl-D-aspartate receptor antagonists rapidly reverse behavioral and synaptic deficits caused by chronic stress exposure. Biol. Psychiatry, 2011;69:754-761. DOI: 10.1016/j.biopsych.2010.12.015.

[22] Yen CF, Hsu SY, Cheng CP. Polysubstance use and its correlates in adolescent ecstasy users in Taiwan. Addict. Behav., 2007;32:2286-2291. DOI: 10.1016/j.addbeh.2007.01.022.

[23] Orhurhu VJ, Vashisht R; Claus LE, Cohen SP. Ketamine toxicity. In: StatPearls [Internet]. Treasure Island (FL): StatPearls Publishing; 2021. Available from: https://www.ncbi.nlm.nih.gov/books/NBK541087/ {accessed: 2021-08-04]

[24] Home Office (2014) The misuse of drugs act 1971 (ketamine etc.) (amendment) order 2014. SI 2014 No. 1106. Available from: http://www.legislation.gov.uk/uksi/2014/1106/pdfs/uksi_20141106_en.pdf [Accessed: 2021-08-01]

[25] Winstock A. Mixmag global drug survey 2013 [Internet]. 2013. Available from: https://issuu.com/mixmagfashion/docs/mm_may13_drug_survey [Accessed: 2021-07-27]

[26] Winstock A, Barratt M, Ferris J, Maier L. Global drug survey 2016: What we learned from GDS2016 – An overview of our key findings [Internet]. 2016. Available from: https://www.globaldrugsurvey.com/wp-content/uploads/2016/06/TASTER-KEY-FINDINGS-FROM-GDS2016.pdf [Accessed: 2021-08-14]

[27] ONS. Deaths related to drug poisoning involving specific substances, England and Wales, deaths registered in 2016 [Internet]. 2017. Available from: https://www.ons.gov.uk/peoplepopulationandcommunity/birthsdeathsandmarriages/deaths/bulletins/deatsrelatedtodrugpoisoningi nenglandandwales/2016registration [Accessed: 2021-07-23]

[28] Peacock A, Price O, Dietze P, et al. Impacts of COVID-19 and associated restrictions on people who use illicit stimulants in Australia: Findings from

the ecstasy and related drugs reporting system 2020. Drug Trends Bulletin Series. Sydney: National Drug and Alcohol Research Centre, UNSW [Internet]. 2020. Available from: https://ndarc.med.unsw.edu.au/sites/default/files/ndarc/resources/COVID%20EDRS%20bulletin_National_20200917.pdf. [Accessed: 2021-08-23]

[29] Sutherland R, Baillie G, Memedovic S, et al., Key findings from the 'Australians' drug use: adapting to pandemic threats (ADAPT)' study. ADAPT Bulletin No. 1. Sydney: National Drug and Alcohol Research Centre, UNSW [Internet]. 2020. Available from: https://6d4c02d1-3362-4c6f-a837-b46833d5b1a5.filesusr.com/ugd/8a9f74_c264d95a82f14b0fbd68031668d6d77b.pdf [Accessed: 2021-08-01]

[30] EMCDDA. Impact of COVID-19 on patterns of drug use and drug-related harms in Europe. June 2020, Lisbone: Publications Office of the European Union [Internet]. 2020. Available from: https://www.emcdda.europa.eu/publications/ad-hoc-publication/impact-covid-19-patterns-drug-use-and-harms_en [Accessed: 2021-08-01]

[31] National Institute on Drug Abuse. Monitoring the future study: trends in prevalence of various drugs [Internet]. 2020. Available from: https://www.drugabuse.gov/drug-topics/trends-statistics/monitoring-future/monitoring-future-study-trends-in-prevalence-various-drugs [Accessed: 2021-07-28] [Accessed: 2021-07-28]

[32] Lhoog M. People are using ketamine at home to escape their pandemic reality [Internet]. 2020. Available from: https://www.vice.com/en/article/akddya/people-are-using-ketamine-to-escape-pandemic-reality-covid-19

[33] Corkery JM, Hung WC, Claridge H, Goodair C, Copeland CS, Schifano F. Recreational ketamine-related deaths notified to the National Programme on Substance Abuse Deaths, England, 1997-2019. J. Psychopharmacol., 2021;5:2698811211021588. DOI: 10.1177/02698811211021588.

[34] Preuss CV, Kalava A, King KC. Prescription of controlled substances: benefits and risks. In: StatPearls [Internet]. Treasure Island (FL): StatPearls Publishing; 2021. Available from: https://pubmed.ncbi.nlm.nih.gov/30726003/ [Accessed: 2021-08-20]

[35] UNODC. World Drug Report United Nations publication [Internet]. 2021. Available from: https://www.unodc.org/unodc/en/frontpage/ketamine-sweeps-the-rave-scene.html [Accessed: 2021-07-25]

[36] Kalsi SS, Wood DM, Dargan PI. The epidemiology and patterns of acute and chronic toxicity associated with recreational ketamine use. Emerg. Health Threats J., 2011;4:7107. DOI: 10.3402/ehtj.v4i0.7107.

[37] Jansen KL. A review of the nonmedical use of ketamine: use, users and consequences. J. Psychoactive Drugs., 2000;32:419-433. DOI: 10.1080/02791072.2000.10400244.

[38] Gable RS. Acute toxic effects of club drugs. J. Psychoactive Drugs, 2004;36:303-313. DOI: 10.1080/02791072.2004.10400031.

[39] Shram MJ, Sellers EM, Romach MK. Oral ketamine as a positive control in human abuse potential studies. Drug Alcohol Depend., 2011;114:185-193. DOI: 10.1016/j.drugalcdep.2010.10.002.

[40] EMCDDA. Report on the risk assessment of ketamine in the framework of the joint action on new synthetic drugs. June 2020, Lisbone: Publications Office of the European Union [Internet]. 2002. Available from: https://www.emcdda.europa.eu/publications/risk-assessments/ketamine_en [Accessed: 2021-08-13]

[41] Nicol AU, Morton AJ. Characteristic patterns of EEG oscillations in sheep (Ovis aries) induced by ketamine may explain the psychotropic effects seen in humans. Sci. Rep., 2020;10:9440. DOI: 10.1038/s41598-020-66023-8.

[42] Blundell M, Dargan P, Wood D. A cloud on the horizon - a survey into the use of electronic vaping devices for recreational drug and new psychoactive substance (NPS) administration. QJM, 2018;111:9-14. DOI: 10.1093/qjmed/hcx178.

[43] Thurtle N, Abouchedid R, Archer JR, Ho J, Yamamoto T, Dargan PI, Wood DM. Prevalence of use of electronic nicotine delivery systems (ENDS) to vape recreational drugs by club patrons in South London. J. Med. Toxicol., 2017;13:61-65. DOI: 10.1007/s13181-016-0583-3.

[44] Siegel RK. Phencyclidine and ketamine intoxication: a study of four populations of recreational users. NIDA Res Monogr., 1978;21:119-147. PMID: 101865.

[45] Malhotra A, Pinals D, Weingartner H, Sirocco MA, Missar CD, Pickar D, Breier A. NMDA receptor function and human cognition: The effects of ketamine in healthy volunteers. Neuropsychopharmacol., 1996;14: 301-307. DOI: 10.1016/0893-133X(95)00137-3.

[46] Hansen G, Jensen SB, Chandresh L, Hilden T. The psychotropic effect of ketamine. J. Psychoactive Drugs., 1988;20:419-425. DOI: 10.1080/02791072.1988.10472511.

[47] Lahti AC, Holcomb HH, Medoff DR, Tamminga CA. Ketamine activates psychosis and alters limbic blood flow in schizophrenia. Neuroreport, 1995;6:869-872. DOI: 10.1097/00001756-199504190-00011.

[48] Javitt D. Glutamate as a therapeutic target in psychiatric disorders. Mol. Psychiatry, 2004;9:984-997. DOI: 10.1038/sj.mp.4001551.

[49] Javitt DC, Zukin SR. Recent advances in the phencyclidine model of schizophrenia. Am. J. Psychiatry, 1991;148:1301-1308. DOI: 10.1176/ajp.148.10.1301.

[50] Curran HV, Morgan C. Cognitive, dissociative and psychotogenic effects of ketamine in recreational users on the night of drug use and 3 days later. Addiction, 2000;95:575-590. DOI: 10.1046/j.1360-0443.2000.9545759.x.

[51] Zhang C, Xu Y, Zhang B, Hao W, Tang WK. Cognitive impairment in chronic ketamine abusers. Psychiatry Res., 2020;291:113206. DOI: 10.1016/j.psychres.2020.113206.

[52] Curran HV, Monaghan L. In and out of the K-hole: a comparison of the acute and residual effects of ketamine in frequent and infrequent ketamine users. Addiction, 2001;96:749-760. DOI: 10.1046/j.1360-0443.2001.96574910.x.

[53] Morgan CJ, Muetzelfeldt L, Curran HV. Consequences of chronic ketamine self-administration upon neurocognitive function and psychological wellbeing: a 1-year longitudinal study. Addiction, 2010;105:121-133. DOI: 10.1111/j.1360-0443.2009.02761.x.

[54] Moghaddam B, Adams B, Verma A, Daly D. Activation of glutamatergic neurotransmission by ketamine: a novel step in the pathway from NMDA receptor blockade to dopaminergic and cognitive disruptions associated with the prefrontal cortex. J. Neurosci., 1997;17:2921-2927. DOI: 10.1523/JNEUROSCI.17-08-02921.1997.

[55] Duan TT, Tan JW, Yuan Q, Cao J, Zhou QX, Xu L. Acute ketamine induces hippocampal synaptic depression and

spatial memory impairment through dopamine D1/D5 receptors. Psychopharmacology (Berl)., 2013;228:451-461. DOI: 10.1007/s00213-013-3048-2.

[56] Morgan CJ, Perry EB, Cho HS, Krystal JH, D'Souza DC. Greater vulnerability to the amnestic effects of ketamine in males. Psychopharmacology (Berl)., 2006;187:405-414. DOI: 10.1007/s00213-006-0409-0.

[57] Li JH, Vicknasingam B, Cheung YW, Zhou W, Nurhidayat AW, Jarlais DC, Schottenfeld R. To use or not to use: an update on licit and illicit ketamine use. Subst. Abuse Rehabil., 2011;2:11-20. DOI: 10.2147/SAR.S15458.

[58] Wong OF, Tsui KL, Lam TS, Sze NN, Wong SC, Lau FL, Liu SH. Prevalence of drugged drivers among non-fatal driver casualties presenting to a trauma centre in Hong Kong. Hong Kong Med. J., 2010;16:246-251. PMID: 20683065.

[59] Durieux ME. Inhibition by ketamine of muscarinic acetylcholine receptor function. Anesth. Analg., 1995;81:57-62. DOI: 10.1097/00000539-199507000-00012.

[60] Rabiner EA. Imaging of striatal dopamine release elicited with NMDA antagonists: is there anything there to be seen? J. Psychopharmacol., 2007;21:253-258. DOI: 10.1177/0269881107077767.

[61] Anis NA, Berry SC, Burton NR, Lodge D. The dissociative anaesthetics, ketamine and phencyclidine, selectively reduce excitation of central mammalian neurones by N-methyl-aspartate. Br. J. Pharmacol., 1983;79:565-575. DOI: 10.1111/j.1476-5381.1983.tb11031.x.

[62] Irifune M, Sato T, Kamata Y, Nishikawa T, Dohi T, Kawahara M. Evidence for GABA(A) receptor agonistic properties of ketamine: convulsive and anesthetic behavioral models in mice. Anesth. Analg., 2000;91:230-236. DOI: 10.1097/00000539-200007000-00043.

[63] Kovelman JA, Scheibel AB. A neurohistological correlate of schizophrenia. Biol. Psychiatry., 1984;19:1601-1621. PMID: 6518211.

[64] Ikonomidou C, Bosch F, Miksa M, Bittigau P, Vöckler J, Dikranian K, Tenkova TI, Stefovska V, Turski L, Olney JW. Blockade of NMDA receptors and apoptotic neurodegeneration in the developing brain. Science, 1999;283:70-74. DOI: 10.1126/science.283.5398.70.

[65] Green SM, Coté CJ. Ketamine and neurotoxicity: clinical perspectives and implications for emergency medicine. Ann. Emerg. Med., 2009;54:181-190. DOI: 10.1016/j.annemergmed.2008.10.003.

[66] Walker SM, Westin BD, Deumens R, Grafe M, Yaksh TL. Effects of intrathecal ketamine in the neonatal rat: evaluation of apoptosis and long-term functional outcome. Anesthesiology, 2010;113:147-159. DOI: 10.1097/ALN.0b013e3181dcd71c.

[67] Walker SM, Yaksh TL. Neuraxial analgesia in neonates and infants: a review of clinical and preclinical strategies for the development of safety and efficacy data. Anesth. Analg., 2012;115:638-662. DOI: 10.1213/ANE.0b013e31826253f2.

[68] Davidson A, Flick RP. Neurodevelopmental implications of the use of sedation and analgesia in neonates. Clin. Perinatol., 2013;40:559-573. DOI: 10.1016/j.clp.2013.05.009.

[69] Liao Y, Tang J, Corlett PR, Wang X, Yang M, Chen H, Liu T, Chen X, Hao W, Fletcher PC. Reduced dorsal prefrontal gray matter after chronic ketamine use. Biol. Psychiatry, 2011;69:42-48. DOI: 10.1016/j.biopsych.2010.08.030.

[70] Wang C, Zheng D, Xu J, Lam W, Yew DT. Brain damages in ketamine addicts as revealed by magnetic resonance imaging. Front. Neuroanat., 2013;7:23. DOI: 10.3389/fnana.2013.00023.

[71] Farber NB, Hanslick J, Kirby C, McWilliams L, Olney JW. Serotonergic agents that activate 5HT2A receptors prevent NMDA antagonist neurotoxicity. Neuropsychopharmacology, 1998;18:57-62. DOI: 10.1016/S0893-133X(97)00127-9.

[72] Sofuoglu M. Cognitive enhancement as a pharmacotherapy target for stimulant addiction. Addiction, 2010;105:38-48. DOI: 10.1111/j.1360-0443.2009.02791.x.

[73] Chang H, Huang MC, Chen LY. Major Depressive Disorder induced by chronic ketamine abuse: A case report. Prim. Care Companion CNS Disord., 2016;18:10.4088/PCC.15l01881. DOI: 10.4088/PCC.15l01881.

[74] McGirr A, Berlim MT, Bond DJ, Fleck MP, Yatham LN, Lam RW. A systematic review and meta-analysis of randomized, double-blind, placebo-controlled trials of ketamine in the rapid treatment of major depressive episodes. Psychol. Med., 2015;45:693-704. DOI: 10.1017/S0033291714001603.

[75] aan het Rot M, Collins KA, Murrough JW, Perez AM, Reich DL, Charney DS, Mathew SJ. Safety and efficacy of repeated-dose intravenous ketamine for treatment-resistant depression. Biol. Psychiatry, 2010;67:139-145. DOI: 10.1016/j.biopsych.2009.08.038.

[76] Trujillo KA, Smith ML, Sullivan B, Heller CY, Garcia C, Bates M. The neurobehavioral pharmacology of ketamine: implications for drug abuse, addiction, and psychiatric disorders. ILAR J., 2011;52:366-78. DOI: 10.1093/ilar.52.3.366.

[77] Fan N, Xu K, Ning Y, Rosenheck R, Wang D, Ke X, Ding Y, Sun B, Zhou C, Deng X, Tang W, He H. Profiling the psychotic, depressive and anxiety symptoms in chronic ketamine users. Psychiatry Res., 2016;237:311-315. DOI: 10.1016/j.psychres.2016.01.023.

[78] Tang WK, Liang HJ, Lau CG, Tang A, Ungvari GS. Relationship between cognitive impairment and depressive symptoms in current ketamine users. J. Stud. Alcohol Drugs., 2013;74:460-468. DOI: 10.15288/jsad.2013.74.460.

[79] Liang HJ, Tang KL, Chan F, Ungvari GS, Tang WK. Ketamine users have high rates of psychosis and/or depression. J. Addict. Nurs., 2015;26:8-13. DOI: 10.1097/JAN.0000000000000060.

[80] Tang WK, Morgan CJ, Lau GC, Liang HJ, Tang A, Ungvari GS. Psychiatric morbidity in ketamine users attending counselling and youth outreach services. Subst. Abuse, 2015;36:67-74. DOI: 10.1080/08897077.2014.935560.

[81] Chen LY, Chen CK, Chen CH, Chang HM, Huang MC, Xu K. Association of craving and depressive symptoms in ketamine-dependent patients undergoing withdrawal treatment. Am. J. Addict., 2020;29:43-50. DOI: 10.1111/ajad.12978.

[82] de Win MM, Reneman L, Jager G, Vlieger EJ, Olabarriaga SD, Lavini C, Bisschops I, Majoie CB, Booij J, den Heeten GJ, van den Brink W. A prospective cohort study on sustained effects of low-dose ecstasy use on the brain in new ecstasy users. Neuropsychopharmacology, 2007;32:458-470. DOI: 10.1038/sj.npp.1301225.

[83] Watts M. Understanding the coexistence of alcohol misuse and depression. Br. J. Nurs.,

2008;17:696-699. DOI: 10.12968/bjon.2008.17.11.29614.

[84] Palomo T, Archer T, Kostrzewa RM, Beninger RJ. Comorbidity of substance abuse with other psychiatric disorders. Neurotox. Res., 2007;1217-27. DOI: 10.1007/BF03033898.

[85] Bonnet U. Long-term ketamine self-injections in Major Depressive Disorder: focus on tolerance in ketamine's antidepressant response and the development of ketamine addiction. J. Psychoactive Drugs, 2015;47:276-285. DOI: 10.1080/02791072.2015.1072653.

[86] Cumming JF. The development of an acute tolerance to ketamine. Anesth. Analg., 1976;55:788-791. DOI: 10.1213/00000539-197611000-00008.

[87] Meliska CJ, Trevor AJ. Differential effects of ketamine on schedule-controlled responding and motility. Pharmacol. Biochem. Behav., 1978;8:679-683. DOI: 10.1016/0091-3057(78)90266-6.

[88] Gerb SA, Cook JE, Gochenauer AE, Young CS, Fulton LK, Grady AW, Freeman KB. Ketamine tolerance in Sprague-Dawley rats after chronic administration of ketamine, morphine, or cocaine. Comp. Med., 2019;69:29-34. DOI: 10.30802/AALAS-CM-18-000053.

[89] Monaghan DT, Bridges RJ, Cotman CW. The excitatory amino acid receptors: their classes, pharmacology, and distinct properties in the function of the central nervous system. Ann. Rev. Pharmacol. Toxicol., 1989;29:365-402. DOI: 10.1146/annurev.pa.29.040189.002053.

[90] Yang C, Hashimoto K. Rapid antidepressant effects and abuse liability of ketamine. Psychopharmacology (Berl)., 2014;231:2041-2042. DOI: 10.1007/s00213-014-3543-0.

[91] Critchlow DG. A case of ketamine dependence with discontinuation symptoms. Addiction, 2006;101:1212-1213. DOI: 10.1111/j.1360-0443.2006.01494.x.

[92] Lim DK. Ketamine associated psychedelic effects and dependence. Singapore Med. J., 2003;44:31-34. PMID: 12762561.

[93] Lerner A, Klein M. Dependence, withdrawal and rebound of CNS drugs: an update and regulatory considerations for new drugs development. Brain Commun., 2019;1:fcz025. DOI: 10.1093/braincomms/fcz025.

[94] Schifano N, Chiappini S, Castiglione F, Salonia A, Schifano F. Is medicinal ketamine associated with urinary dysfunction issues? Assessment of both the European Medicines Agency (EMA) and the UK Yellow Card Scheme pharmacovigilance database-related reports. Low Urine Tract Sympt., 2021;13:230-237. DOI: 10.1111/luts.12355.

[95] Baker SC, Shabir S, Georgopoulos NT, Southgate J. Ketamine-induced apoptosis in normal human urothelial cells: A direct, N-Methyl-D-Aspartate receptor-independent pathway characterized by mitochondrial stress. Am. J. Pathol., 2016;186:1267-1277. DOI: 10.1016/j.ajpath.2015.12.014.

[96] Winstock, AR, Barratt, MJ, Maier, LJ, et al. GDS2018 key findings report, 9 May. London: Global Drug Survey [Internet]. 2018. Available at: https://www.globaldrugsurvey.com/gds-2018/ [Accessed: 2021-09-01].

[97] Shahani R, Streutker C, Dickson B, Stewart RJ. Ketamine-associated ulcerative cystitis: a new clinical entity. Urology, 2007;69:810-812. DOI: 10.1016/j.urology.2007.01.038.

[98] Bokor G, Anderson PD. Ketamine: an update on its abuse. J. Pharm. Pract.,

2014;27:582-586. DOI: 10.1177/0897190014525754.

[99] Chu PS, Kwok SC, Lam KM, Chu TY, Chan SW, Man CW, Ma WK, Chui KL, Yiu MK, Chan YC, Tse ML, Lau FL. 'Street ketamine'-associated bladder dysfunction: a report of ten cases. Hong Kong Med. J., 2007;13:311-313. PMID: 17592176.

[100] Chu PS, Ma WK, Wong SC, Chu RW, Cheng CH, Wong S, Tse JM, Lau FL, Yiu MK, Man CW. The destruction of the lower urinary tract by ketamine abuse: a new syndrome? BJU Int., 2008;102:1616-1622. DOI: 10.1111/j.1464-410X.2008.07920.x.

[101] Chen CH, Lee MH, Chen YC, Lin MF. Ketamine-snorting associated cystitis. J. Formos. Med. Assoc., 2011;110:787-791. DOI: 10.1016/j.jfma.2011.11.010.

[102] Hopcroft SA, Cottrell AM, Mason K, Abrams P, Oxley JD. Ureteric intestinal metaplasia in association with chronic recreational ketamine abuse. J. Clin. Pathol., 2011;64:551-552. DOI: 10.1136/jcp.2010.087171.

[103] Tsai TH, Cha TL, Lin CM, Tsao CW, Tang SH, Chuang FP, Wu ST, Sun GH, Yu DS, Chang SY. Ketamine-associated bladder dysfunction. Int. J. Urol., 2009;16:826-829. DOI: 10.1111/j.1442-2042.2009.02361.x.

[104] Wang J, Chen Y, Gu D, Zhang G, Chen J, Zhao J, Wu P. Ketamine-induced bladder fibrosis involves epithelial-to-mesenchymal transition mediated by transforming growth factor-β1. Am. J. Physiol. Renal Physiol., 2017;313: F961-F972. DOI: 10.1152/ajprenal.00686.2016.

[105] Mason K, Cottrell AM, Corrigan AG, Gillatt DA, Mitchelmore AE. Ketamine-associated lower urinary tract destruction: a new radiological challenge. Clin. Radiol., 2010;65:795-800. DOI: 10.1016/j.crad.2010.05.003.

[106] Middela S, Pearce I. Ketamine-induced vesicopathy: a literature review. Int. J. Clin. Pract., 2011;65:27-30. DOI: 10.1111/j.1742-1241.2010.02502.x.

[107] Castellani D, Pirola GM, Gubbiotti M, Rubilotta E, Gudaru K, Gregori A, Dellabella M. What urologists need to know about ketamine-induced uropathy: A systematic review. Neurourol. Urodyn., 2020;39:1049-1062. DOI: 10.1002/nau.24341.

[108] Cheung RY, Chan SS, Lee JH, Pang AW, Choy KW, Chung TK. Urinary symptoms and impaired quality of life in female ketamine users: persistence after cessation of use. Hong Kong Med. J., 2011;17:267-273. PMID: 21813893.

[109] Dick D, Torrance C. 'Mixmag drugs survey', Mixmag, 2010;225:44-53 [Internet]. 2010. Available from: https://issuu.com/mixmagfashion/docs/drug_survey_2010 [Accessed: 2021-08-29]

[110] Poon TL, Wong KF, Chan MY, Fung KW, Chu SK, Man CW, Yiu MK, Leung SK. Upper gastrointestinal problems in inhalational ketamine abusers. J. Dig. Dis., 2010;11:106-110. DOI: 10.1111/j.1751-2980.2010.00424.x.

[111] Selby NM, Anderson J, Bungay P, Chesterton LJ, Kolhe NV. Obstructive nephropathy and kidney injury associated with ketamine abuse. NDT Plus, 2008;1:310-312. DOI: 10.1093/ndtplus/sfn054.

[112] Ng SH, Lee HK, Chan YC, Lau FL. Dilated common bile ducts in ketamine abusers. Hong Kong Med. J., 2009;15: 157. PMID: 19342747.

[113] Wong SW, Lee KF, Wong J, Ng WW, Cheung YS, Lai PB. Dilated common bile ducts mimicking choledochal cysts in ketamine abusers. Hong Kong Med. J., 2009;15:53-56. PMID: 19197097.

[114] Zielmann S, Grote R. Auswirkungen der Langzeitsedierung auf die intestinale Funktion [The effects of long-term sedation on intestinal function]. Anaesthesist, 1995;44Suppl3:S549-58. PMID: 8592966.

[115] Yu WL, Cho CC, Lung PF, Hung EH, Hui JW, Chau HH, Chan AW, Ahuja AT. Ketamine-related cholangiopathy: a retrospective study on clinical and imaging findings. Abdom. Imaging., 2014;39:1241-1246. DOI: 10.1007/s00261-014-0173-2.

[116] Lo RS, Krishnamoorthy R, Freeman JG, Austin AS. Cholestasis and biliary dilatation associated with chronic ketamine abuse: a case series. Singapore Med. J., 2011;52:e52-55. PMID: 21451916.

[117] Lo JN, Cumming JF. Interaction between sedative premedicants and ketamine in man in isolated perfused rat livers. Anesthesiology, 1975;43:307-312. DOI: 10.1097/00000542-197509000-00007.

[118] Domino EF, Domino SE, Smith RE, Domino LE, Goulet JR, Domino KE, Zsigmond EK. Ketamine kinetics in unmedicated and diazepam-premedicated subjects. Clin. Pharmacol. Ther., 1984;36:645-653. DOI: 10.1038/clpt.1984.235.

[119] Sweeney BP, Bromilow J. Liver enzyme induction and inhibition: implications for anaesthesia. Anaesthesia, 2006;61:159-177. DOI: 10.1111/j.1365-2044.2005.04462.x.

[120] Domino EF, Chodoff P, Corssen G. Pharmacologic effects of CI-581, a new dissociative anesthetic, in man. Clin. Pharmacol. Ther., 1965;6:279-291. DOI: 10.1002/cpt196563279.

[121] Lilius TO, Jokinen V, Neuvonen MS, Niemi M, Kalso EA, Rauhala PV. Ketamine coadministration attenuates morphine tolerance and leads to increased brain concentrations of both drugs in the rat. Br. J. Pharmacol., 2015;172:2799-2813. DOI: 10.1111/bph.12974.

[122] Lalovic B, Kharasch E, Hoffer C, Risler L, Liu-Chen LY, Shen DD. Pharmacokinetics and pharmacodynamics of oral oxycodone in healthy human subjects: role of circulating active metabolites. Clin Pharmacol Ther., 2006;79:461-479. DOI: 10.1016/j.clpt.2006.01.009.

[123] Lilius T, Kangas E, Niemi M, Rauhala P, Kalso E. Ketamine and norketamine attenuate oxycodone tolerance markedly less than that of morphine: from behaviour to drug availability. Br. J. Anaesth., 2018;120:818-826. DOI: 10.1016/j.bja.2017.11.081.

[124] Fuhr U. Drug interactions with grapefruit juice. Extent, probable mechanism and clinical relevance. Drug Saf., 1998;18:251-272. DOI: 10.2165/00002018-199818040-00002.

[125] Peltoniemi MA, Saari TI, Hagelberg NM, Laine K, Neuvonen PJ, Olkkola KT. S-ketamine concentrations are greatly increased by grapefruit juice. Eur. J. Clin. Pharmacol., 2012;68:979-986. DOI: 10.1007/s00228-012-1214-9.

[126] Rao LK, Flaker AM, Friedel CC, Kharasch ED. Role of Cytochrome P4502B6 polymorphisms in ketamine metabolism and clearance. Anesthesiology, 2016;125:1103-1112. DOI: 10.1097/ALN.0000000000001392.

[127] Carrier N, Kabbaj M. Sex differences in the antidepressant-like

effects of ketamine. Neuropharmacology, 2013;70:27-34. DOI: 10.1016/j.neuropharm.2012.12.009.

[128] Zoupa E, Gravanis A, Pitsikas N. The novel dehydroepiandrosterone (DHEA) derivative BNN27 counteracts behavioural deficits induced by the NMDA receptor antagonist ketamine in rats. Neuropharmacology, 2019;151:74-83. DOI: 10.1016/j.neuropharm.2019.04.001.

[129] Roytblat L, Katz J, Rozentsveig V, Gesztes T, Bradley EL Jr, Kissin I. Anaesthetic interaction between thiopentone and ketamine. Eur. J. Anaesthesiol., 1992;9:307-312. PMID: 1628634.

[130] Hong W, Short TG, Hui TW. Hypnotic and anesthetic interactions between ketamine and midazolam in female patients. Anesthesiology, 1993;79:1227-1232. DOI: 10.1097/00000542-199312000-00013.

[131] Andrashko V, Novak T, Brunovsky M, Klirova M, Sos P, Horacek J. The antidepressant effect of ketamine is dampened by concomitant benzodiazepine medication. Front. Psychiatry, 2020;11:844. DOI: 10.3389/fpsyt.2020.00844.

[132] Ford N, Ludbrook G, Galletly C. Benzodiazepines may reduce the effectiveness of ketamine in the treatment of depression. Aust. N.Z. J. Psychiatry, 2015;49:1227. DOI: 10.1177/0004867415590631.

[133] Irifune M, Sato T, Kamata Y, Nishikawa T, Nomoto M, Fukuda T, Kawahara M. Inhibition by diazepam of ketamine-induced hyperlocomotion and dopamine turnover in mice. Can. J. Anaesth., 199;45:471-478. DOI: 10.1007/BF03012584.

[134] Krystal JH, Karper LP, Bennett A, D'Souza DC, Abi-Dargham A, Morrissey K, Abi-Saab D, Bremner JD, Bowers MB Jr, Suckow RF, Stetson P, Heninger GR, Charney DS. Interactive effects of subanesthetic ketamine and subhypnotic lorazepam in humans. Psychopharmacology (Berl)., 1998;135:213-229. DOI: 10.1007/s002130050503.

[135] Tobin HA. Low-dose ketamine and diazepam. Use as an adjunct to local anesthesia in an office operating room. Arch. Otolaryngol., 1982;108:439-440. DOI: 10.1001/archotol.1982.00790550043011.

[136] Erdmann W, Salt PJ, Agoston S, Langrehr D. Antagonism of the cardiovascular effects of ketamine by diazepam in volunteers. Acta Anaesthesiol. Belg., 1979;30:239-245. PMID: 549439.

[137] Morse Z, Sano K, Kanri T. Effects of a midazolam-ketamine admixture in human volunteers. Anesth. Prog., 2004;51:76-79. PMID: 15497296.

[138] Arruda MDOV, Soares PM, Honório JER, Lima RCDS, Chaves EMC, Lobato RDFG, Martin ALDAR, Sales GTM, Carvalho KDM, Assreuy AMS, de Brito EM, Vasconcelos SMM. Activities of the antipsychotic drugs haloperidol and risperidone on behavioural effects induced by ketamine in mice.Scientia Pharmaceutica, 2008;76:673-688. DOI: 10.3797/scipharm.0810-11.

[139] Smith DJ, Bouchal RL, deSanctis CA, Monroe PJ, Amedro JB, Perrotti JM, Crisp T. Properties of the interaction between ketamine and opiate binding sites in vivo and in vitro. Neuropharmacology, 1987;26:1253-1260. DOI: 10.1016/0028-3908(87)90084-0.

[140] Trujillo KA, Akil H. Inhibition of opiate tolerance by non-competitive N-methyl-D-aspartate receptor antagonists. Brain Res., 1994;633:

178-188. DOI: 10.1016/0006-8993(94)91538-5.

[141] Williams NR, Heifets BD, Blasey C, Sudheimer K, Pannu J, Pankow H, Hawkins J, Birnbaum J, Lyons DM, Rodriguez CI, Schatzberg AF. Attenuation of antidepressant effects of ketamine by opioid receptor antagonism. Am. J. Psychiatry, 2018;175:1205-1215. DOI: 10.1176/appi.ajp.2018.18020138.

[142] Marton T, Barnes DE, Wallace A, Woolley JD. Concurrent use of buprenorphine, methadone, or naltrexone does not inhibit ketamine's antidepressant activity. Biol. Psychiatry, 2019;85:e75-e76. DOI: 10.1016/j.biopsych.2019.02.008.

[143] Sarton E, Teppema LJ, Olievier C, Nieuwenhuijs D, Matthes HW, Kieffer BL, Dahan A. The involvement of the mu-opioid receptor in ketamine-induced respiratory depression and antinociception. Anesth. Analg., 2001;93:1495-1500.DOI:10.1097/00000539-200112000-00031.

[144] Global Drug Survey. The high-way code: Ketamine [Internet]. 2014. Available from: https://www.globaldrugsurvey.com/wp-content/uploads/2014/04/The-High-Way-Code_Ketamine.pdf [Accessed: 2021-08-03]

[145] Kwatra NV, Morris ME. Toxicokinetic/toxicodynamic interaction studies in rats between the drugs of abuse γ-Hydroxybutyric acid and ketamine and treatment strategies for overdose. Pharmaceutics, 2021;13:741. DOI: 10.3390/pharmaceutics13050741.

[146] Koek W, France CP. Cataleptic effects of gamma-hydroxybutyrate (GHB) and baclofen in mice: mediation by GABA(B) receptors, but differential enhancement by N-methyl-d-aspartate (NMDA) receptor antagonists. Psychopharmacology (Berl)., 2008;199:191-198. DOI: 10.1007/s00213-008-1160-5.

[147] Liang Z, Yin P, Zhao L. Effects of combined toxicity of methamphetamine and ketamine on apoptosis, oxidative stress and genotoxicity in HepG2 cells. Food Chem. Toxicol., 2019;132:110653. DOI: 10.1016/j.fct.2019.110653.

[148] Hayase T, Yamamoto Y, Yamamoto K. Behavioral effects of ketamine and toxic interactions with psychostimulants. BMC Neurosci., 2006;7:25. DOI: 10.1186/1471-2202-7-25.

[149] Xu DD, Mo ZX, Yung KK, Yang Y, Leung AW. Individual and combined effects of methamphetamine and ketamine on conditioned place preference and NR1 receptor phosphorylation in rats. Neurosignals, 2006-2007;15(6):322-331. DOI: 10.1159/000127492.

[150] Dong H, Yang C, Shen Y, Liu L, Liu M, Hao W. Effects of ketamine use on psychotic disorders and symptoms in male, methamphetamine-dependent subjects. Am. J. Drug Alcohol Abuse, 2019;45:276-284. DOI: 10.1080/00952990.2018.1559849.

[151] Rofael HZ. Effect of ketamine pretreatment on cocaine-mediated hepatotoxicity in rats. Toxicol. Lett., 2004;152:213-222. DOI: 10.1016/j.toxlet.2004.04.035.

[152] Slomski A. Ketamine to help treat cocaine use disorder. JAMA, 2019;322:717. DOI: 10.1001/jama.2019.12352.

[153] Kohrs R, Durieux ME. Ketamine: teaching an old drug new tricks. Anesth. Analg., 1998;87:1186-1193. DOI: 10.1097/00000539-199811000-00039.

[154] Contreras CM, Marvan ML, Mexicano G, Puente A, Morfin A. Ketamine antagonizes toxic action of

anticholinesterase agents. Bol. Estud. Med. Biol., 1990;38:10-15. PMID: 2291776.

[155] Toro-Matos A, Rendon-Platas AM, Avila-Valdez E, Villarreal-Guzman RA. Physostigmine antagonizes ketamine. Anesth. Analg., 1980;59:764-767. PMID: 6999946.

[156] Balmer HGR. The reversal of ketamine sedation by physostigmine. In: Proc. Sixth World Congress of Anaesthesiology, 24-30 April 1976; Mexico City. p. 222-223

[157] Drummond JC, Brebner J, Galloon S, Young PS. A randomized evaluation of the reversal of ketamine by physostigmine. Can. Anaesth. Soc. J., 1979;26:288-295. DOI: 10.1007/BF03006289.

[158] Hess L. Is the combination of alpha2 agonist-ketamine suitable for human anaesthesia? Anesteziologie Intenz. Med., 2004;15:74-80 [Internet]. Available from: https://www.aimjournal.cz/en/artkey/aim-200402-0003_is-the-combination-of-alpha2-agonist-ketamin-suitable-for-human-anaesthesia.php [Accessed: 2021-08-03]

[159] Zhang GF, Liu WX, Qiu LL, Guo J, Wang XM, Sun HL, Yang JJ, Zhou ZQ. Repeated ketamine administration redeems the time lag for citalopram's antidepressant-like effects. Eur. Psychiatry, 2015;30:504-510. DOI: 10.1016/j.eurpsy.2014.11.007.

[160] Sheikh S, Sonone P, Verma V, Tripathi CD, Karim BA, et al. Ketamine, a better antidepressant? An animam study evaluating the efficacy of citalopram, ketamine and their combination in animal models of depression. J. Neurol. Neurol. Sci. Disord., 2021;7:019-023. DOI: 10.17352/jnnsd.000043

[161] Langston WT, Wathen JE, Roback MG, Bajaj L. Effect of ondansetron on the incidence of vomiting associated with ketamine sedation in children: a double-blind, randomized, placebo-controlled trial. Ann. Emerg. Med., 2008;52:30-34. DOI: 10.1016/j.annemergmed.2008.01.326.

[162] Melo A, Kokras N, Dalla C, Ferreira C, Ventura-Silva AP, Sousa N, Pêgo JM. The positive effect on ketamine as a priming adjuvant in antidepressant treatment. Transl. Psychiatry, 2015;5:e573. DOI: 10.1038/tp.2015.66.

[163] Frizza J, Chesher GB, Jackson DM, Malor R, Starmer GA. The effect of delta 9-tetrahydrocannabinol, cannabidiol, and cannabinol on the anaesthesia induced by various anaesthetic agents in mice. Psychopharmacology (Berl)., 1977;55:103-107. DOI: 10.1007/BF00432824.

[164] Hallak JE, Dursun SM, Bosi DC, de Macedo LR, Machado-de-Sousa JP, Abrão J, Crippa JA, McGuire P, Krystal JH, Baker GB, Zuardi AW. The interplay of cannabinoid and NMDA glutamate receptor systems in humans: preliminary evidence of interactive effects of cannabidiol and ketamine in healthy human subjects. Prog. Neuropsychopharmacol. Biol. Psychiatry, 2011;35:198-202. DOI: 10.1016/j.pnpbp.2010.11.002.